R. Engemann R. Holzheimer A. Thiede (Eds.)

Immunology and Its Impact on Infections in Surgery

With 33 Tables and 71 Figures

Springer-Verlag
Berlin Heidelberg New York London Paris
Tokyo Hong Kong Barcelona Budapest

Prof. Dr. RAINER ENGEMANN
Dr. med. RENE HOLZHEIMER
Prof. Dr. med. A. THIEDE

Universität Würzburg
Chirurgische Universitäts- und Poliklinik
Josef-Schneider-Str. 2
97080 Würzburg
Germany

ISBN 3-540-58145-6 Springer-Verlag Berlin Heidelberg New York
ISBN 0-387-58145-6 Springer-Verlag New York Berlin Heidelberg

Library of Congress Cataloging-in-Publication Data – Immunology and its impact on infections in surgery/ R. Engemann, R. Holzheimer, A. Thiede (eds.). P. cm. Includes bibliographical references and index. ISBN 0-387-58145-6 (alk. paper). – ISBN 3-540-58145-6 (alk. paper): 1. Surgical wound infections – Immunological aspects – Congresses. 2. Surgical wound infections – Immunotherapy – Congresses. 3. Surgical wound infections – Prevention – Congresses. I. Engemann, Rainer. II. Thiede, Arnulf. III. Holzheimer, R. (René), 1954– . IV. International Congress "Recent Developments in Immunology: Potential Clinical Impact on Surgery and the Treatment of Infections" (1993: Würzburg, Germany) [DNLM: 1. Surgical Wound Infection – immunology – congresses. 2. Burns – immunology – congresses. 3. Immunotherapy – methods – congresses. WO 185 I33 1994] RD98.3.I47 1994 617'.01 – dc20 94-28825

Typesetting: Best-set Typesetter Ltd., Hong Kong

SPIN: 10127008 24/3130/SPS – 5 4 3 2 1 0 – Printed on acid-free paper

Preface

The growing body of information in immunology and aspects of molecular biology related to it and the beginning interest of clinicians prompted the idea of organizing a discussion forum which was different from the usual meetings with leading experts in the field. Despite all the progress which has been made in intensive care, the powerful antibiotics, and skillful surgical techniques, there is still a very high rate of 60%–80% of severe surgical infections such as peritonitis. One aspect of the international congress "Recent Developments in Immunology. Potential Clinical Impact on Surgery and the Treatment of Infections" jointly organized by the Surgical Department of Würzburg University, the Association of European Young Medical Scientists e.V. (AEYMS), and the Surgical Infection Society (SIS) and held on 3–4 September 1993 in Würzburg, Germany, was to bridge the gap between basic science and clinical application; we need more clinicians who unterstand the importance of immunology and molecular biology for future therapy and diagnosis in surgery and infections. The congress participants came from the United States of America and 14 European countries as well as from several German universities. International scientists and clinicians presented the state of the art to young European scientists, discussed the presentations of young scientists with young scientists, and gave direction to future research. The fulminant discussions have shown that this was a wise guideline.

The seminar-like meeting ended with presentations of recent developments in immunology and their potential clinical impact by reputable scientists. Patients with major burn injuries usually die of infection. Recent mouse model results (J.A. Mannick, Boston, MA, USA) showed that severe burn injuries induced immunosuppression, as expressed by reduced interleukin-2 production. This immunosuppression would also explain why such patients have no resistance to infection. The mouse model also showed that the deficiency is not traceable on the interleukin-2-receptor level or in the interleukin-2-receptor mRNA expression, but that it takes place before transcription. The animal model inspired Boston scientists to start treating patients with a low-dose interleukin-2 substitution. Pilot examinations with the growth factor GM-CSF (R. Molloy, Edinburgh, UK) with this model are very encouraging. Animal models are indispensable for the study of gram-negative infections (I. Autenrieth, Würzburg, Germany) and intraabdominal abscesses (W.G. Steinmetz, Würzburg, Germany).

Macrophages have a key function in multiple organ failure (C.C. Baker, Chapel Hill, NC, USA). They recognize and present antigens and influence the cascade of infectious mediators such as interleukin-1, interleukin-6, TNF, and prostagland in E_2. The successful immunomodulation by anti-endotoxin antibodies, monoclonal antibodies against TNF-α, or interleukin-1 receptor antagonists are influenced by macrophage hyperactivity, "angry macrophage" (R. Maier, Seattle, WA, USA). In addition to macrophages, neutrophil granulocytes have been detected recently to be important factors in mediator release (M. Rodrick, Boston, MA, USA; E. Faist, Munich, Germany) after trauma and sepsis. Early states of sepsis already induce an interaction of activated cells such as PMN, monocytes, and endothelium via so-called adhesion molecules (A. Aasen, Oslo, Norway). The activation of the endothelium and subsequent endothelial lesion influencing the cascade of inflammation by producing eicosanoids, platelet activating factor, and cytokines seems to be decisive for the sepsis process (C. Aprahamian, Milwaukee, WI. USA), and reduced blood circulation and a lack of oxygenation was recognized to induce tissue damage (F. Gottrup, Copenhagen, Denmark).

In addition to the aforementioned possibility of immunomodulation with antiendotoxin antibodies, anti-TNF antibodies, interleukin-1-receptor antagonist, inhibitors of the cyclooxygenase pathway (Indomethacin, Ibuprofen), immunoglobulin therapy which can normalize suppressed phagocytosis, if given in high doses, proved to be very effective in treating infections (L. Dominioni, Varese, Italy). This was also demonstrated by preliminary clinical results after coronary bypass operations, where immunoglobulin therapy was effective in preventing the inflammation cascade and possible postoperative infections (H.G. Kress, Vienna, Austria). Antibiotic therapy, which is still one of the mainstays of infection treatment, can have immunosuppressive effects by influencing the phagocytosis of neutrophils and macrophages. Certain antibiotics seem to favor endotoxin release into the blood circulation (O. Wittmann, Milwaukee, WI, USA; R. Urbaschek, Mannheim, Germany).

A new tool for evaluating epidemic processes, genomic fingerprinting, indicated the growing importance of molecular biology for future clinical diagnosis (H. Karch, Würzburg, Germany).

We were happy to welcome Christopher C. Baker (Chapel Hill, NC, USA) and Ronald Maier (Seattle, WA, USA), the past and present presidents of the US Society of University Surgeons, who followed the invitation to Würzburg.

Thanks to the generous support of German and international companies, we were able to keep the congress fees low, which, together with special funds, made it possible for young scientists from Eastern Europe to attend this meeting.

Würzburg, Germany,
August 1994

R. ENGEMANN
R. HOLZHEIMER
A. THIEDE

Contents

Risk Factors

Therapy Modalities (1)

Therapy Modalities (2)

List of Contributors

AASEN, A.O.
Institute for Surgical Research, Rikshospitalet,
University of Oslo, 0027 Oslo, Norway

ANDREE, C.
Brigham/Children's/Havard Division of Plastic Surgery, 75, Francis
Street, Boston, MA 02115, USA

ALCALDE, J.A.
Hopital General de Galicia, Department of Surgery, Calle Galeras s/n,
Santiago de Compostela, Spain

APECECHEA, A.
Laboratorio de Cirurgia Experimental Facultad de Medicina y Odontologia,
Universitad del Pais Vasco, B Sarriena s/n, 48940 Lejona,
Vizcaya, Spain

AUTENRIETH, I.B.
Institut für Hygiene und Mikrobiologie der Universität Würzburg,
Josef-Schneider-Strasse 2, 97080 Würzburg, Germany

BAKER, C.C.
Department of Surgery, Head Trauma Section, University of North
Carolina at Chapelhill, 131 Burnett Womack Bld., Chapelhill,
NC 37514, USA

BAIER, J.
Chirurgische Universitätsklinik der Ruhr-Universität, St. Josef
Hospital, Gudrunstrasse 56, 44791 Bochum, Germany

BARBARISI, A.
Instituto di Patologia Generale e Oncologia, II Universita degli Studi, Via
S. Andrea delle Dame 2, 80138 Napoli, Italy

BECKER, K.-P
Institut für Med Mikrobiologie und Hygiene, Klinikum Mannheim, Theodor-Kutzer-Ufer, 68167 Mannheim, Germany

BEER, M.
Institut für Hygiene und Mikrobiologie der Universität Würzburg, Josef-Schneider-Strasse 2, 97080 Würzburg, Germany

BERENTEY, G.
Department of Traumatology, Semmelweis University of Medical Sciences, Peterfy Hospital, P.O. Box 76, 1441 Budapest, Hungary

BERGER, D.
Department of General Surgery, University of Ulm, Steinhövelstrasse 9, 89075 Ulm, Germany

BERGHMANS, R.
see R.F. DE JONGH

BIELECKI, K.
see U. KUBICKA

BILBAO, J.E.
Laboratorio de Cirurgia Experimental Facultad de Medicina y Odontologia, Universitad del Pais Vasco, B Sarriena s/n, 48940 Lejona, Vizcaya, Spain

BODEN, K.
Klinik und Poliklinik für Chirurgie, Fr.-Loeffler-Strasse 23, 17487 Greifswald, Germany

BÖHM, H.
Institut für Hygiene und Mikrobiologie der Universität Würzburg, Josef-Schneider-Strasse 2, 97080 Würzburg, Germany

BOHN, E.
Institut für Hygiene und Mikrobiologie der Universität Würzburg, Josef-Schneider-Strasse 2, 97080 Würzburg, Germany

BOSMANS, E.
see R. DE JONGH

BRESCIANO, E.
Instituto di Patologia Generale e Oncologia, II Universita degli Studi, Via S. Andrea delle Dame 2, 80138 Napoli, Italy

Broll, R.
Institut für Mikrobiologie, Medizinische Universität zu Lübeck, Ratzeburger Allee 160, 23562 Lübeck, Germany

Bruch, H.-P.
Klinik für Chirurgie, Medizinische Universität zu Lübeck, Ratzeburger Allee 160, 23562 Lübeck, Germany

Buø, L.
Institute for Surgical Research, Rikshospitalet, University of Oslo, 0027 Oslo, Norway

Bustamante, M.
Hopital General de Galicia, Department of Surgery, Calle Galeras s/n, Santiago de Compostela, Spain

Cainzos, M.
Department of Surgery, Hopital General de Galicia, Galeras s.n., Calle Galeras s/n, Santiago de Compostela, Spain

Carnicero, J.A.
Laboratorio de Cirurgia Experimental Facultad de Medicina y Odontologia, Universitad del Pais Vasco, B Sarriena s/n, 48940 Lejona, Vizcaya, Spain

Chen U.
Max-Planck-Gesellschaft, Klinische Arbeitsgruppe für Rheumatologie, Schwabachanlage 10, 91054 Erlangen, Germany

Cholakov, D.S.
Immunology Laboratory, Medical University, 9002 Varna, Bulgaria

Collins, K.
Department of Surgery, Havard Medical School, Brigham and Women's Hospital, 75, Francis Street, Boston, MA 02115, USA

Curley, P.J.
Surgical Immunology, Brigham and Women's Hospital, 75, Francis Street, Boston, MA 02115, USA

De Jongh, R.F.
Department of Anesthesia, Sint Jansziekenhuis, Schiepse Bos 2, 3500 Genk, Belgium

DIONIGI, R.
Department of Surgery, Universita di Pavia,
Viale L. Borri 57, 21100 Varese, Italy

DOMINIONI, L.
Department of Surgery, Universita di Pavia,
Viale L. Borri 57, 21100 Varese, Italy

EILERS, J.
Klinik für Chirurgie, Medizinische Universität zu Lübeck, Ratzeburger Allee 160, 235362 Lübeck, Germany

EMPARAN, C.
Laboratorio de Cirurgia Experimental Facultad de Medicina Y Odontologia, Universitad del Pais Vasco, B Sarriena s/n, 48940 Lejona, Vizcaya, Spain

ENGEMANN, R.
Chirurgische Universitäts- und Poliklinik,
Josef-Schneider-Strasse 2, 97080 Würzburg, Germany

ERIKSSON, E.
Department of Surgery, Havard Medical School, Brigham and Women's Hospital, 75, Francis Street, Boston, MA 02115, USA

FRATTA, M.
Instituto di Patologia, Generale e Oncologia, II Universita degli Studi, Via S. Andrea delle Dame 2, 80138 Napoli, Italy

GANEVA, M.
Dept. of Pharmacology, Metodii Kusev Str. N 1-B, 13, 6000 Stara Zagora, Bulgaria

GASSEL, A.M.
Pathologisches Institut der Universität,
Josef-Schneider-Strasse 2, 97080 Würzburg, Germany

GASSEL, H.-J.
Chirurgische Universitäts- und Poliklinik,
Josef-Schneider-Strasse 2, 97080 Würzburg, Germany

GATERMANN, S.
Klinik für Chirurgie, Medizinische Universität zu Lübeck, Ratzeburger Allee 160, 23562 Lübeck, Germany

GAZZERRO, P.
Instituto di Patologia Generale e Oncologia, II Universita degli Studi, Via S. Andrea delle Dame 2, 80138 Napoli, Italy

GENNARI, R.
Department of Surgery, Universita di Pavia,
Viale L. Borri 57, 211000 Varese, Italy

GOTTRUP, F.
Surgery and Gasteroenterology Dept. 235, Hvidovre University Hospital, Kettegaard Alle 30, 2550 Hvidovre, Denmark

GULUBOVA, M.
Metodii Kusev Str. N 1-B, 13, 6000 Stara Zagora, Bulgaria

HANTSCHMANN, P.
Institut für Hygiene und Mikrobiologie der Universität,
Josef-Schneider-Strasse 2, 97080 Würzburg, Germany

HARINGS, T.
Chirurgische Universitätsklinik der Ruhr-Universität, St. Josef Hospital, Gudrunstrasse 56, 44791 Bochum, Germany

HATZIS, D.
Brigham/Children's/Harvard Division of Plastic Surgery,
Boston, MA 02115, USA

HAUPTMANN, S.
Pathologisches Institut, RWTHA, Pauwelsstrasse 30, 52074 Aachen, Germany

HEYLEN, R.
Department of Anesthesia, Sint Jansziekenhuis, Schiepse Bos 2,
3500 Genk, Belgium

HEESEMANN, J.
Institut für Hygiene und Mikrobiologie der Universität,
Josef-Schneider-Strasse 2, 97080 Würzburg, Germany

HOLZHEIMER, R.
Chirurgische Universitäts- und Poliklinik,
Josef-Schneider-Strasse 2, 97080 Würzburg, Germany

HOLZHEIMER, R.G.
Surgical Immunology, Brigham and Women's Hospital, 75, Francis Street Boston, MA 02115, USA

HOMANN, H.-H.
Chirurgische Universitätsklinik der Ruhr-Universität, St. Josef Hospital, Gudrunstrasse 56, 44791 Bochum, Germany

HORGAN, A.F.
Department of Surgery, Havard Medical School, Brigham and Women's Hospital, 75, Francis Street, Boston, MA 02115, USA

HUNSICKER, A.
Klinik und Poliklinik für Chirurgie, Fr.-Loeffler-Strasse 23, 17487 Greifswald, Germany

IELPO, M.T.
Instituto di Patologia Generale e Oncologia, II Universita degli Studi, Via S. Andrea delle Dame 2, 80138 Napoli, Italy

IMPERATORI, A.
Department of Surgery, Universita di Pavia,
Viale L. Borri 57, 21100 Varese, Italy

ITURBURU, I.
Laboratorio de Cirurgia Experimental, Facultad de Medicina y Odontologia, Universitad del Pais Vasco, B Sarriena s/n, 48940 Lejona,
Vizacya, Spain

JONAS, S.
Klinik für Chirurgie, Medizinische Universität zu Lübeck, Ratzeburger Allee 160, 23562 Lübeck, Germany

KAPRELYAN, A.G.
Immunology Laboratory, Medical University, 9002 Varna, Bulgaria

KARCH, H.
Institut für Hygiene und Mikrobiologie der Universität,
Josef-Schneider-Strasse 2, 97080 Würzburg, Germany

KATTENBECK, K.
Klinik für Chirurgie, Medizinische Universität zu Lübeck, Ratzeburger Allee 160, 23562 Lübeck, Germany

KEMEN, M.
Chirurgische Universitätsklinik der Ruhr-Universität, St. Josef Hospital, Gudrunstrasse 56, 44791 Bochum, Germany

KIRKPATRICK, C.J.
Pathologisches Institut, Johannes Gutenberg-Universität Mainz, Langenbeckstrasse 1, 55131 Mainz, Germany

KLOSTERHALFEN, B.
Unfallchirurgie, Chirurgische Klinik, RWTHA, Pauwelsstrasse 30, 52074 Aachen, Germany

KLÖTING, I.
Fachkrankenhaus für Diabetes, Abt. für Versuchstiere, Greifswalder Strasse 11, 17495 Karlsburg, Germany

KOOISTRA, A.
Klinik für Chirurgie, Medizinische Universität zu Lübeck, Ratzeburger Allee 160, 23562 Lübeck, Germany

KRESS, H.G.
Department B of Anaesthesia and General Intensive Care Medicine, Universität Wien, Währinger Gürtel 18-20, 1090 Wien, Austria

KUBICKA, U.
Department for Surgical Research and Transplantology, Medical Research Center, Polish Academy of Sciences, 5 Chalubinskiego Strasse, 02-004 Warsaw, Poland

KUHN, M.
Basel Institute for Immunology, Grenzacherstrasse 487, 4005 Basel, Switzerland

KULLICH, W.
Ludwig -Boltzmann-Institut, Thorer Strasse 26, 5760 Saalfelden, Austria

LEBEAU, A.
see A. WOLTMANN

LORENZ, D.
Rudolfinerhaus Billrothstrasse 78, 1190 Wien, Austria

MAIER, R.V.
Department of Surgery, ZA-16, Harbor View Medical Center, 325, Ninth Avenue, Seattle, WA 98104, USA

MANCINO, D.
Instituto di Patologia Generale e Oncologia, II Universita degli Studi, Via S. Andrea delle Dame 2, 80138 Napoli, Italy

MANNICK, J.A.
Surgical Immunology, Brigham and Women's Hospital, 75, Francis Street, Boston, MA 02115, USA

MANNICK, J.R.
Surgical Immunology, Brigham and Women's Hospital, 75, Francis Street, Boston, MA 02115, USA

MAZZOCCOLI, V.
Institute of Surgery and Surgical Therapy, School of Medicine and Surgery, Second University of Naples, 80138 Napoli Italy

MCCUSKEY, R.S.
Institut für Med Mikrobiologie und Hygiene, Klinikum Mannheim, Theodor-Kutzer-Ufer, 68167 Mannheim, Germany

MENDEZ, J.
Laboratorio de Cirurgia Experimental Facultad de Medicina y Odontologia, Universitad del Pais Vasco, B Sarriena s/n, 48940 Lejona, Vizcaya, Spain

MENDEZ, M.
Department of Surgery, Havard Medical School, Brigham and Women's Hospital, 75, Francis Street, Boston, MA 02115, USA

MENDEZ, M.V.
Department of Surgery, Havard Medical School, Brigham and Women's Hospital, 75, Francis Street, Boston, MA 02115, USA

MESZAROS, T.
Department of Traumatology, Semmelweis University of Medical Sciences, Peterfy Hospital, P.O. Box 76, 1441, Budapest, Hungary

METODIEV, K.T.
Immunology Laboratory, Medical University, 9002 Varna, Bulgaria

MINCHEV, D.M.
Immunology Laboratory, Medical University, 9002 Varna, Bulgaria

MINCHEVA, N.M.
Immunology Laboratory, Medical University, 9002 Varna, Bulgaria

MOK, H.
Basel Institute for Immunology, Grenzacherstrasse 487, 4005 Basel, Switzerland

MOLLOY, R.G.
Department of Surgery, Victoria Hospital, Hayfield Road, Kirkcaldy, FIFE SCOTLAND, KY2 5AH, United Kingdom

MOSTI M.
Instituto di Patologia Generale e Oncologia, II Universita degli Studi, Via S. Andrea delle Dame 2, 80138 Napoli, Italy

MOZES, T.
Department of Traumatology, Semmelweis University of Medical Sciences, Peterfy Hospital, P.O. Box 76, 1441, Budapest, Hungary

MULLIGAN, R.
Department of Surgery, Havard Medical School, Brigham and Women's Hospital, 75, Francis Street, Boston, MA 02115, USA

NESTOR, M.
Surgical Immunology, Brigham and Women's Hospital, 75, Francis Street, Boston, MA 02115, USA

OLSZEWSKI, W.L.
Department for Surgical Research and Transplantology, Medical Research Center, Polish Academy of Sciences, 5 Chalubinskiego Strasse, 02-004 Warsaw, Poland

OMBELET, W.
Department of Anesthesia, Sint Jansziekenhuis, Schiepse Bos 2, 3500 Genk, Belgium

O'RIORDAN, D.S.
Department of Surgery, Havard Medical School, Brigham and Women's Hospital, 75, Francis Street, Boston, MA 02115, USA

PANZIG, B.
Universität Greifswald, Institut für Mikrobiologie, Lutherstrasse 06, 17487 Greifswald, Germany

PETERMANN, J.
Klinik und Poliklink für Chirurgie, Fr.-Loeffer-Strasse 23, 17487 Greifswald, Germany

PORTUGAL, V.
Laboratorio de Cirurgia Experimental Facultad de Medicina y Odontologia, Universitad del Pais Vasco, B Sarriena s/n, 48940 Lejona, Vizcaya, Spain

POTEL, J.
Department of Surgery, Hospital General de Galicia, Galeras, s.n., Alcalde, Santiago de Compostela, Spain

PUENTE, J.L.
Department of Surgery, Hospital General de Galicia, Galeras, s.n., Alcalde, Santiago de Compostela, Spain

PUYLAERT, M.J.
Department of Anesthesia, Sint Jansziekenhuis, Schiepse Bos 2, 3500 Genk, Belgium

RODRICK, M.L.
Surgical Immunology, Brigham and Women's Hospital, Boston, MA 02115, USA

ROEDER, R.G.
see U. CHEN

ROKOS, H.
Henning Berlin GmbH, Abt. für chemische Forschung, Komturstrasse 58-62, 12099 Berlin, Germany

SAPOROSCHETZ., I.
Surgical Immunology, Brigham and Women's Hospital, Boston, MA 02115, USA

SCHADE, U.
Forschungsinstitut Borstel, Medizinische Universität zu Lübeck, Ratzeburger Allee 160, 23562 Lübeck, Germany

Schmidt, H.
Institut für Hygiene und Mikrobilogie der Universität, Josef-Schneider-Strasse 2, 97080 Würzburg, Germany

SCHNEIDER, J.
Chirurgische Universitäts- und Poliklinik, Josef-Schneider-Strasse 2, 97080 Würburg, Germany

SCHULT, M.
Klinik für Chirurgie, Medizinische Universität zu Lübeck, Ratzeburger Allee 160, 23562 Lübeck, Germany

SCHWARZKOPF, A.
Institut für Hygiene und Mikrobiologie der Universität, Josef-Schneider-Strasse 2, 97080 Würzburg, Germany

SCHWESINGER, G.
Universität Greifswald, Institut für Pathologische Anatomie, Fr.-Loeffler-Strasse 23, 17487 Greifswald, Germany

SENKAL, M.
Chirurgische Universitätsklinik der Ruhr-Universität, St. Josef Hospital, Gudrunstrasse 56, 44791 Bochum, Germany

SILBER, R.
Dept. of Thoracic and Cardiovascular Surgery, Universität Würzburg, Josef-Schneider-Strasse 2, 97080 Würzburg, Germany

STAUBACH, K.-H.
Klinik für Chirurgie, Medizinische Universität zu Lübeck, Ratzeburger Allee 160, 23562 Lübeck, Germany

STEINMETZ, W.-G.
Chirurgische Universitäts- und Poliklinik, Josef-Schneider-Strasse 2, 97080 Würzburg, Germany

SUZUKI, H.
see R.F. DE JONGH

TARNOWSKI, W.
Department for Surgical Research and Transplantology, Medical Research Center, Polish Academy of Sciences, 5, Chalubinskiego Strasse, 02-004 Warsaw, Poland

TAYLOR, E.W. ESQ.
Consultant Surgeon, Vale of Leven, District General Hospital, Department of Surgery, Alexandria, Dunbartonshire G83 OUA, England

THIEDE, A.
Pathologisches Institut der Universität, Josef-Schneider-Strasse 2, 97080 Würzburg, Germany

THOMPSON, S.
Brigham/Children's/Harvard Division of Plastic Surgery, Boston, MA 02115, USA

THORPE, D.
Basel Institute for Immunology, Grenzacherstrasse 487, 4005 Basel, Switzerland

TIMMERMANN, W.
Chirurgische Universitäts- und Poliklinik, Josef-Schneider-Strasse 2, 97080 Würzburg, Germany

TODOROVA, K.
Department of Internal Medicine, Higher Medical Institute, 11, Armeiska Street, 6003 Stara Zagora, Bulgaria

URBASCHEK, B.
Department of Cell Biology and Anatomy, College of Medicine, University of Arizona, 1501 N. Campbell Ave. Tucson, AZ 85724, USA

URBASCHEK, R.
Institut für Med. Mikrobiologie und Hygiene, Klinikum Mannheim, Theodor-Kutzer-Ufer, 68167 Mannheim, Germany

VANDEPUT, H.
Department of Anesthesia, Sint Jansziekenhuis, Schiepse Bos 2, 3500 Genk, Belgium

VASILEV, I.
Department of Pathology, 11, Armeiska Street, 6003 Stara Zagora, Bulgaria

VOGT, P.
Klinik fur Plastische Chirurgie und Schwerbrandverlezte, BG-Kliniken "Bergmannsheil", Universitätsklinik der Ruhr-Universität Bochum, Gilsingstrasse 14, 44789 Bochum, Germany

VOLK, H.W.
University Hospitals of Würzburg, Department of Surgery, Josef-Schneider-Strasse 2, 97080 Würzburg, Germany

VUOTTO, M.L.
Instituto di Patologia Generale e Oncologia, II Universita degli Studi, Via S. Andrea delle Dame 2, 80138 Napoli, Italy

WEISSENHOFER, W.
Rudolfinerhaus, Billrothstrasse 78, 1190 Wien, Austria

WILLE, J.
Department of Traumatology, Semmelweis University of Medical Sciences, Peterfy Hospital, P.O. Box 76, 1441 Budapest, Hungary

WITTMANN, D.H.
Department of Surgery, Medical College of Wisconsin, 8700 West Wisconsin Avenue, Milwaukee, WI 53226, USA

WOLTMANN, A.
Klinik für Chirurgie, Medizinische Universität zu Lübeck, Ratzeburger Allee 160, 23562 Lübeck, Germany

ZIOLKOWSKA, A.
see U. KUBICKA

ZUMTOBEL, V.
Chirurgische Universitätsklinik der Ruhr-Universität, St. Josef Hospital, Gudrunstrasse 56, 44791 Bochum, Germany

Animal Models

Yersinia enterocolitica Infection in Mice: A Possible Experimental Model for the Immunobiology of Gram-Negative Infections

I.B. Autenrieth, M. Beer, P. Hantschmann, E. Bohn, and J. Heesemann

Yersinia enterocolitica is a member of the Enterobacteriaceae family which causes foodborne diseases designated yersiniosis. Both intestinal (e.g., enteritis, enterocolitis, mesenteric lymphadenitis) and extraintestinal (e.g., reactive arthritis, uveitis, erythema nodosum) manifestations can be associated with infection by *Y. enterocolitica* [1]. Moreover, septicemic yersiniosis including abscesses in multiple organs such as the spleen and liver can occur, particularly in immunocompromised individuals. The virulence of *Y. enterocolitica* is controlled by chromosomal and extrachromosomal determinants [2, 3]. All human pathogenic yersiniae harbor a virulence plasmid which encodes for several putative virulence factors (e.g., outer membrane proteins and released proteins). These factors mediate pathogenic functions such as resistance to phagocytosis and complement lysis, cytotoxicity, and tyrosine phosphatase activity which can dephosphorylate host proteins [3].

During the past two decades, several experimental animal models for *Y. enterocolitica* have been established [3]: (a) the rabbit model to study *Yersinia*-induced enterotoxin-mediated enteritis and humoral immune responses, (b) the rat model to investigate the pathogenesis of reactive arthritis, and (c) the mouse model to study the immunobiology of yersiniosis. In contrast to other models for human enteropathogenic microorganisms, experimental yersiniosis in rodents closely resembles yersiniosis in humans. Thus, the *Yersinia* animal models mentioned above may provide a better understanding of the pathogenesis of human yersiniosis and its associated lesions and sequelae. This brief overview will focus on the study results of the immunobiology of *Y. enterocolitica* infection in the experimental mouse model.

Electron microscopic studies have shown substantial evidence that *Y. enterocolitica* is predominantly located extracellularly in host tissues [4]. According to current models of immunity to bacterial infections, extracellular pathogens are eliminated primarily by nonspecific cellular (phagocytes), humoral (complement), and specific humoral (antibodies) mechanisms, whereas intracellular pathogens (e.g., listeriae, mycobacteriae) are eliminated by specific T cells in cooperation with activated macrophages. However, surprisingly, it was demonstrated for the very first time that T cells are involved in and required for resolution of primary *Yersinia* infection. The most salient results of our recent studies are listed and discussed below.

1. Following parenteral *Yersinia* infection the organs most involved as sites of infection are the spleen, the liver, and the lungs. By histomorphological studies it was demonstrated that yersiniae could induce abscesses and granuloma-like lesions (Fig. 1) [5]. This is interesting because abscesses are thought to be the hallmark of infection by extracellular pathogens, whereas granulomas reflect interaction with intracellular pathogens. By immunohistology *Yersinia* antigen was detected within abscesses but not in granulomatous lesions [5]. Moreover, it was shown that phagocytes ($CD11b^+/CD18^+$) as well as T cells ($CD4^+$ and $CD8^+$) were present in *Yersinia*-induced tissue lesions. These results suggest that the cellular immune response is involved and may play an important role in the host response to yersiniae.

2. To investigate whether specific T cells are required for resolution of *Yersinia* infection, the course of the infection was compared in normal and T cell-deficient athymic nude mice [6]. Normal C57BL/6 mice were relatively resistant to yersiniae whereas T cell-deficient nude C57BL/6 mice were found to be highly susceptible. While normal mice developed a short-term transient infection, the T cell-deficient mice developed a biphasic chronic and progressive disease. Thus, in the early phase (days 1–3 p.i.) nude mice partially controlled the infection, which was paralleled by a marked influx of phagocytes and natural killer (NK) cells into the spleen. The late phase was characterized by disease progression and increasing bacterial counts and tissue destruction in liver and spleen. Unlike in normal mice, granulomatous lesions were not found in T cell-deficient mice following *Yersinia* infection. Moreover, T cell-deficient mice lacked production of *Yersinia*-specific

a
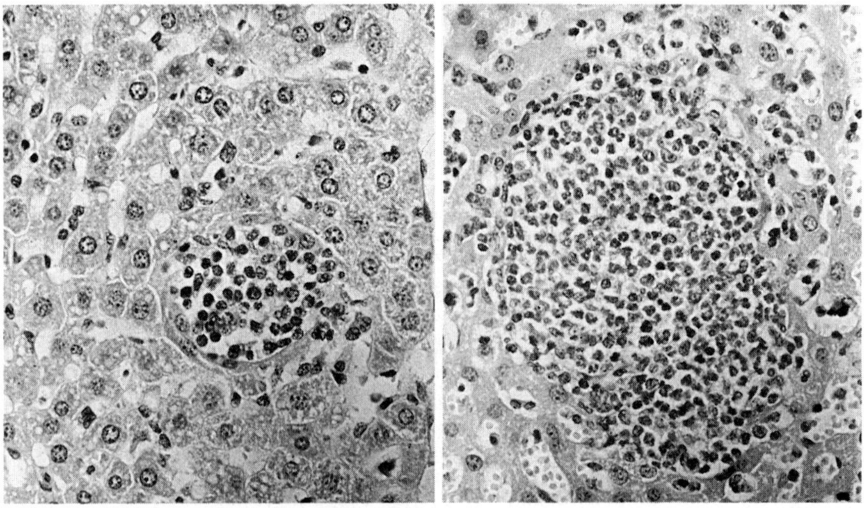
b

Fig. 1. Yersinia-induced granuloma-like lesion (**a**) and pyogenic lesion (abscess; **b**) in the liver of C57BL/6 mice 7 days after infection by *Y. enterocolitica*. HE stain antibodies, suggesting that production of *Yersinia*-specific antibodies strictly depends on the presence of specific T cells.

3. To determine the role of T cells in yersiniosis more precisely, *Yersinia*-specific T cell lines and clones were generated and established [7]. The clones obtained showed the phenotype of cytotoxic ($CD8^+$) and helper ($CD4^+$) α-β T cell-receptor T cells. All T cell clones produced significant quantities of interferon-γ (IFN-γ) but not interleukin-4. When transferred into nonimmune mice, some of the $CD4^+$ as well as $CD8^+$ T cell clones could mediate at least partial protection against the challenge of a lethal dose of *Y. enterocolitica* (Fig. 2). Likewise, adoptive transfer of *Yersinia*-specific T cells into athymic nude mice mediated resistance against yersiniae and restored both granuloma formation and production of specific antibodies.

4. Cytokines are known to be important mediators of the inflammatory host response against infectious pathogens. By the reverse transcription-polymerase chain reaction a rapid increase in expression of tumor necrosis factor-α (TNF-α), IFN-γ, IL-1, IL-6, IL-10, and IL-12 mRNAs after challenge with *Y. enterocolitica* was observed (manuscript in preparation). Consequently, the role of TNF-α and IFN-γ in yersiniosis was investigated. We found that injection of neutralizing anti-TNF-α and/or anti-IFN-γ antibodies prior to or during the infection abrogated resistance to *Y. enterocolitica* and caused fatal yersiniosis [8]. T cells as well as NK cells are the main source of IFN-γ, which in turn activates macrophages; macrophages are the main source of TNF-α. Therefore, from these results we presume

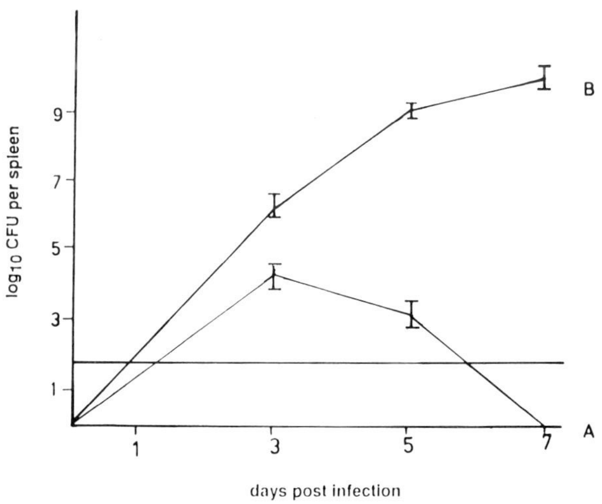

Fig. 2. Adoptive transfer of *Yersinia*-specific T cell line YTL 14.6 (*A*) 1 day prior to infection with *Y. enterocolitica*. Control mice (*B*) received ovalbumin-specific T cells. The *horizontal lines* indicate the limit of detectable yersiniae. CFU, colony-forming units (=viable bacteria)

that T cells in cooperation with activated macrophages play an essential role in the resolution of yersiniosis.

5. $CD4^+$ T cells segregate into two subsets designated Th1 and Th2 cells [9]. It has been suggested that Th1 cells, which characteristically produce IFN-γ and IL-2, assist cell-mediated immune responses while Th2 cells, which typically produce IL-4, IL-5, and IL-10, mediate humoral immune responses. Comparison of immune reponses against yersiniae in *Yersinia*-susceptible BALB/c and *Yersinia*-resistant C57BL/6 mice revealed evidence that resistance to yersiniae may be related to the development of Th1 responses. After specific stimulation, freshly isolated (7 days p.i.) T cells from resistant C57BL/6 mice produced IFN-γ in vitro and exhibited protective properties in adoptive transfer experiments. In contrast, T cells from susceptible BALB/c neither produced IFN-γ in vitro nor mediated protection in vivo (Autenrieth et al., submitted).

6. Finally, the role of antibodies in yersiniosis was investigated [10]. The adoptive transfer of *Yersinia*-specific antibodies mediated resistance against the challenge of a lethal dose of yersiniae. Furthermore, it was shown that the presence of the intact virulence plasmid of *Y. enterocolitica* and expression of the adhesin YadA were essential for induction of a protective humoral immune response by immunization procedures. These results may be an important step in vaccine development for prevention of yersiniosis in patients who are at high risk for *Yersinia* infection and its complications.

Concluding Remarks

Our studies have shown that T cells (CD4 and CD8), phagocytes, and cytokines (IFN-γ and TNF-α) play an important role in yersiniosis. This was surprising since *Y. enterocolitica* is an extracellular pathogen. In contrast to intracellular pathogens such as listeriae, the transfer of specific antibodies against certain surface antigens of yersiniae mediated protection. As mentioned above, *Y. enterocolitica* is an enteropathogenic microorganism involving predominantly the Peyer's patches after intestinal infection. Future studies will therefore focus primarily on the response of the gut-associated lymphoid tissue to intestinal *Yersinia* infection to gain more insight into the pathomechanisms induced via the natural infection route, and possibly to elucidate the pathomechanisms of infection by other enteropathogenic microorganisms.

References

1. Cover TL, Aber RC (1989) *Yersinia enterocolitica*. N Engl J Med 321:16–24
2. Cornelis G, Laroche Y, Balligand G, Sory MP, Wauters G (1987) *Yersinia enterocolitica*, a primary model of bacterial invasiveness. Rev Infect Dis 9:64–87

3. Heesemann J, Gaede K, Autenrieth IB (1993) Experimental *Yersinia enterocolitica* infection in rodents: a model of human yersiniosis. APMIS 101:417–429
4. Hanski C, Kutschka U, Schmoranzer HP, Naumenn M, Stallmach A, Hahn H, Menge H, Riecken EO (1989) Immunohistochemical and electron microscopic study of interaction of *Yersinia enterocolitica* serotype O:8 with intestinal mucosa during experimental enteritis. Infect Immun 57:673–678
5. Autenrieth IB, Hantschmann P, Heymer B, Heesemann J (1993) Immunohistological characterization of the cellular immune response against *Yersinia enterocolitica* in mice: evidence for the involvement of T lymphocytes. Immunobiol 187:1–16
6. Autenrieth IB, Vogel U, Preger S, Heymer B, Heesemann J (1993) Experimental *Yersinia enterocolitica* infection in euthymic and athymic T cell deficient C57BL/6 nude mice: comparison of time course, histomorphology and immune response. Infect Immun 61:2585–2595
7. Autenrieth IB, Tingle A, Reske-Kunz A, Heesemann BJ (1992) T lymphocytes mediate protection to *Yersinia enterocolitica* in mice: characterization of murine T cell clones specific for *Y. enterocolitica*. Infect Immun 60:1140–1149
8. Autenrieth IB, Heesemann J (1992) In vivo neutralization of tumor necrosis factor alpha and gamma interferon abrogates resistance to *Yersinia enterocolitica* in mice. Med Microbiol Immunol 181:333–338
9. Bottomly K (1988) A functional dichotomy in CD4 + T lymphocytes. Immunol Today 9:268–274
10. Vogel U, Autenrieth IB, Berner R, Heesemann J (1993) Role of plasmidencoded antigens of *Yersinia enterocolitica* in humoral immunity against secondary *Y. enterocolitica* infection in mice. Microbial Pathogen 15:23–26

Development of a New Animal Model for Chronic Abscess-Forming Peritonitis

W.-G. STEINMETZ, J. SCHNEIDER, and H.W. VOLK

Introduction

Diffuse intraabdominal infection was described as a disease as far back as 2000 years ago. The first time reasonable concepts of treatment were developed was during the last century, but the prognosis for patients continues to be far from ideal.

Nowadays, we know that, in a simplified way, the course of the disease can be described as consisting of two phases: first, the endotoxin-related phase, when we first recognize symptoms of infection, and second, the more protracted phase, when intraabdominal abscess formation and necrosis prevail.

Most of the advances achieved over the last two or three decades have been due to better antibiotic therapy options and progress in intensive care medicine. These advances are largely based on better control of the deleterious effects the first phase has on the organism. Yet, we still have problems in getting a grip on the second phase, which is why it is necessary to find better ways of studying it.

There is a large variety of small animal models which deal with the septic-endotoxic phase of diffuse peritonitis. Most used and best known are models involving ligation of the gut – mostly the cecum – and artificial perforation of the gut. While this approach obviously mimics the clinical situation very well, there are two major problems associated with this method: (1) Control of the amount and type of bacteria causing the infection is very poor. (2) Usually all or most of the animals die very early in the septic-toxic phase of the disease. If we want to take a closer look at the abscess-forming phase, we need to find a different approach, which eliminates the endotoxin-related first phase.

Even though the bacterial gut flora is rather complex, *E. coli* and *Bacteroides fragilis* are commonly regarded as the main causative pathogens. Since *E. coli* is the source of endotoxin, we have to exclude it in our model.

Material and Methods

As experimental animals we chose young, female Wistar rats with a weight between 200 and 260 g. With the help of the Institute for Microbiology of

Würzburg University we selected the encapsulated *Bacteroides fragilis* strain No. 25285 of the American Type Culture Collection to use for the infection of the animals.

Macrophage activity in rats is extremely high compared to the activity in humans. Therefore, it is necessary to use some agent to protect the bacteria for some period after they are introduced into the abdominal cavity. If this is not done, even large quantities of bacteria have little visible influence on the organism up to a certain concentration, when suddenly the outcome is quickly lethal for the animals.

Practically all of the substances which have previously been used for these protective purposes, when used alone, cause more or less severe inflammatory reactions of the peritoneum or lead to abscess formation. After trying different methods and substances, a special nutrition agar made by Merck appeared to be most suitable for our needs (No. 11471).

We mixed 2 ml of the still warm and liquid agar with 2 ml of bacterial suspension with a concentration of 10^8 CFU of *Bacteroides fragilis* per ml. In this way, we received exactly quantified small bacteria-agar blocks. These blocks were then introduced into the abdomen via a median laparotomy and spread evenly over all four quadrants, after taking a swab first. We treated 46 animals in this way, while 15 animals only received a sterile 4-ml block of the agar. The animals were then randomly stratified into groups, as shown in Table 1.

During the observation period the animals were allowed food and water ad libitum. Weight and "clinical appearance" were recorded daily, but otherwise the animals were not disturbed in any way. On the last day of the observation period the animals were sacrificed. Immediately after opening the abdomen, several swabs were obtained from all four quadrants and also directly from the abscesses. During the section the following items were put into a protocol: (a) vascularization of the peritoneum, (b) localization, number and size of abscesses, (c) enlargement of mesenteric lymph nodes, (d) amount of exudate, and (e) amount of adhesions. Most of the animals'

Table 1. Treatment and observation period in 61 female Wistar rats

Observation period (days)	Inoculated with agar-bacteria clots (n = 46)	Sham operated (n = 15)
3	2	0
7	11	5
10	11	0
14	11	5
21	11	5

blood volume was aspirated and various tissue samples taken for histological workup.

Results

Within the first 2 days after laparotomy the mean body weight of all the animals dropped. After that, the control groups quickly recovered and continued to gain weight until the end of the observation period.

The groups with the bacteria showed a biphasic course. They continued to lose weight until the fifth day, then showed some recovery until day 8, when their weight started to decline again to a low on day 12. This was followed by a slow weight gain with the initial weight restored around day 20 of the observation period. The difference in mean weight between the two groups was significant from day 3 on.

Behavior of the animals reflected the weight curve: During the first 8–12 h the control animals were lethargic and avoided motion; they started to feed after approximately 24 h. In the other group the same lethargic behavior lasted for almost 3 days, with first food intake after more than 48 h following the initial procedure. During the second week of the observation period this group had another phase of reduced activity and food intake. Only after day 12 were no more differences noted between the two groups.

The *macroscopic findings after 3 days* were those of an acute inflammatory reaction. Exudate and thin fibrin layers were present, but no abscesses, yet. On *day 7* all animals were found to have intraabdominal abscesses. Vascular injection had increased and an average amount of 2 ml of exudate was present. Multiple adhesions and enlarged mesenteric lymph nodes were noted, too. At *10 days* the findings were very similar with less exudate. After *14 days* the size of the abscesses had increased significantly, with about half the animals showing abscesses of more than 1 cm diameter. The amount of exudate in these animals was minimal; mesenteric lymph nodes were clearly enlarged in all animals. At *21 days*, only 8 of the 11 animals were found to have abscesses. The redness of the peritoneum, which was noted in all the other groups, was missing. Very little exudate was present and only half of the animals had enlarged mesenteric lymph nodes.

In the animals of the *control group*, pathological changes could not be found after any interval. No remains of the sterile agar could be found.

The *cultures* which were grown from the swabs we took at the time of the section showed the following results: The swabs taken on *day 3* and on *day 7* after inoculation grew not only *Bacteroides fragilis*, but also in various concentrations: *E. coli*, streptococci, *Staph. aureus*, other *Bacteroides* species, *Pasteurella pneumotropica* (specific for the rat gut!), *Pseudomonas aeruginosa*, enterococci, various *Clostridium* species, and various *Proteus* species. After 14 days the swabs taken from the abdominal cavity from half of the animals showed no significant growth; the other half yielded the above-mentioned results. All the abdominal cavity swabs taken on day 21 were negative.

As would have been expected, the swabs taken directly from the abscesses grew large quantities of *Bacteroides fragilis*, but there were also various other species of *Bacteroides* and various enterococci. All swabs taken from the control groups remained negative throughout the observation period. These results strongly indicate a translocation of gut bacteria through the intact bowel wall.

The *histological slides* showed a strong inflammatory response with proliferation of mesothelial cells and fibroblasts with a peak around day 7 after the inoculation. By day 21 the abscesses became fully encapsulated. The peak of inflammatory reaction in the regional lymph nodes was on day 7. The same is true for the changes in the liver, which mainly consisted in activation of Kupffer cells and a widening of liver sinuses.

To verify whether or not this model could be utilized to examine metabolic changes, we checked blood samples for the following items: WBCs, RBCs, hemoglobin, hematocrit, thrombocyte count, pyruvate, 2-oxoglutarate, citrate, lactate, β-OH butyrate, acetoacetate, α_2-macroglobulin, and α_1-antitrypsin.

Because of the small numbers, none of the above values showed significant deviations from the levels in the control groups. However, when looking at the differences in the levels between the different observation periods, some significant changes were evident. Lack of space precludes further discussion of these changes here.

Conclusion

We think that with this model we have a valid tool at hand with which we can further explore physiological changes occurring in chronic abscess-forming peritonitis and in intraabdominal infections in general. Most of the results are sufficiently similar to what we can see in peritonitis patients to draw the conclusion that the model will work for research in that area. Our intention is to use this model (a) to find out more about mechanisms of bacterial translocation in a state of intraabdominal inflammation and (b) to explore the role of endotoxin and various cytokines in this situation.

Tolerance to Endotoxin in an Animal Model of Acute Pancreatitis Is Associated with Improved Cellular Immune Function

P.J. Curley, R.G. Holzheimer, M. Nestor, I. Saporoschetz, J.A. Mannick, and M.L. Rodrick

Introduction

Endotoxin is thought to play a central role in the development of irreversible multi-organ failure in patients with septic shock which is the largest cause of mortality in the intensive care setting [1]. Antiserum to the central core of endotoxin has been shown to reduce mortality in septic patients from 39% to 22% [2] lending further credence to the central role of endotoxin in the pathogenesis of multi-organ failure. There is some evidence that endotoxin is involved in the pathogenesis of necrotizing pancreatitis also. Windsor et al. [3] have demonstrated high endotoxin levels in the serum and ascitic fluid of a majority of patients with pancreatic necrosis. Deitch et al. [4] have shown that the absence of bile from the gut of mice leads to increased bacterial translocation and higher levels of bacterial contamination in the caecum thus lending further support to the concept of disimpaction of gallstones for the urgent treatment of gallstone pancreatitis [5].

Fossard and Kakkar [6] reported the presence of circulating endotoxin in 3 patients with acute pancreatitis. Foulis et al. [7] confirmed this finding as did Kivilaakso et al. [8], Pierrakakis et al. [9], Fugger et al. [10] and Exley et al. [11]. Not only was the presence of endotoxaemia documented but, more importantly, levels of endotoxin were correlated with outcome. Florholmen et al. [12] have reported histological evidence of pancreatic injury after infusion of endotoxin in pigs including disruption of cellular plasma membranes. More recent work demonstrates consumption of protective anti-core glycolipid antibodies in patients with acute pancreatitis, an indication of recent exposure to endotoxin. Exposure to endotoxin would account for the increased tumour necrosis factor (TNF) levels reported by Banks et al. [13] and by Exley et al. [11] in patients with acute pancreatitis and for the increased interleukin-6 (IL-6) levels found by Leser et al. [14] and Heath et al. [15] in similar patients.

One approach to countering endotoxin-mediated effects is to produce tolerance in the host. Sanchez-Cantu et al. [16] studied the effects of endotoxin tolerance in rats and found that repeated injection of sublethal doses of endotoxin conferred protection against a lethal challenge in the same animal. Furthermore, such protection was attended by reduced TNF release. He et al. [17] confirmed these findings and demonstrated abrogation of TNF release after 3 days of tolerance and of IL-6 release after 7 days tolerance. These blunted cytokine responses to LPS reverted to normal 72 and 96 h after repeated LPS challenge was stopped. Endotoxin tolerance was also associated with significantly increased survival after a septic challenge in the form of an infected thermal injury, suggesting that tolerance is of clinical as well as experimental interest.

We have previously reported decreased interleukin-2 (IL-2) production in mice with choline-deficient, ethionine supplemented dietinduced acute pancreatitis. These animals are exquisitely susceptible to septic chanllenge in the form of intraperitoneal lipopolysaccharide (LPS) injection. The aim of this study was to examine the effect of LPS tolerance upon both IL-2 production and mortality in this murine model.

Methods

Acute Pancreatitis Model

Adult 6–8 week old female Swiss-Webster mice weighing 20–25 g (Taconic Farms, New York) were allowed to acclimatise for 1 week and were then given either a choline-deficient diet supplemented with 0.5% ethionine (ICN Biochemicals, Cleveland, Ohio) or standard laboratory chow. Animals were randomised to either placebo or treatment. Tolerance to endotoxin was produced by daily injection of small quantities of endotoxin intraperitoneally to the treatment group (0.1 mg/100 g body weight). On day 10 mice were either killed and splenocyte function analysed, or entered into survival studies after injection of 0.25 mg/kg LPS.

Mice were killed by carbon monoxide asphyxiation and spleens were harvested via a left subcostal incision. Spleens were minced with forceps and cells were washed 3 times in RPMI 1640 (GIBCO Grand Island, New York USA) containing 2 m*M* 1-glutamine, $5 \times 10^{-5} M$ 2-mercaptoethanol, 1% antibiotic/antimycotic (penicillin 5000 units, streptomycin 5000 μg and amphotericin 2.5 μg/ml) and 2 m*M* HEPES buffer. After the third wash cells were resuspended in complete medium (CM: RPMI, penicillin/streptomicin/fungizone, HEPES, 2-mercaptoethanol, 5% foetal calf serum) counted using Turk's solution and diluted to a concentration of 2×10^6 mononuclear cells/ml. 100 μl of cell suspension was added to 96-well plates and cultured in a total volume of 200 μl in the presence or absence of concanavalin A (Con A, Sigma Chemical Co., St. Louis, Missouri) at 5 μg/ml final concentration.

Supernatants were harvested after 48 h and frozen at −70°C until assayed for IL-2 activity.

IL-2 Assay

The assay used was a modification of the method of Gillis et al. [18]. Briefly, 50-μl samples were added in serial dilutions from 1:2 to 1:128 to 96-well plates. CTLL-2 cells were washed 3 times to remove T cell growth factor, diluted to a concentration of 5×10^4 cells/ml and 50-μl added to each well. Standards were run on each plate and comprised 25 μl of a 20 U/ml solution of rhIL-2 (Genzyme, Cambridge, Massachusetts). At 20 h, 25 μl of MTT (5 mg/ml in PBS, Sigma Chemical Co., St. Louis, Missouri) was added and 4 h later 150 μl of 10% SDS was added. The development of blue formazan colour was detected on an ELISA plate reader (Molecular Devices) at 570 nm with 690 nm reference.

One unit of IL-2 activity was defined as that producing half-maximal stimulation of the CTLL cells. The optical density curves generated were analysed by probit analysis using a computer program kindly supplied by Dr. Brian Davis.

Proliferation

Splenocytes were plated at a final concentration of 1×10^6 and stimulated with Con A, 5 μg/ml final concentration and incubated at 37°C in a 5% CO_2 atmosphere. At 30 h 1 μCi tritiated thymidine (New England Nuclear, Boston, Massachusetts) was added to each well and the plates were frozen 18 h later. The well contents were harvested onto glass-fibre filter paper in an automated cell harvester (Cambridge Technology, Cambridge, Massachusetts) and incorporation of thymidine was measured using a beta counter (LKB Rackbeta Gaithersburg, Maryland).

Statistical analysis was performed using the Mann-Whitney U test for differences between groups and the Wilcoxon-Gehan statistic for survival curve data.

Determination of Fatal LPS Dose

Normal mice were challenged with varying doses of LPS on day 10 (Fig. 1). No mortality was seen at doses of 1.0 mg/kg, 2.5 mg/kg or 25 mg/kg. However, a dose of 40 mg/kg was associated with a mortality of 70%. The LD_{50} was therefore between 2.5 and 4.0 mg/kg body weight.

Results

Acute pancreatitis was associated with significant reduction in both proliferation and IL-2 production compared to control animals ($n = 6$). By contrast, induction of LPS tolerance with daily injections of small, non-toxic LPS doses was associated with significantly increased proliferation (Fig. 2) and IL-2 (Fig. 3), both of which returned almost to normal levels.

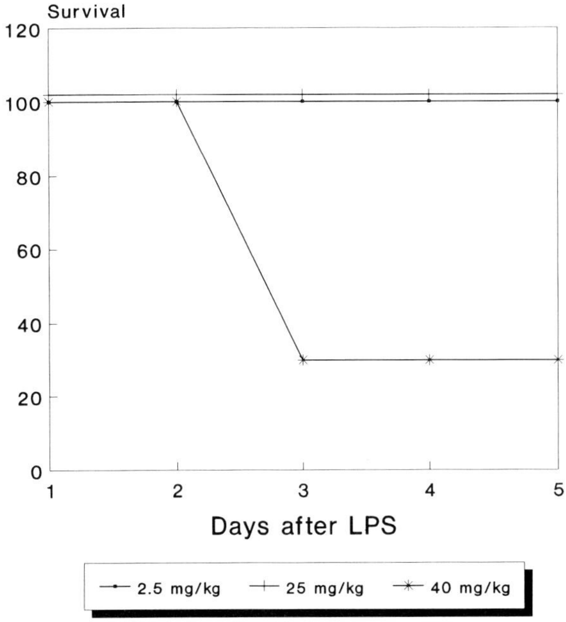

Fig. 1. Fatal LPS dose in normal mice

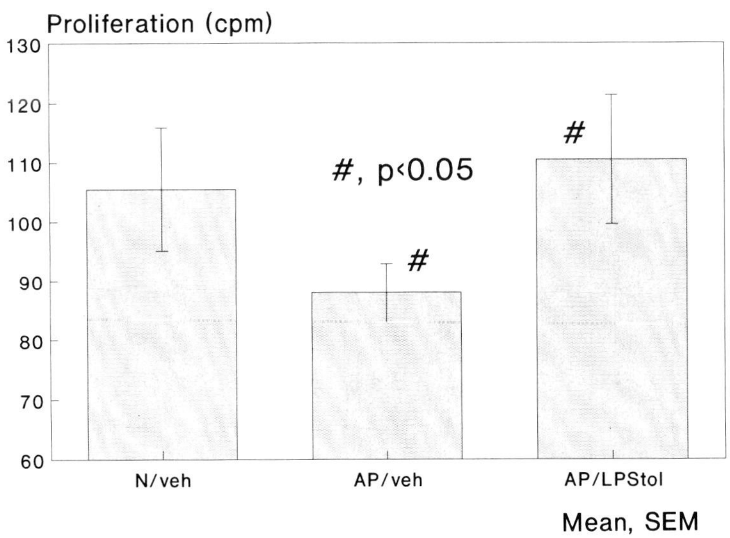

Fig. 2. Proliferation (cpm) in normal mice (*N/veh*), mice with acute pancreatitis (*AP/veh*) and mice with acute pancreatitis and LPS tolerance (*AP/LPStol*)

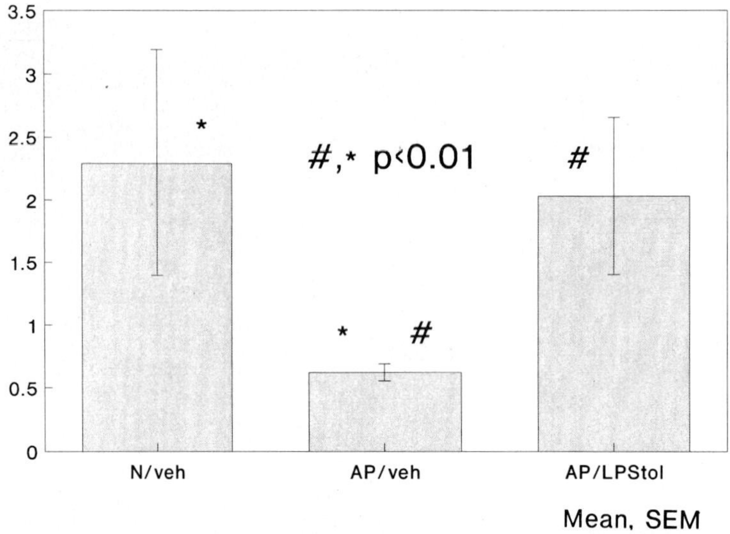

Fig. 3. Interleukin-2 in normal mice (*N/veh*), mice with acute pancreatitis (*AP/veh*) and mice with acute pancreatitis and LPS tolerance (*AP/LPStol*)

In addition, induction of LPS tolerance was not associated with any mortality when animals were challenged on day 10 with intraperitoneal LPS (0.25 mg/kg). Animals treated daily with vehicle had, however, a 48% mortality ($P < 0.05$, Wilcoxon-Gehan statistic, $n = 8$) (Fig. 4).

Discussion

In 1965 Apostolou et al. [19] reported an apparent induction of tolerance in dogs when cross circulation was established between an animal with acute pancreatitis and one without. The second animal had a much milder course of the disease if pancreatitis was subsequently induced some time later. Indeed compared to an initial mortality of 90%, no "inoculated" animal died of acute pancreatitis induced 6 weeks later. Further evidence of immunological "tolerance" in acute pancreatitis can be invoked from the common finding of the less aggressive nature of recurrent pancreatitis with a much lower mortality than primary events [20]. In 1980 Antal et al. [21] reported his findings of immunological abnormalities in patients during and after acute pancreatitis. Elevated immune complex levels were found in addition to decreased active T cells as determined by sheep erythrocyte rosette formation. These abnormalities paralleled his findings in chronic pancreatitis and furthermore were evident up to 14 months after the acute event.

It has been widely reported that the immune system is compromised by a number of insults such as burns, sepsis, trauma and surgery [22]. It is not

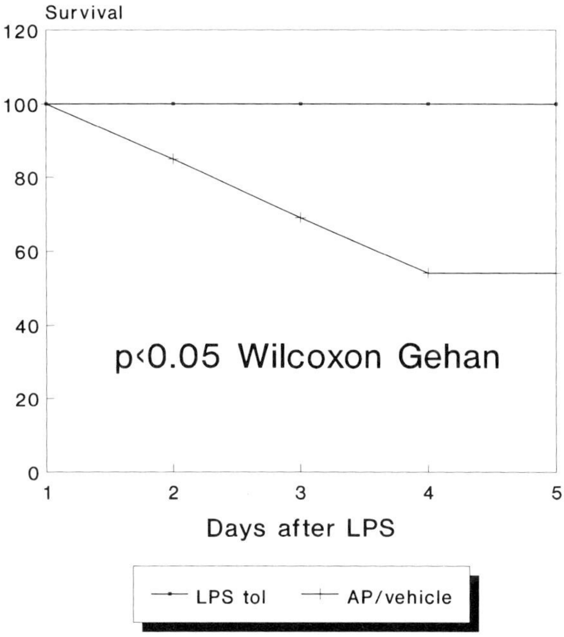

Fig. 4. Relation between LPS tolerance and mortality

surprising then that patients in the postoperative period who develop acute pancreatitis have a higher mortality than any other group [20, 23, 24]. Peterson et al. [20] showed mortality was double the overall rate when occurring in the postoperative period (36% vs 18%). He also demonstrated the protective effect of a previous attack of pancreatitis with a zero mortality in that group. Garcia-Sabrido et al. [25] have correlated the delayed hypersensitivity reaction of patients with acute pancreatitis with the clinical course. As has previously been shown in burns, sepsis and trauma they demonstrated an increased mortality in patients with skin anergy. On admission 35% of patients with a mild attack were anergic compared to 92% of those with severe disease. In addition, patients with necrotising pancreatitis were all anergic on admission. Anergic patients had a higher incidence of complications and of death than reactive patients. The close relationship between endotoxaemia and abnormal cellular immune function [26] led us to examine the potential for endotoxin tolerance as a therapy in this murine model of acute pancreatitis.

The effects of tolerance on IL-2 production and proliferation are important. Gough et al. [27] investigated the role of immunostimulation with IL-2 therapy in a murine model of burn injury. Decreased IL-2 production was shown to correlate strongly with mortality from a septic challenge in burned animals and administration of recombinant IL-2 daily for 5 days prior to septic challenge reduced mortality significantly from 100% to 55%. Later, recognition of the importance of prostaglandin E_2 (PGE_2) as a downregulator of IL-2 synthesis led to investigation of a lower dose of IL-2 combined with indomethacin (negative regulator of PGE_2 production) in the same model [28]. Similar improvements in survival were reported to those using high dose IL-2 with evidence of upregulation of the native production of IL-2 in treated animals. Further evidence of the importance of IL-2 in normal host defences comes from the finding that IL-2 causes Kupffer cell activation [29] and Kupffer cell blockade increases septic mortality in an animal model [30].

The experimental in vitro and in vivo actions of LPS tolerance therapy is of particular interest. There is a large body of evidence implicating endotoxin in severe acute pancreatitis. Since patients with acute pancreatitis often exhibit the sepsis syndrome in the absence of demonstrable infection [31], endotoxin exposure may be the key to controlling multi-organ system failure. If this is the case then induction of endotoxin tolerance is a treatment modality which may be useful in human disease. Upregulation of IL-2 production and protection against endotoxin-related mortality by administration of low-dose endotoxin may prove to be a practical immunomodulatory strategy in this disease.

References

1. Parillo JE (1990) Septic shock in humans: advances in the understanding of pathogenesis, cardiovascular dysfunction and therapy. Annals Intern Med 113: 227–242
2. Ziegler EJ, McCutchan JA, Fierer J et al. (1982) Treatment of gram negative bacteremia and shock with human antiserum to a mutant Escherichia coli. N Engl J Med 307:1225–1230
3. Windsor SA, Fearon KC, Boss JA, Barclay GR, Smyth E et al. (1993) Role of serum endotoxin and antiendotoxin core antibody levels in predicting the development of multiple organ failure in acute pancreatitis. Br J Surg 88:1942–1946
4. Deitch EA, Sittig K, Li M, Berg R et al. (1990) Obstructive jaundice promotes bacterial translocation from the gut. Am J Surg 159:79–84
5. Neoptolemos JP, Carr-Locke DL, Leese T, James D (1987) Acute cholangitis in association with acute pancreatitis: incidence, clinical features and outcome in relation to ERCP and endoscopic sphincterotomy. Br J Surg 74:1103–1106
6. Fossard DP, Kakkar VV (1974) The Limulus test in experimental and clinical endotoxaemia. Br J Surg 61:798–804
7. Foulis AK, Murray WR, Galloway D, McCartney AC et al. (1982) Endotoxaemia and complement activation in acute pancreatitis in man. Gut 23:656–661
8. Kivilaakso E, Valtonen VV, Malkamaki M, Palmu A et al. (1984) Endotoxaemia and acute pancreatitis: correlation between the severity of the disease and the anti-bacterial common antigen antibody titre. Gut 25:1065–1070
9. Pierrakakis S, Xepapadakis G, Mega AM, Megas T et al. (1990) Studio sull'-endotossinemia nella pancreatite acuta con l'impiego del limulus amebocyte lysate test (LAL test). Minerva Chir 45:295–301
10. Fugger R, Hamilton G, Rogy M, Herbst F et al. (1990) Prognostic significance of endotoxin determination in patients with severe intraabdominal infection. J Infect Dis 161:1314–1315

11. Exley AR, Leese T, Holliday MR, Swann RA, Cohen J (1992) Endotoxaemia and serum tumour necrosis factor as prognostic markers in severe acute pancreatitis. Gut 1992;33(8):1126–1128
12. Florholmen J, Lindal S, Rokke O, Olsen R et al. (1988) Effects of endotoxin on the pancreatic ultrastructure APMIS 96:991–996
13. Banks RE, Evans SW, Alexander D, McMahon MJ et al. (1990) Is fatal acute pancreatitis a consequence of excessive leukocyte stimulation? Cytokine 3: 1–6
14. Leser HG, Gross V, Scheinbenbogen C, Heinisch A, Salm R et al. (1991) Elevation of serum interleukin-6 concentration precedes acutephase response and reflects severity in acute pancreatitis. Gastroenterology 101:782–785
15. Heath DI, Cruickshank A, Gudgeon M, Jehanli A et al. (1993) Role of interleukin-6 in mediating the acute phase protein response and potential as an early means of severity assessment in acute pancreatitis. Gut 34:41–45
16. Sanchez-Cantu L, Rode HN, Christou NV (1989) Endotoxin tolerance is associated with reduced secretion of tumour necrosis factor. Arch Surg 124:1432–1436
17. He W, Fong Y, Marano MA, Gershenwald JE et al. (1992) Tolerance to endotoxin prevents mortality in infected thermal injury: association with attenuated cytokine responses. J Infect Dis 165:859–864
18. Gillis B, Ferm MM, Ou W, Smith KA (1978) T-cell growth factor: parameters of production and a quantitative microassay for activity. J Immunol 120:2027–2032
19. Apostolou K, Nasbeth DC, Shapiro DH, Ryak P (1965) Immunity to the lethal effects of acute pancreatitis. Surg Forum 16:382–384
20. Peterson LM, Collins JJ, Wilson RE (1968) Acute pancreatitis occurring after operation. Surg Gynecol Obstet 23–28
21. Antal L, Kavai M, Szabo G, Sonkoly I et al. (1980) Immunological investigations in acute and chronic human pancreatitis. Digestion 20:100–105
22. Burleson DG, Mason AD, McManus AT, Pruitt BA (1988) Lymphocyte phenotype and function changes in burn patients after intravenous IgG therapy. Arch Surg 123:1379–1382
23. White TT, Morgan A, Hopton D (1970) Postoperative pancreatitis: a study of seventy cases. Am J Surg 120:132–135
24. Bragg LE, Thompson JS, Burnett DA, Hodgson PE et al. (1985) Increased incidence of pancreas-related complications in patients with postoperative pancreatitis. Am J Surg 150:694–697
25. Garcia-Sabrido JL, Valdecantos E, Bastida E, Tellado JM (1989) The anergic state as a predictor of pancreatic sepsis. Zentralbl Chir 114:114–120
26. Richardson RP, Rhyne CD, Fong Y, Hesse DG, Tracey KJ et al. (1989) Peripheral blood leukocyte kinetics following in vivo lipopolysaccharide (LPS) administration to normal human subjects. Ann Surg 210(2):239–245
27. Gough DB, Moss NM, Jordan AA, Grbic JT, Rodrick ML, Mannick JA (1988) Recombinant interleukin-2 (rIL-2) improves immune response and host resistance to septic challenge in thermally injured mice. Surgery 104:292–299
28. Horgan PG, Mannick JA, Dubravec DB, Rodrick ML (1990) Effect of low dose recombinant interleukin-2 plus indomethacin on mortality after sepsis in a murine burn model. Br J Surg 77:401–404
29. Curran RD, Billiar TR, West MA, Bentz BG et al. (1988) Effect of interleukin 2 on Kupffer cell activation. Arch Surg 123:1373–1378
30. Callery MP, Kamei T, Flye W (1990) Kupffer cell blockade increases mortality during intra-abdominal sepsis despite improving systemic immunity. Arch Surg 125:36–41
31. Karimgani I, Porter KA, Langevin E, Banks PA (1992) Prognostic factors in sterile pancreatic necrosis. Gastroenterology 103:1636–1640

Prolonged and Recurrent Endotoxemia in Domestic Pigs: A First Step Toward a Porcine Model of Human Multiple Organ Failure?

B. Klosterhalfen, S. Hauptmann, and C.J. Kirkpatrick

Today septic shock and multiple organ failure research require animal models which allow in-depth investigation of the pathophysiology of these diseases and conclusions relevant to the human situation. The basis of such a model should be the use of animals with a similar pathophysiology to man, an experimental design identical ot critical care unit conditions, long observation periods, and the administration of LPS or bacteria in recurrent quantities reported in septic patients [1–3]. Although septic shock or organ failure is clinically characterized by hemodynamic and biochemical changes, the best diagnostic criteria are specific pathomorphological findings, which in most cases are only found at autopsy. Consequently, animal models of human septic shock or organ failure must show identical microscopic and ultrastructural lesions.

Materials and Methods

Animal Model

Domestic pigs (28–32 kg) were quarantined for at least 1 week and treated with an antibiotic (100 mg doxycycline/day; Vibravenös) to prevent infections of the respiratory tract. Experimentation was carried out in a sterile surgical room at 22°C. All manipulations and surgical procedures were done under sterile conditions. Animals were divided into two groups: a test group (n = 6) with two endotoxin applications (0.5 μg/kg over 60 min) at t = 1 h and t = 22 h during a 48-h experimental duration, and a control group (n = 3) which received the same amount of physiologic saline solution. Additionally, the experimental design was such that each animal of the test group served as its own control. After an overnight fast, the pigs were premedicated with 3 mg/kg azaperon (Stresnil) intramuscularly, followed by induction using 5 mg/kg etomidate (Hypnodil) and intratracheal intubation. Anesthesia was maintained with a mixture of etomidate (Hypnodil, 0.06 mg/kg h), pancuronium (Pancuronium Organon, 0.4 mg/kg h), and piritramide (Dipidolor; 0.5 mg/kg h). To maintain an arterial PCO_2 of 35–40 mmHg, the pigs were ventilated with room air using a volume-cycled respirator (Dräger

AV1) at a tidal volume of 10–15 ml/kg and a respiratory rate of between 15 and 20 1/min.

After 48 h the animals were killed with i.v. KCl. In all animals tissue samples of all organs were immediately removed and processed for morphologic investigations.

Light and Electron Microscopy

Tissue samples were fixed in 10% formalin, embedded in paraffin, and sections were stained with hematoxylin and eosin (H&E), as well as periodic-acid Schiff (PAS) plus diastase. For transmission electron microscopy (TEM), tissue specimens were fixed in 3% cacodylate-buffered glutaraldehyde for 30 min. After postfixation in osmium, buffered in 0.1 *M* cacodylate, they were dehydrated in ethanol and embedded in epon. Semithin sections (1.0 μm) were stained with methylene blue-azure II. Ultrathin sections were mounted on copper grids, stained with uranyl acetate and lead citrate, and examined with a transmission electron microscope (Philips, EM400T). For scanning electron microscopy (SEM), specimens were fixed with 3% glutaraldehyde in 0.1 *M* sodium cacodylate, pH 7.5 for 30 min, postfixed in 1% OsO_4 in 0.1 *M* cacodylate, rinsed in water, and dehydrated through graded ethanol. They were then critically point dried from absolute ethanol in a critical point dryer using CO_2 as the transition medium. The dried preparations were coated with 20 nm gold in a sputter coater, and viewed on a Philips SEM 515 scanning electron microscope at 15 or 30 kV.

Computer Tomography

Computed tomography (CT) of the lungs was performed at several time points during the experiment. CT studies were performed on a Somatom DR scanner (Siemens, FRG). The scanning parameters included 1 mm slice thickness, 4 mm table incrementation, 550 mAS, 960 projections, and 125 kV. The pigs were investigated in the prone position and were mechanically ventilated; each exposure was obtained in deep inspiration.

Results

Histology

Compared with the controls, histopathologic specimens of the lungs of the endotoxin group demonstrated pulmonary edema within scattered alveoli and the alveolar interstitium, as well as an increased cellularity within the capillaries, in the interstitium, and around vascular structures. Small amounts of red cell extravasation could also be detected. All animals of the test group showed some chronic changes including interstitial fibrosis and a clubbing of the alveoli. In the thickened parts of the alveolar septa proliferating capillaries could be detected. Thrombus formation in pulmonary arteries and veins could be detected in some sections. Lymph vessels seemed to be dilated. No signs of pneumonia could be observed.

Morphological alterations noted elsewhere in the septic group included thrombotic vegetations on the mitral and aortic heart valves ("abacterial endocarditis"), scattered necrotic hepatocytes in the centrilobular zones of the liver, scattered necrotic cells of the renal tubules, skeletal muscles, and heart muscle, and patchy hemorrhagic lesions of the small intestine.

Transmission and Scanning Electron Microscopy

In the test group widespread interstitial edema was seen in the alveolar walls, as well as proliferating fibroblasts, fibrin strands, cell debris, and degenerative changes in elastic fibers. The alveoli contained erythrocytes, small numbers of granulocytes and macrophages, amorphous edema, and strands of fibrin. Type I pneumocytes showed a range of degenerative changes; in particular, the thinnest regions of these cells were damaged or detached from the basement membrane. Type II pneumocytes were present in increased numbers in the alveolar lumina. The basement membrane remained intact. The number of alveolar vessels in the thickened parts of the alveolar wall was increased. The vessels were filled with red blood cells and granulocytes, a confirmation of the findings in light microscopy. In the pulmonary microvasculature, endothelial cells showed a spectrum of degenerative changes up to complete endothelial cell necrosis.

Scanning electron microscopy of the medium-sized and small pulmonary vessels, as well as the heart valves, demonstrated general damage of pulmonary endothelial cells (Fig. 1B) and the endothelium of the heart valves, in particular of the mitral and aortic valves. The margins of the valves were almost completely denuded. Discrete lesions were found in the ascending, thoracic, and abdominal aorta, as well as in the common iliac, femoral, and common carotid arteries. No defects could be observed in the portal vein or in other small arteries and in veins of the test group. Animals of the control group showed no defects (Fig. 1A).

Computed Tomography

Five animals of the test group developed dystelectasis of the lower lung lobes, especially in paracardiac locations. The overall density of the lung parenchyma was markedly increased in all lung lobes. The air bronchogram was visible in all regions, but was more pronounced in central areas (Fig. 2).

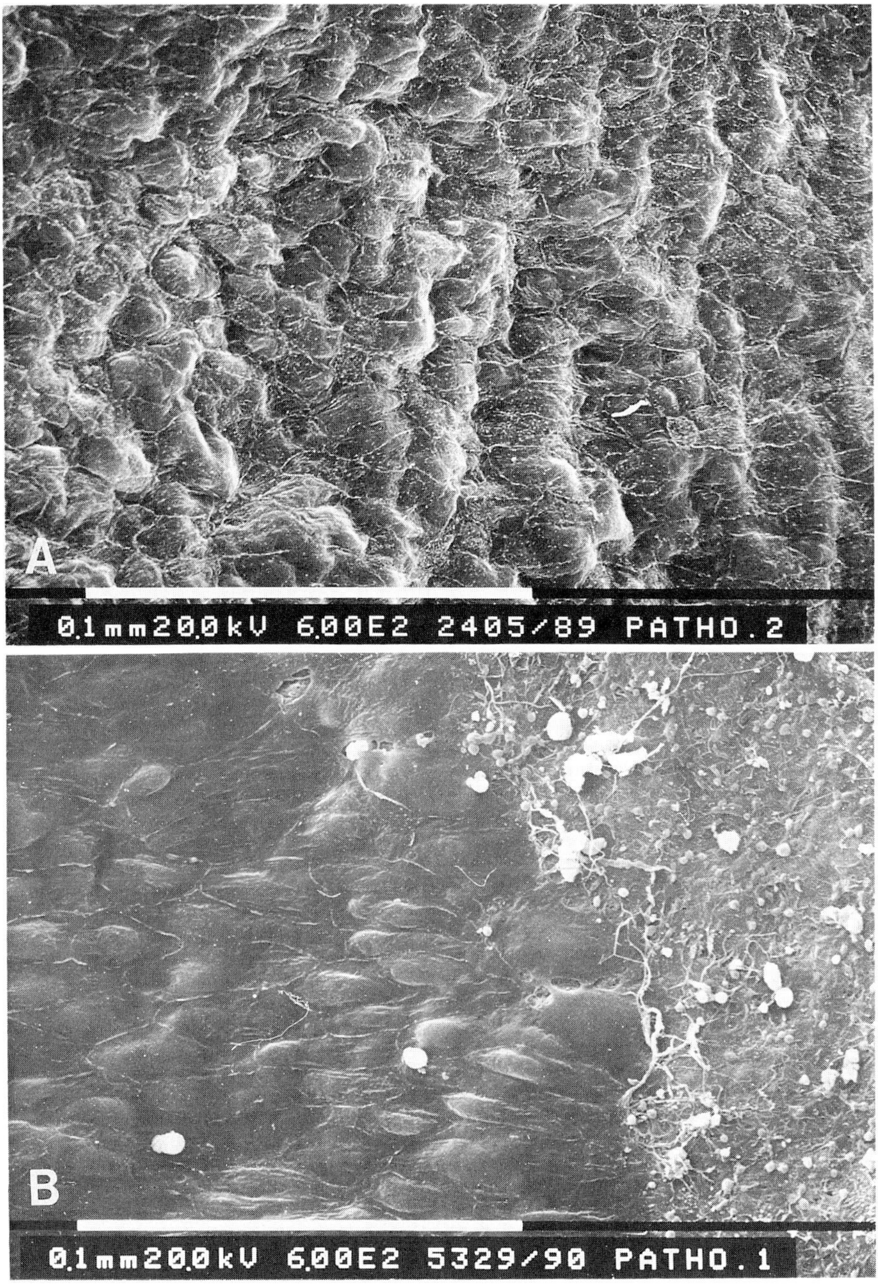

Fig. 1A, B. SEM study. **A** Intact pulmonary endothelial cell layer of control animals with protruding cell margins and superficial microvilli. ×1000. **B** Detached endothelial cells in a small pulmonary artery with exposure of the subendothelial components. Strands of fibrin and platelets are deposited. ×940

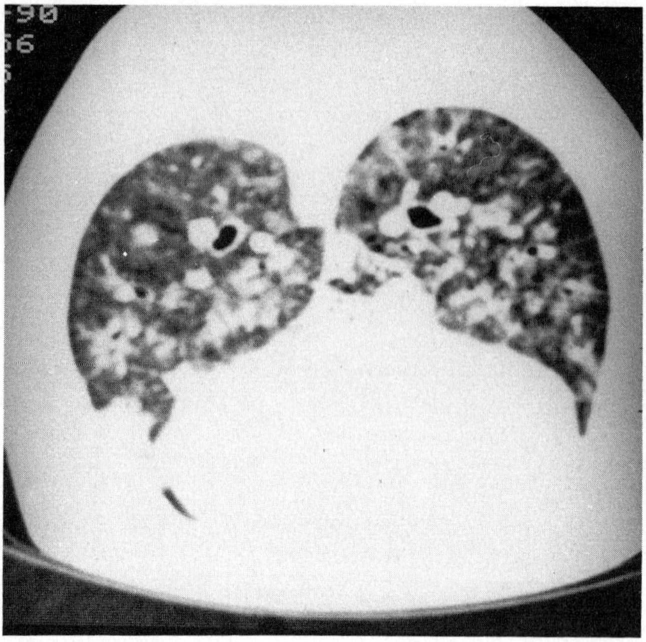

Fig. 2. CT of test animal, after 18 h experimental duration, with severe pulmonary edema, indicated by numerous opacities

One animal with clinically mild ARDS only presented accentuated interstitial opacities predominantly in ventral and paracardiac regions.

Discussion

The presented experimental model shows typical morphological alterations known from early human multiple organ failure. The histopathologic and ultrastructural changes seen in the test animals were similar to early and chronic changes in man [4] and to changes in other animal models [5, 6]. CT of lungs affected by severe interstitial edema (as confirmed by histopathologic findings) showed mainly in basal segments severe opacities similar to the changes seen in X-rays or CTs of human ARDS patients [7, 8].

The functional and structural impairment of the endothelial cell layer appears to be responsible for the permeability defects in the microvasculature. The question of whether this cell damage is a direct effect of endotoxin or indirectly mediated by other factors has been answered in a controversial way in the literature. Endotoxins have been extensively used to cause endothelial injury and several reports claim endothelial cell loss and injury in blood vessels [9, 10]. Parameters influencing the degree of injury seem to be the length of the observation period, the type and origin of the endothelial cells, and the amount and type of the applied endotoxins. In vitro experiments by Brigham and Meyrick [11] indicate that bovine pulmonary artery cells show necrosis under the influence of endotoxin concentrations of 1 μg/ml in the absence of serum. In the presence of 10% fetal calf serum endothelial cell damage can be elicited by concentrations as low as 0.001 μg/ml. From our studies porcine pulmonary artery endothelial cells do not appear to possess this sensitivity to endotoxin. But besides endotoxin other underlying pathobiochemical alterations in plasma during the course of septic shock have to be considered to influence endothelial cells: the dramatic increase in eicosanoid production [12] and PAF acether [13], release of cytokines, in particular of IL-1, IL-6, and TNE-α [14–16], formation of oxygen-derived free radicals from granulocytes and macrophages [17], release of leukocyte elastase [18] accompanied by oxidative inactivation of serum protease inhibitors, activation of the plasmatic coagulation cascade, fibrinolysis [19], and complement activation [20].

The results of our in vivo studies stress that in septic shock the endothelial cells are variably affected and probably the family of the endothelial cells can be subdivided into different groups with individual pathophysiological and -morphological reaction patterns. Severe endothelial cell damage was only found in medium-sized and small pulmonary vessels, the heart valves, and the whole microvasculature. Endothelium of other vessel sites showed no or discrete lesions. Tritiated thymidine autoradiography of the endothelium samples demonstrated that cell replication did increase in regions with endothelial cell injury, indicating that these endothelial lesions are not artifacts of preparation. These findings signify a balance or imbalance between endothelial cell injury and replication in different stages of septic shock.

In conclusion, we developed a porcine model of recurrent and prolonged endotoxemia. The morphological specimen showed early changes of cell failure and cell dysfunction. The uniform reaction pattern in all organs is characterized by generalized edema, cell degeneration, and cell death, in particular of the endothelial cells. Future experiments with longer experimental durations than 48 h have to show whether this porcine animal model is able to imitate the pathomorphology of chronic human multiple organ failure or not.

References

1. Shenep JL, Barrett FF, Stidham Gl, Westenkirchner DF, Flynn P (1985) Endotoxin liberation during therapy for gram-negative sepsis. Crit Care Med 13:298
2. Pearson FC, Dubczak J, Weary M, Bruszer G, Donohue G (1985) Detection of endotoxin in the plasma of patients with gram-negative bacterial sepsis by the limulus amoebocyte lysate assay. J Clin Microbiol 21(6):865–868

3. Ramsay G, Newman PM, McCartney AC, Ledingham IM (1988) Endotoxemia in multiple organ failure due to sepsis. Prog Clin Biol Res 272:237–246
4. Haselton PS (1983) Adult respiratory distress syndrome – a review. Histopathology 7:307–332
5. Craig I, Judges D, Gnidec A, Lefcoe M, Paterson N, Finley R, Sibbald W (1987) Pulmonary permeability edema in a large animal model of nonpulmonary sepsis. Am J Pathol 128:241–251
6. Hangen DH, Bloom RJ, Stevens JH, O'Hanley P, Ranchod M, Collins J, Raffin TA (1987) Adult respiratory distress syndrome – a live *E. coli* septic primate model. Am J Pathol 126:396–400
7. Gattinoni L, Pesenti A, Bombino M, Baglioni S, Rivolta M, Rossi F, Rossi G, Fumagalli R, Marcolin R, Mascheroni D, Torresin A (1988) Relationships between lung computed tomographic density, gas exchange, and PEEP in acute respiratory failure. Anesthesiology 69:824–832
8. Gattinoni L, Pesenti A, Avalli L, Rossi F, Bombino F (1987) Pressure-volume curve of total respiratory system in acute respiratory failure. Am Rev Respir Dis 136:730–736
9. Reidy MA, Schwartz SM (1983) Endothelial injury and regeneration IV. Endotoxin: a nondenuding injury to aortic endothelium. Lab Invest 48:25–34
10. Meyrick B, Johnson JE, Brigham KLAD (1989) Endotoxin-induced pulmonary endothelial injury. Prog Clin Biol Res 308:91–99
11. Brigham KL, Meyrick B (1986) Endotoxin and lung injury. Am Rev Respir Dis 133:913–927
12. Lefer AM (1989) Significance of lipid mediators in shock states. Circ Shock 27:3–12
13. Doebber TW, Wu MS, Robbins JC, Choy BM, Chang MN, Shen TY (1985) Platelet-activating factor (PAF) involvement in endotoxin-induced hypotension. Studies with PAF receptor antagonist kadsurenone. Biochem Biophys Res Commun 127:799–808
14. Dinarello CA (1988) Biology of interleukin 1. FASEB J 2:108–115
15. Haak CE, De Groot ER, Felt-Bersma JR, Nuijens JH, Strack van Schijndel RJM, Erenberg-Belmer AJM, Thijs LG, Aardden LA (1989) Increased plasma levels of interleukin-6 in sepsis. Blood 74:1704–1710
16. Cannon JG, Tompkins RG, Gelfand JA, Michie HR, Stanford GG, van der Meer JWM, Endres S, Lonnemann G, Corsetti J, Chernow B, Wilmore DW, Wolff SM, Burke JF, Dinarello CA (1990) Circulating interleukin-1 and tumor necrosis factor in septic shock and experimental endotoxin fever. J Infect Dis 161:79–84
17. Flohe L, Giertz H (1988) Endotoxins, arachidonic acid and superoxide formation. In: Urbascheck B (ed) Perspectives on bacterial pathogenesis and host defense. The University of Chicago Press, Chicago, pp 123–131
18. Fritz H, Jochum M, Daswald KH, Dittmer H, Kortmann H, Neumann S, Lang H (1986) Granulocyte proteinases as mediators of unspecific proteolysis in inflammation: a review in proteinases. In: Tschesche H (ed) Inflammation and tumor invasion. de Gruyter, Berlin, pp 1–23
19. West RL, Elovitz MJ, Hardaway RM (1966) Blood coagulation factors activity in experimental endotoxemia. Ann Surg 163:567–572
20. Snedegard G, Lui L, Hugli TE (1989) Endotoxin induced shock in the rat. A role of C5a. Am J Pathol 135:489–497

Endotoxin, Interferon-γ, Biopterin, Serum Phospholipase A_2 Activity and β-Endorphin as Differentiation Factors and Their Correlations in the Acute Immune Response During Lethal Gram-Negative Sepsis in LEW Rats

A. Hunsicker, W. Kullich, W. Weissenhofer, D. Lorenz, J. Petermann, K. Boden, I. Klöting, B. Panzig, G. Schwesinger, and H. Rokos

Aim of the Study

The purpose of our study was to establish a standardized reproducible animal model of intraperitoneal sepsis, induced by *E. coli* endotoxinaemia in LEW.1W rats, in order to investigate early immunoserological responses with a view to identifying a mediator-based evaluation system for such sepsis. In the pilot phase of this study we evaluate some mediators like endotoxin, phospholipase A_2 and neopterin (biopterin) as possible markers for the outcome, i.e., the prognosis of a peritonitis infection.

Introduction

Approximately 40% of patients with gram-negative sepsis undergo shock development, with a mortality of about 90% (DiPiro 1990; Neugebauer et al. 1987; Nyström et al. 1990). Endotoxin plays a central part in this process. Redl et al. (1989) describe endotoxin as the central mediator in the septic process. This potent bacterial antigen has toxic effects on all organ systems, even amounting to multiple organ failure. The process takes place by the systemic activation of cascade reactions of biological or inflammatory mediators of cellular and humoral immune defence (DiPiro 1990; Hardie and Kruse-Elliot 1990; Philippe and De Buyzere 1988). In this process macrophages produce a broad spectrum of markers, which represent the immune activation (Redl et al. 1989). Thus the cytokine interferon-γ (IFN-γ), released by the T lymphocytes, stimulates macrophages which secrete the tumour necrosis factor and interleukin-1 (IL-1). The macrophage-mediated stimulation of the eicosanoid metabolism with the activation of phospholipase A_2 (PLA_2) releases lipid mediators (Hardie and Kruse-Elliot 1990), and PLA_2 serum concentration correlates with the duration and severity of the septic event (Vadas 1984; Vadas et al. 1988). The pteridin derivative neopterin is distinguished as a further sensitive marker for the macrophage stimulation (Hausen et al. 1989; Kellermann et al. 1989). It is produced in the tetrahydro-biopterin (BH_4) cycle after an IFN-γ stimulus

(Huber 1984). Neopterin may be measured in humans and primates only (Duch et al. 1984; Ohlenschläger and Berger 1989; Kammüller et al. 1991); rats produce neopterin only in an intermediate stage in their metabolisation of the BH_4. Therefore it is necessary to estimate biopterin concentrations in rat models.

Materials and Methods

Diffuse peritonitis was induced by means of an intraperitoneal injection of a mixture of *E. coli* and haemoglobin, in accordance with the methods of Hau and Simmons (1978, 1981), Pruett et al. (1984, 1985) and Kullich and Weissenhofer (1988).

The animals studied were 42 male LEW.1W rats with a weight of 318 ± 44 g and an age of 10.1 ± 1.7 weeks.

E. coli were obtained from a patient who suffered from severe diffuse peritonitis: K1 : H^+, MR-HA negative; haemolysin negative; colicine positive; dulcitol-fermentation negative.

A control group received an intraperitoneal injection of 6.0 ml physiological saline solution. Animals in the peritonitis group were injected with 6.0 ml of a mixture consisting of 0.1 ml of a suspension containing 10^{10} *E. coli*/ml, 2.9 ml of diluted haemolytic autogenous blood with a haemoglobin concentration of 3% and 3.0 ml of a 0.9% NaCl solution.

E. coli Preparation. This strain, identified as *E. coli* (API 20 E, bio Merieux), was spread thickly with a spatula on Columbia agar (Oxoid), incubated for 18 h at 35°C and then rinsed with a sterile 0.9% NaCl solution free of pyrogen (Delta Pharma Co.). The microbial suspension was homogenised and suspended at a density of 1×10^{10} organisms/ml (McFarland-Standard; Vitec Systems ATB 1550, bio Merieux).

Preparation of the Haemoglobin Solution. To produce the Hb solution, autogenic rat blood was used. This was extracted after intraperitoneally anaesthetising the animals with thiopental (Nycomed Arzneimittel, Munich, FRG; 40 mg/100 g body weight) by means of cardiac puncture under sterile conditions. The blood was deep frozen 3 times at −30°C under sterile conditions to cause haemolysis. Before use, the haemolysed blood was adjusted to a Hb content of 3% using in a 0.9 NaCl solution.

As a consequence of the results of the initial experiments, the duration of this experiment was limited to 6 h. At the end of this period the animals were subjected to general intraperitoneal anaesthesia (thiopental). All the blood was extracted from the animals within 3 min by means of intracardiac puncture under aseptic conditions. Then the animals were dissected and the organs inspected.

Endotoxin. The measurement of the endotoxin content in the rat was performed by means of a quantitative chromogenic limulus-amoebocyte-lysate test, which was checked and approved by the FDA (QCL 1000, Whittaker Bioproducts Inc., Walkersville, Md., USA). This genuine, quantitative endotoxin test can identify endotoxin concentrations from 0.01 to 10 EU/ml. The measurement of the staining reaction was carried out using a microtitre plate photometer with an extinction at 405 nm (SLT EAR 400 FW, SLT, Austria) (Kullich et al. 1993).

Biopterin. The total biopterin in the serum was determined by means of radioimmunoassay (double antibody method) (Rokos 1989). Firstly, the acid oxidation of the insabile BH_4 to biopterin was brought about in 15 min by using manganese dioxide (6 mg in 20 μl 1 N HCl/100 μl serum). After neutralisation with diluted NaOH solution, addition of the specific biopterin antibodies and subsequent centrifugation, the residue was subjected directly to a radioimmunoassay.

Phospholipase A_2. To determine the phospholipase A_2 in the serum the test set was used to supplement the test combination "free fatty acids" and the enzymatic staining test to determine free fatty acids for use (Boehringer Mannheim Biochemica). PLA_2 causes lecithin to split into lysolecithin and free fatty acids. The fatty acids thus formed were then measured quantitatively using the fully enzymatic staining test. The coloured matter formed was measured with a spectral photometer, SUMAL PE2 (Carl Zeiss, Jena), at a wavelength of 512 nm. The activity is calculated from the amount of free fatty acids released per unit of time.

Interferon-γ. In the plasma, interferon-γ was measured by means of a solid-phase enzyme-linked immunosorbent assay, based on the sandwich principle (rat interferon-gamma ELISA, Cell Biology Products HBT Holland, Biotechnology; supplier for Austria: Biomedica Vienna). The test uses two monoclonal antibodies specific to rat IFN-γ. The enzyme reaction was determined at 405 nm (Kullich et al. 1993).

β-Endorphin. β-Endorphin was determined by means of direct measurement utilizing a solid phase, two-site immunoradiometric assay (IRMA) based on the "sandwich" principle. (Alle gro β-Endorphin, human beta-endorphin; Nichols Institute, San Juan Capistrano, Calif., USA). The radioactivity bound to the solid phase was measured with a gamma scintillation counter.

Statistics. The statistical calculation (descriptive statistics, Mann-Whitney U-test, correlations with Pearson R; linear discriminant analysis) was made on a personal computer using the software package SPSS –PC+, Vers. 4.01 (SPSS Inc., USA).

Results

In contrast to the sham-treated rats, the peritonitis animals showed significant differences in the concentrations of endotoxin, IFN-γ, biopterin and PLA_2 activity. There were no differences in the β-endorphin levels.

For the peritonitis group strong correlations were found between the degree of endotoxinaemia and elevated levels of IFN-γ ($r_p = 0.72$, $P < 0.0001$; Fig. 1) and biopterin synthesis ($r_p = 0.80$, $P < 0.00001$; Fig. 2).

The increase in IFN-γ levels was correlated to the regulatory synthesis of the pteridin derivate biopterin ($r_p = 0.73$, $P < 0.0001$; Fig. 3) and to the PLA_2 activity ($r_p = 0.50$, $P < 0.005$; Fig. 4).

The biopterin synthesis correlated slightly with the PLA_2 activity ($r_p = -0.38$; $P < 0.05$). In the peritonitis animals, the mean serum PLA_2 activity rose to 62.8% of normal serum activity in the control group, but was characterized by a weak level of significance ($P < 0.01$) during the prefinal phase of the septic shock process.

In the animals with peritonitis, it was impossible to demonstrate any significant correlation between the prefinal serum PLA_2 activities and the degree of endotoxinaemia ($r_p = 0.24$).

Using only the parameters of endotoxin, IFN-γ levels, biopterin and the PLA_2 activity, the statistical procedure of the linear discriminant analysis

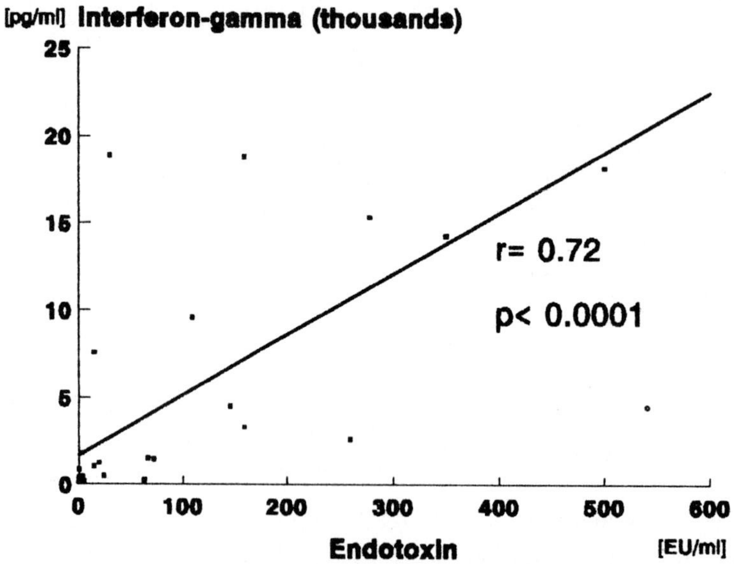

Fig. 1. Correlation between the degree of endotoxinaemia and the enhanced levels of IFN-γ in the prefinal phase of the septic shock process. The correlation coefficient of linear regression ($r_P = 0.72$) was highly significant ($P < 0.0001$)

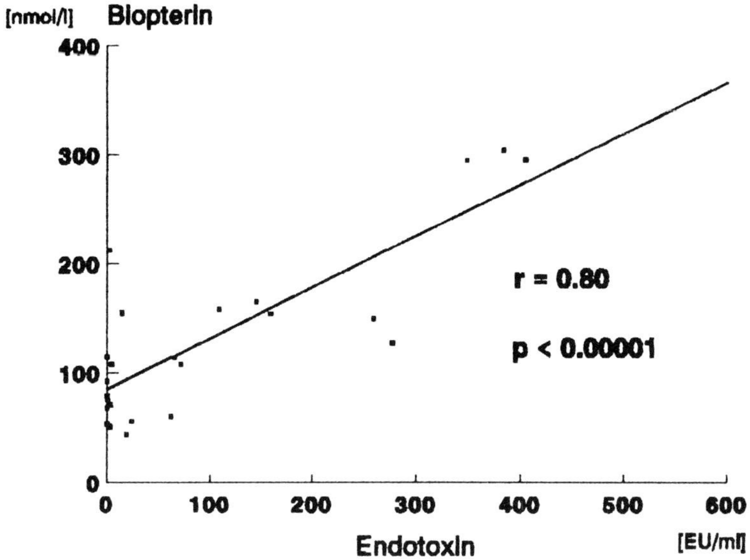

Fig. 2. Correlation between the degree of endotoxinaemia and the enhanced synthesis of biopterin in the prefinal phase of the septic shock process. The correlation coefficient of linear regression ($r_P = 0.80$) was highly significant ($P < 0.00001$)

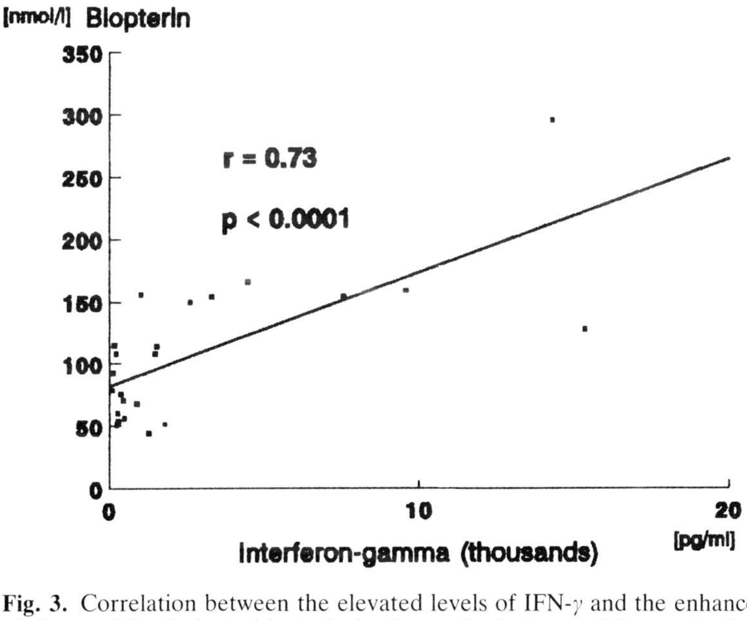

Fig. 3. Correlation between the elevated levels of IFN-γ and the enhanced synthesis of the pteridin derivate biopterin in the prefinal phase of the septic shock process. The correlation coefficient of linear regression ($r_P = 0.73$) was highly significant ($P < 0.0001$)

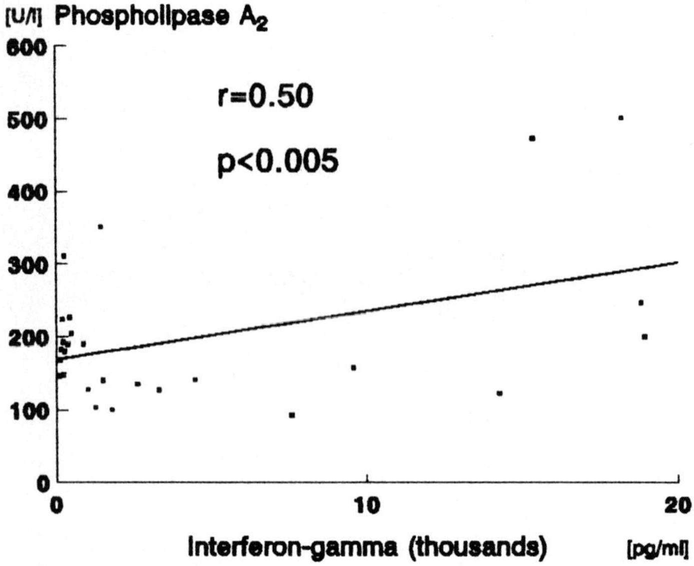

Fig. 4. Correlation between the elevated levels of IFN-γ and the enhanced serum phospholipase A_2 activity during the prefinal phase of the septic shock process. The correlation coefficient of linear regression ($r_P = 0.50$) was statistically significant ($P < 0.005$)

makes it possible to distinguish between non-septic animals and septic animals correctly at a rate of 87%.

Discussion

We used LEW.1W rats for a standardized reproducible animal model because of their good immunological responsiveness (Greenhouse et al. 1990; Hedrich 1990). The sepsis in these LEW.1W rats was induced by a haemoglobin/*E. coli* suspension, which is an accepted and well-tried model. After intraperitoneal injection of the Hb.-*E.coli* mixture, all animals suffered from fulminant peritonitis and died within 6 h.

Our experiments also confirm that the course of peritonitis correlates with level of endotoxin, both quantitatively and qualitatively (Gögler and Meckes 1989).

As section of endotoxin concentrations in the peripheral blood is always pathological and the limulus-amoebocyte-lysate test also allows highly sensitive, specific and rapid detection of endotoxin (Smalley et al. 1986), we suggest the practicability of serological monitoring of the peritonitis.

Phospholipases of the A_2 type are released mainly in the presence of, and following, a generalized septic infection in nearly all tissues or circulating cell populations, including monocytes/macrophages (Kellermann et al. 1989; Büchler 1989). As a result of the formation of arachidonic acid, phospholipases play an important regulatory role in the release of inflammatory mediators (Bastian et al. 1991). PLA_2 concentrations in humans show a marked increase 5–6h after the beginning of endotoxinaemia. The maximal enzyme activities were found after 24h (Vadas et al. 1991). In rats an increase in serum PLA_2 activity was found to be present 6h after the induction of peritonitis. Kellermann et al. (1989) found a slight correlation between PLA_2 activity and neopterin concentrations in human sepsis. In contrast to these findings, we were not able to demonstrate such a relation in the LEW rat model.

In the initial stages of the immune response, a situation comparable to that of experimental peritonitis in this animal model, T lymphocytes recognize microbial antigens and by the release of IFN-γ activate the monocyte/macrophage system (Kullich et al. 1993). Huber (1984) and Bitterlich et al. (1988) showed that IFN-γ selectively stimulates the mononuclear phagocytes to produce pteridines like neopterin. Since rats do not produce detectable neopterin (Duch et al. 1984), we considered the related pteridine biopterin as a marker for increased synthesis of pteridines in activated phagocytic cells.

Neopterin is suitable for differentiating between patients suffering from sepsis or non-septic disease, and neopterin is especially helpful in the clinical follow-up of patients with septic disease (Hausen et al. 1989). It was demonstrated in patients that neopterin seems to be a suitable marker for monocyte and macrophage stimulation in septic shock and organ failure (Redl et al. 1991).

The correlation of biopterin to endotoxin levels and to the release of IFN-γ also revealed clearly significant relationships between them. This result hints at the possibility that the secretion of biopterin from activated macrophages is induced by IFN-γ as well as by a direct impact of endotoxin (Kullich et al. 1993).

Conclusion

Endotoxin, IFN-γ, biopterin and PLA_2 measurements are sufficient for early recognition and estimation of the extent of the immunological activation process in peritonitis. These parameters allow differentiation between septic and non-septic disorders with high probability.

References

Bastian BC, Römisch J, Paques E-P, Burg G (1991) Lipokortine und Phospholipasen: Neue Aspekte in der Physiologie der Glukokortikosteroidwirkung. Hautarzt 42: 417–423

Bitterlich G, Szabo G, Werner ER, Larchner C, Fuchs D, Hausen A, Reibnegger G, Schultz TF, Troppmeier J, Wachter H, Dierich MP (1988) Selective induction of monouclear phagocytes to produce neopterin by interferons. Immunobiology 176: 228–235

Dipiro JT (1990) Pathophysiology and treatment of gram-negative sepsis. Am J Hosp Pharm 47(3):6–10

Duch S, Browers SW, Woolf JH, Nichol CA (1984) Biopterin cofactor biosynthesis: GTP cyciohydroiase, neopterin and biopterin in tissues and body fluids of mammalian species. Life Sci 35:1895–1901

Gögler H, Meckes P (1983) Peritonitis, septischer Schock und Endotoxin – elne tierexperimentelle studie. Z Exp Chir Transplant Künstliche Organe 22(3): 159–167

Greenhouse DD, Festing MFW, Hasan S, Cohen AL (1990) Catalogue of inbred strains of rats. In: Hedrich HJ (ed) Genetic monitoring of inbred strains of rats. Fischer, Stuttgart, pp 433–434

Hausen A, Fuchs D, Reibnegger G, Werner ER, Wachter H (1989) Neopterin in clinical use. Pteridines 1:3–10

Hedrich HJ (1990) List of congenic and segregating inbred strains. In: Hedrich HJ (ed) Genetic monitoring of inbred strains of rats. Fischer, Stuttgart, pp 481–486

Huber O (1984) Immune response-associated production of neopterin. J Exp Med 160:310

Kammüller ME, van Rooijen HJM, Seinen W, Bloksma N (1991) Urinary biopterin levels in mice during graft-versus-host reactions and during exposure to 5,5-diphenylhydantoin. Int J Immunopharmacol 13(5):463–471

Kellermann W, Frentzel-Beyme R, Welte M, Jochum M (1989) Phospholipase A in acute lung injury after trauma and sepsis: its relation to the inflammatory mediators PMN-elastase, C3a and neopterin. Klin Wochenschr 67:190–195

Kullich W, Weissenhofer W (1988) Thyroid function and endotoxinemia in experimental peritonitis. Surg Res Commun 3:159–164

Kullich W, Weissenhofer W, Hunsicker A, Rokos H (1993) Immune stimulation of the interferon-gamma and biopterin synthesis with endotoxin in animal-experimental peritonitis. Pteridines

Nyström PO, Bax R, Patchen Dellinger E, Dominioni L, Knaus AW, Meakins JL, Ohmann C, Solomkin JS, Wacha H, Wittmann H (1990) Proposed definitions for diagnosis, severity scoring, stratification, and outcome for trials on intraabdominal infections. World J Surg 14(2):148–158

Ohlenschläger G, Berger I (1989) Biochemische und klinische Beobachtungen zu den immunmodulatoren: Interferone (IFN), Interleukin-2 (IL-2), Tumornekrose-Faktor (TNF) und dem immunmarker Neopterin (Teil I). Biol Med 4:496–508

Philippe JJ, De Buyzere ML (1988) Endotoxin: detection and clinical significance. Acta Clin Belg 43(6):429–436

Pruett TL, Rotstein OD, Fiegel VD, Sorenson JJ, Nelson RD, Simmons RL (1984) Mechanism of the adjuvant effect of hemoglobin in experimental peritonitis. VIII. Surgery 96(2):375–382

Pruett TL, Rotstein OD, Wells CL, Sorenson JJ, Simmons RL (1985) Mechanism of the adjuvant effect of hemoglobin in experimental peritonitis. IX. Surgery 96(3): 371–377

Redl H, Strohmaier W, Schlag G, Pacher R, Woloszczuk W, Inthorn D, Troppmair J, Huber C (1989) Possible use of the monocyte/macrophage activation marker neopterin for clinical monitoring of sepsis-related multiorgan fallure. In: Immune consequences of trauma, hock and sepsis. Springer, Berlin Heidelberg Now York, pp 109–113

Redl H, Schlag G, Bahrami S, Dinges HP, Schade U, Ceska M (1991) Markers of endotoxin related leucocyte activation and injury mechanisms. Prog Clin Biol Res 367:83–100

Rokos H (1989) Radioimmunoassay for determination of biopterin. Pteridines 1(4): 224

Smalley DL, Baddour LM, Kraus AP Jr (1986) Rapid detection of gram-negative bacterial peritonitis by the limulus amoebocyte lysate assay. J Clin Microbiol 24(5):882–883

Vadas P (1984) Elevated phospholipase A_2 levels: correlation with the haemodynamic and puimonary changes in gram-negative septic shock. J Lab Clin Med 104:873

Vadas P, Pruzanski W, Stefanski E, Sternby B, Mustard R, Bohnen J, Fraser I, Farewell V, Bombardier C (1988) Pathogenesis of hypotension in septic shock. Crit Care Med 16:1

Vadas P, Pruzanski W, Farewell V (1991) A predictive model for the clearance of soluble phospholipase A_2 during septic shock. J Lab Clin Med 118:471–475

Gene Expression

The Effects of Burn Injury on Cytokine Production and Gene Expression

A.F. Horgan, J.A. Mannick, D.S. O'Riordan, M.V. Mendez, R.C. Holzheimer, K. Collins, and M.L. Rodrick

Introduction

Severe thermal injury leads to a depression of cell mediated immunity with abnormalities of T-lymphocyte activation and proliferation in response to antigenic or mitogenic stimuli [1–3]. Our laboratory has previously shown that one of the major immunologic abnormalities in this setting is decreased production of interleukin-2 (IL-2) in response to mitogenic stimulation [4]. IL-2 plays a central role in immunoregulation supporting lymphocyte proliferation, promoting helper cell activity and augmenting cytotoxicity.

The earliest events in T-cell activation from the stimulation of the T-cell receptor to IL-2 gene transcription have been the subject of intense investigation in recent years. At least two separate stimuli are necessary for T-cell activation and the production of lymphokines, one of which acts through the T-cell receptor and the other through activation of the CD28 molecule on the T-cell surface or through other accessory cell signalling mechanisms, including the production of interleukin-1 (IL-1). Among the early events which result from the triggering of T-cell surface receptors is activation of phospholipase C leading to hydrolysis of phosphatidylinositol 4,5-bisphosphate and the generation of two important second messengers inositol tris-phosphate and diacylglycerol [5]. Diacylglycerol, in turn, stimulates protein kinase C (pkC) activation and release of inositol tris-phosphate results in increased intracellular calcium ion concentration through mobilization of intracellular calcium and increased membrane calcium uptake [6]. These signals communicate by ill-defined mechanisms with the cell nucleus and control a set of transcription factors that interact with the regulatory regions of genes such as the IL-2 promotor, thus regulating transcription.

T-lymphocyte activation and proliferation also require the binding of IL-2 to receptor proteins on the cell's surface. This autocrine mechanism is of critical importance and is dependent on the expression of functional IL-2 receptors as well as the production and secretion of IL-2 protein. Structurally, the IL-2 receptor consists of a number of polypeptide chains. Of these, the principal two are a 55-kDa IL-2Rα chain and the 70- to 75-kDa IL-2Rβ chain. The β chain is of intermediate affinity and is expressed on resting cells. The α chain, on the other hand, is not expressed in the resting state, is of low affinity when expressed alone, but together with the IL-2Rβ forms the high affinity IL-2 receptor [7]. Expression of high affinity IL-2R and thus cell proliferation, is therefore significantly regulated by IL-2Rα gene expression [7, 8].

Alterations in macrophage/monocyte function also occur following thermal injury [9]. Macrophages isolated from major trauma and burn patients exhibit enhanced production of inflammatory cytokines [10]. However, there has been little systematic study of the timing of this phenomenon and its association with cytokine gene activation.

The presently reported studies were designed to study the production of IL-2 and the pro-inflammatory cytokines IL-1, IL-6, and tumor necrosis factor-α (TNF-α) as well as the expression of the IL-2 receptor in splenic mononuclear cells following thermal injury in an animal model. A further goal was to relate cytokine production and IL-2R receptor expression with the expression of mRNAs for these proteins as a first step in relating abnormalities of cytokine production and receptor expression with activation of the genes responsible for the synthesis of these molecules.

Methods

Animal Model

All animal studies were performed with the approval of and under the guidance of Harvard Medical School's Standing Committee on Animal Research and the National Institutes of Health. As previously described [2], male A/J mice, 7–8 weeks old (Jackson Laboratories, Bar Harbor, Maine), were caged in groups of five in a controlled environment with water and mouse food ad libitum for acclimatization for 1 week. Animals were randomized into study groups and anesthetized with pentobarbital sodium, and their dorsa were shaved. Animals were placed in a plastic template, and a burn injury of 20% body surface area or sham burn was produced by immersion for 9 s in water at 90°C or room temperature, respectively. The former produced a localized, full thickness burn. Animals were resuscitated with 1 ml 0.9% saline, recaged under the same conditions, and killed in groups of 11 or more burns and 11 or more sham burns 4, 7, 10, 14, or 21 days later. Spleens were harvested for in vitro studies.

Organ Harvesting and Cell Culture

Spleens were teased apart, and single cell suspensions were produced. Cells were washed 3 times in RPMI-1640 with 2 mmol/l L-glutamine, 10 mmol/l HEPES buffer, 5×10^{-2} mmol/l 2-mercaptoethanol, and a 1% antibiotic/antimycotic solution which contained 10 000 units of penicillin, 10 mg streptomycin, and 25 μg amphotericin B per ml. All reagents were obtained from

Grand Island Biological Company, New York. The mononuclear cells were counted in Turk's solution and diluted to 2×10^6/ml in the described medium with added 5% heat inactivated fetal calf serum (complete medium). For measurement of IL-2 production and IL-2 mRNA expression, cells were cultured on 96-well microtiter plates with 200 μl per well of a solution containing 1×10^6 cells/ml at 37°C in 5% CO_2 and stimulated in one of two ways. Concanavalin A (Con A) (Sigma Chemical Co., St Louis, Mo.) was used at a final well concentration of 2.5 µg/ml Con A or, alternatively, cells were stimulated with a combination of the phorbol ester PMA (Sigma Chemical Co.) at 20 ng/ml and the calcium ionophore A23187 (Sigma) at 40 ng/ml. For measurement of IL-1β, IL-6, and TNF-α production and mRNA expression, cells were stimulated with *Escherichia coli* 026:B6 lipopolysaccharide (LPS) (1 μg/ml) (Sigma Chemical Co.).

Measurement of Proliferative Response

After 30 h of stimulation 1 μCi of tritiated thymidine (^{3}HTdr; New England Nuclear, Boston, Mass.) was added to each well, and plates were rapidly frozen 18 h later. Plates were subsequently harvested with a multiautomated sample harvester (Cambridge Technology, Cambridge, Mass.) and ^{3}HTdr incorporation was counted for 1 min in a liquid scintillation counter (LKB Instruments, Gaithersburg, Md.). Mitogen responses were calculated by subtracting ^{3}HTdr incorporation in unstimulated cultures.

IL-2 Bioassay

Splenocytes from individual mice were cultured and stimulated with Con A or PMA/A23187, as described above. At 48 h supernatants were harvested and frozen at −20°C for later assay. Supernatants were diluted from 1:2 to 1:128 in 100 μl of complete medium, incubated for 1 h at 37°C and 5% CO_2 and CTLL-2 cells added (100 μl at 5×10^4 cells/ml). Cultures were incubated for 20 h at 37°C in 5% CO_2 and proliferation assessed by uptake of 3-(4,5-dimethylthiazol-2-yl)-2,5-diphenyltetrazolium bromide (MTT) (Sigma). MTT was added (125 μg per well) and after 4 h, cells were solubilized by the addition of 10% acidified sodium dodecyl sulfate (SDS). Uptake and conversion of MTT to formazan was determined in an automated enzyme-linked immunosorbent assay (ELISA) reader (Molecular Devices, Mountain View, Calif.) at 570 nm, using 650 nm as reference. IL-2 production was then calculated from standard curves using probit analysis (computer software generously provided by Dr. Brian Davis of Immunex Corp, Seattle, Wash.).

IL-1 Bioassay

Supernatants of splenocytes stimulated with *E. coli* LPS for 48 h were tested for IL-1 using a CTLL-2/NOB-1 bioassay. Briefly 1×10^5 NOB-1 cells and 5×10^3 CTLL-2 cells were added in $100\,\mu l$ media per well to 96 well plates as above. Supernatants were added to wells in serial dilutions from 1:2 to 1:128. Plates were incubated for 20 h at 37°C in the presence of 5% CO_2, pulsed with ^{3}HTdr (New England Nuclear, Boston, Mass.) $1\,\mu$Ci/well, and incorporation of ^{3}HTdr determined using a liquid scintillation counter (LKB instruments, Gaithersburg, MD). IL-1 was then calculated using probit analysis.

IL-6 Bioassay

IL-6 production was determined using the IL-6 dependent B9 cell line (with kind permission of Dr. Aarden). IL-6 was the generous gift of Genetics Institute, Cambridge, Mass. Supernatants were serially diluted as above, and after equilibration at 37°C and 5% CO_2 for 1 h, 5×10^3 B9 cells per well were added. Plates were incubated for 68 h, followed by the addition of $125\,\mu$g/well of MTT for 4 h. Cells were then solubilized by the addition of 10% acidified SDS, and uptake of MTT determined in the automated ELISA reader. IL-6 production was calculated from standard curves.

TNF ELISA

TNF was measured using a "sandwich" ELISA technique as modified from Sheehan et al. [11]. Briefly adherent cell supernatants were incubated in 96 well ELISA plates coated with hamster monoclonal anti-murine-TNF antibody (Genzyme, Boston, Mass.). The plates were washed and incubated sequentially with rabbit polyclonal anti-TNF antibody (Genzyme), and alkaline phosphatase-conjugated goat anti-rabbit IgG (Boehringer Mannheim, Indianapolis, Ind.). The alkaline phosphatase linked antibody was then detected at 400 nm after incubation with the phosphatase substrate *p*-nitrophenyl phosphate disodium (Sigma, St. Louis, Mo.).

RNA Isolation and Northern Blot Analysis

Northern blot analysis for cytokine mRNA expression was performed on days 7, 10, and 14 following injury. After 8 h of stimulation in vitro with Con A or LPS, cells from animals in each group were pooled, lysed in guanidium isothiocyanate, and stored at −70°C. Total cellular RNA from 1

$\times$ 10^8 cells per sample was isolated using a phenol/chloroform extraction. RNA samples were electophoresed on 1% agarose/formaldehyde gels and transferred to nylon membranes by capillary action. RNA was fixed to membranes by ultraviolet crosslinking.

cDNA Probes

cDNA probes were produced from plasmids for murine IL-2, murine p55 IL-2 receptor, murine IL-1β, murine TNF-α, and chicken β-actin and radiolabelled with [a^{32}P]deoxycytidine triphosphate (New England Nuclear) with random sequence hexanucleotide priming [12]. Briefly, 25 ng of the cDNA probe was denatured at 100°C for 10 min and then incubated with Klenow enzyme, a mixture of dATP, dGTP, and dTTP (Boehringer Mannheim), and 50 μCi [a^{32}P]dCTP for 120 min at 37°C. The reaction was terminated with ethylenediaminetetraacetate (EDTA). Labelling was measured in a liquid scintillation counter (LKB Instruments) and specific activity calculated. Specific activity ranged from 5×10^8– 5×10^9 cpm/μg. Probes were denatured using sodium hydroxide and fish sperm DNA was added to decrease nonspecific binding.

Hybridization

Prehybridization was at 42°C for 1–2 h in a solution containing 0.1% SDS, 50 m*M* Tris, 1 *M* NaCl, and 1 m*M* EDTA in a rotating glass bottle. Radiolabelled murine cDNA (25 ng) was hybridized with the membranes for 18 h under the following conditions: 50% formamide, 1 $\times$ Denhardt's solution, 0.1% SDS, 10 m*M* phosphate buffer, 5 $\times$ SSC (0.15 *M* NaCl, 15 m*M* sodium citrate), 20 μg/ml denatured salmon sperm DNA (Sigma) at 42°C. Membranes were washed 4 times for 30 min each: two washes at room temperature, 2 $\times$ SSC, and 0.1% SDS and the last two washes at 55°C, 0.1 $\times$ SSC, 0.1% SDS. Membranes were wrapped in plastic and autoradiographed using Kodak XAR-5 film (Sigma) and intensifying screens at −70°C. The probe was later stripped from the membrane in a 1% glycerol solution at 80°C for 10 min and hybridization using β-actin cDNA was subsequently performed.

Quantification and Standardization of mRNA Expression

Autoradiographs were quantified using a laser densitometer (Molecular Dynamics, 300 Series computing densitometer). Signal intensity for cytokine and IL-2R mRNA expression was normalized using the β-actin signal and expressed as a ratio of cytokine to β-actin mRNA expression.

Interleukin-2 Receptor p55 Protein Expression in CD3+ Cells

Splenocytes were harvested and cultured in the presence of Con A, as described above, for 48 h, after which viability was assessed with trypan blue stain. 10^6 viable cells were incubated for 45 min at 4°C in the presence of fluorescein conjugated monoclonal murine anti-CD3 antibody (Boehringer Mannheim, Indianapolis, Ind.) and phycoerythrin conjugated anti-IL-2R p55 chain antibody (Boehringer Mannheim) and then fixed in formaldehyde. Samples were processed using an Epics C flow cytometer with a single 488-nm argon laser, counting 5000 cells per sample. Forward and 90° two-color analysis was used and the data were processed by computer using Howard Shapiro 4cyte software. Nonspecific fluorescence and background staining was accounted for using appropriate controls including normal murine IgG and staining of unstimulated cells.

Cellular Interleukin-2 Binding

Splenocytes were stimulated with Con A (2.5 μg/ml) for 48 h, after which 10^6 viable cells were incubated for 1 h at 4°C with biotinylated recombinant human interleukin-2 (Boerhinger Mannheim), then washed and incubated for 45 min in the presence of an avidin-fluorescein complex. Samples were again processed by flow cytometric analysis as above. Nonspecific fluorescence and background staining were accounted for using an irrelevant first step antibody followed by the same second step reagent.

Statistical Analysis

Control and burn animals were compared and results expressed as percentage change in the burn group compared to the sham group. Proliferation and cytokine production between the different groups were compared using the Mann-Whitney U test. Results were considered significant if $P \leqslant 0.05$.

Results

IL-2 Production and Mitogenic Response to Con A Stimulation

Initially, cells from burn and sham burn animals were stimulated with the mitogenic lectin Con A which directly activates the CD3/T cell receptor complex, mimicking the effects of antigen presentation. T-cell suppression was confirmed by reduction of the proliferative response to mitogenic stimulation in burn animals, by 50%, 37%, and 23% on days 4, 7, and 10, respectively, following injury (Table 1). Significant suppression of IL-2

Table 1. In vitro proliferation of mouse splenocytes in response to stimulation with Con A expressed in counts per minute

	Day after burn				
	4	7	10	14	21
Sham	40 864	51 029	47 154	78 281	89 409
Burn	20 499	31 904	36 189	74 238	78 978
Percent change[a]	−50*	−37*	−23	−5	−12

* $P < 0.05$
[a] Percent change is the percent difference in burns compared with controls

production in burn mice compared to controls occurred at days 7 (40% suppression), 10 (36%), and 14 (30%) following burn injury ($P < 0.05$) (Fig. 1).

IL-2 Production and Mitogenic Response to PMA/A23187 Stimulation

To determine whether abnormalities in the initiating events of the T-cell activation pathway played a significant role in abnormal activation, cells were stimulated with phorbol myristate acetate (PMA) and with the calcium ionophore A23187. By directly activating pkC and increasing $[Ca^{2+}]_i$, PMA/A23187 bypasses these early events. In comparison to the sham burns, cells from burned mice showed a consistent suppression of IL-2 production when stimulated with PMA/A23187 (Fig. 2). This suppression was of a similar magnitude to, and showed good temporal correlation with, that seen following Con A stimulation, ranging between 30% and 41% on days 7 through 21 ($P < 0.05$, all days). The proliferative response was also consistently suppressed in burn animals stimulated in this manner but on no day did this reach statistical significance.

IL-2 mRNA Expression

Having established that the abnormalities in IL-2 production following burn injury are primarily downstream of the early transmembrane signalling events we then examined IL-2 mRNA expression to determine whether these abnormalities were pre- or post-transcriptional. Cells from burned mice, whether stimulated with Con A or with PMA/A23187, demonstrated suppression of IL-2 mRNA expression compared to the control animals on all days (Fig. 3). When quantified by densitometry and standardized to β-actin mRNA, IL-2 mRNA suppression in burn animals compared to controls

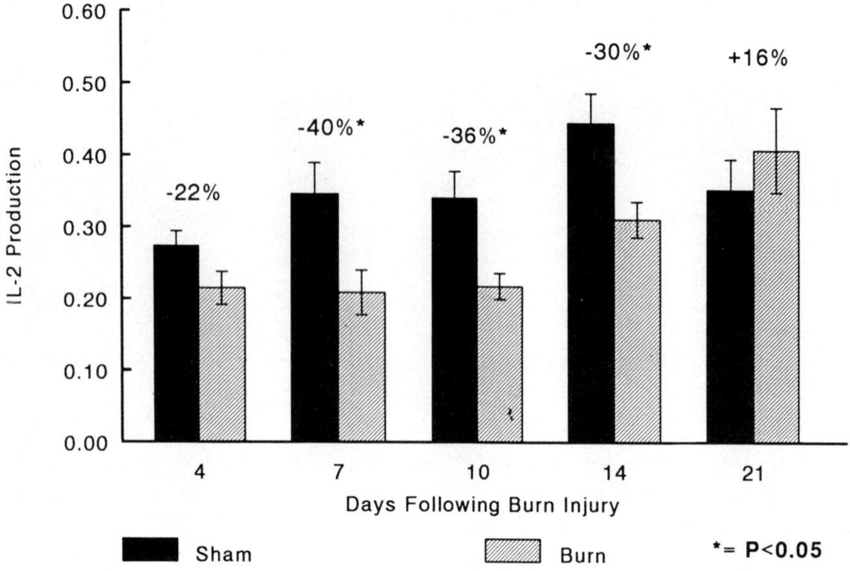

Fig. 1. IL-2 production of Con A-stimulated splenocytes of sham burn and burned animals on days 4, 7, 10, 14, and 21 after injury. *Numbers above error bars* represent percent change in burned animals compared with sham burns. $^*P < 0.05$. (Reprinted with permission of Surgery)

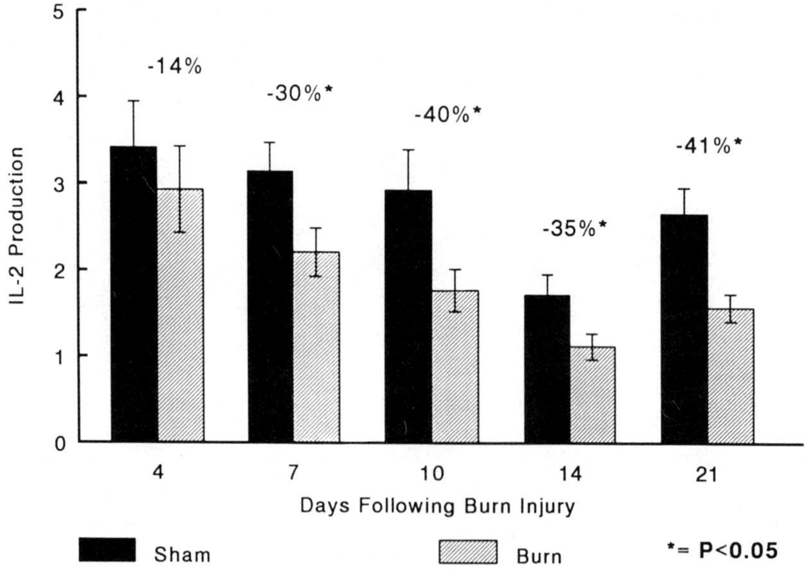

Fig. 2. IL-2 production of splenocytes of sham burn and burned animals on days 4–21 stimulated with PMA and the calcium ionophore A23187. *Numbers above error bars* represent percent change in burned animals compared with sham burns. $^*P < 0.05$. (Reprinted with permission of Surgery)

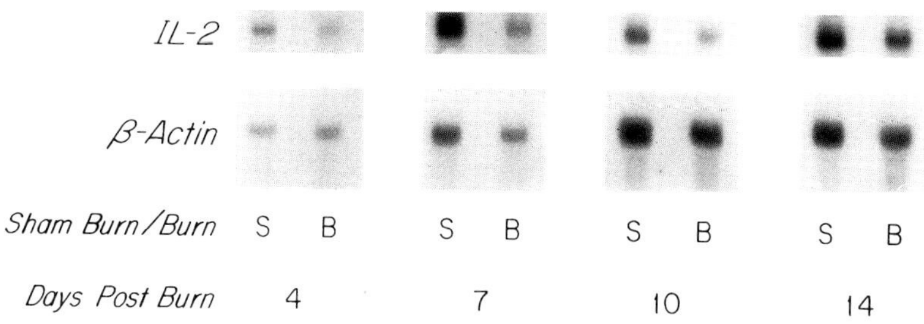

Fig. 3. Northern blot shows IL-2 mRNA expression in PMA + A23187-stimulated splenocytes of sham burn and burned animals on days 4, 7, 10, and 14 after injury. IL-2 message is shown above and β-actin control below. (Reprinted with permission of Surgery)

was 74%, 46%, 38%, and 29% on days 4, 7, 10, and 14 respectively for cells stimulated with Con A (Fig. 4) and 11%, 67%, 46%, and 31% on days 4, 7, 10, and 14 respectively with PMA/A23187 stimulation (Fig. 5).

IL-2R Expression

Cell surface IL-2R p55 chain expression in mitogen stimulated $CD3^+$ cells was not changed in the burn animals compared to the control animals at any day measured between day 4 and 21 (Table 2). The percentage of Con A stimulated, CD3+ cells expressing IL-2R p55 measured between 50% and 80% at different time points, and at any given time point results in burn and control groups were very similar, varying by no more than 9% on day 7.

IL-2 Receptor Functional Studies

Binding of fluorescein labelled IL-2 was unchanged in burned animals compared with sham burned mice on days 4, 7, and 21 but was increased by 117% ($P < 0.01$) and 22% (P = n.s.) on days 10 and 14, respectively (Table 2).

Addition of IL-2 to cultures of cells from burned mice caused a significant increase in the proliferative response on all days following injury, indicating the presence of functional cellular IL-2 receptors. On each day IL-2 restored the response of the burn cells to that of the control cells.

IL-2R mRNA Expression

IL-2R p55 chain mRNA expression in response to in vitro stimulation, as measured by Northern blot analysis, showed no consistent change in ther-

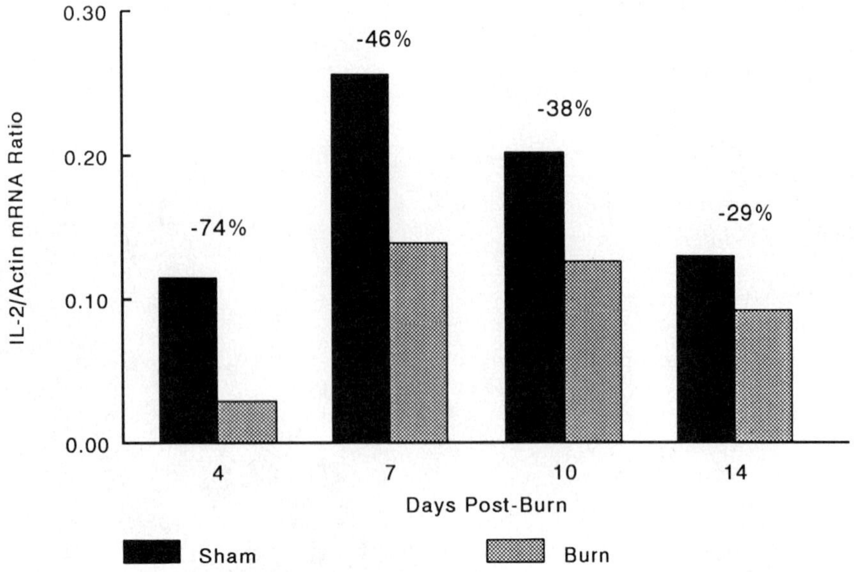

Fig. 4. Results of quantification by laser densitometry and standardization to β-actin control of IL-2 mRNA expression in Con A stimulated splenocytes of sham burn and burned animals on days 4, 7, 10, and 14 after injury. *Numbers above bars* represent percent change in burned animals compared with sham burns. (Reprinted with permission of Surgery)

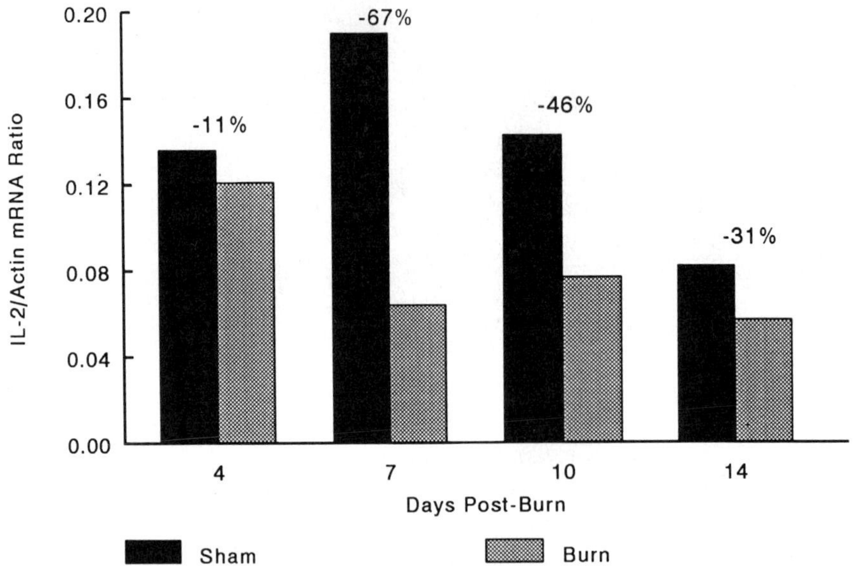

Fig. 5. Results of quantification by laser densitometry and standardization to β-actin control of IL-2 mRNA expression in PMA + A23187-stimulated splenocytes of sham burn and burned animals on days 4, 7, 10, and 14 after injury. *Numbers above bars* represent percent change in burned animals compared with sham burns

Table 2. Results of in vitro studies of IL-2R expressed as percentage change in the burned mice compared to the sham burn animals

	Day 4	Day 7	Day 10	Day 14	Day 21
IL-2R expression in CD3+ cells	−6%	+9%	+1%	+7%	−5%
Splenocyte Il-2 binding	−3%	+2%	+117%*	+22%	−7%

* $P < 0.01$

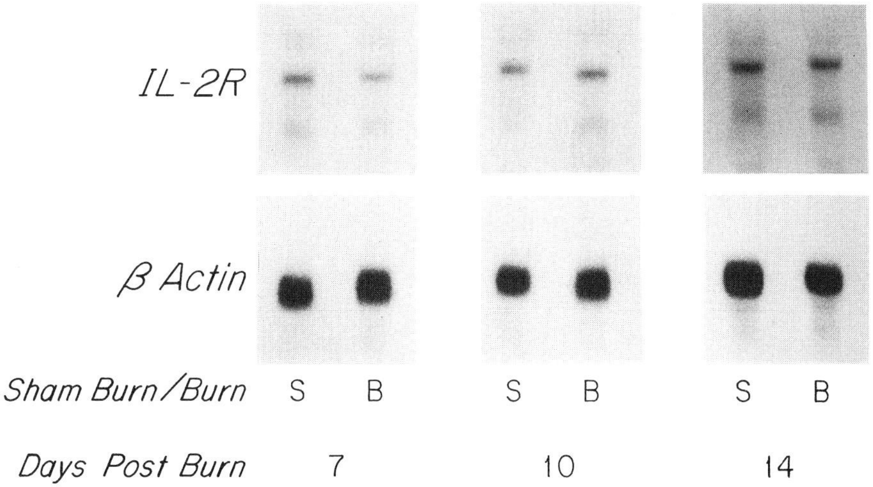

Fig. 6. IL-2 receptor p55 chain mRNA expression in mitogen stimulated murine splenocytes on days 7, 10, and 14 following burn or sham burn injury

mally injured animals compared to controls when measured on days 7, 10, or 14 (Fig. 6). Quantification by laser densitometry revealed changes in IL-2R p55 mRNA expression in the burn animals of −23%, +6%, and −12% respectively on days 7, 10, and 14.

Monokine Secretion

IL-1, IL-6, and TNF production by LPS-stimulated adherent splenocytes were all significantly increased by day 10 in the burned mice when compared with sham burn mice (Fig. 7). Median IL-1 production by cells from burned mice was 12.5 units/ml (P = 0.0001), TNF production 1582 pg/ml (P = 0.002), and IL-6 production 0.565 units/ml (P = 0.0007) compared with sham burned values (median IL-1 1.43 units/ml, TNF 155 pg/ml, and IL-6 0.01 units/ml).

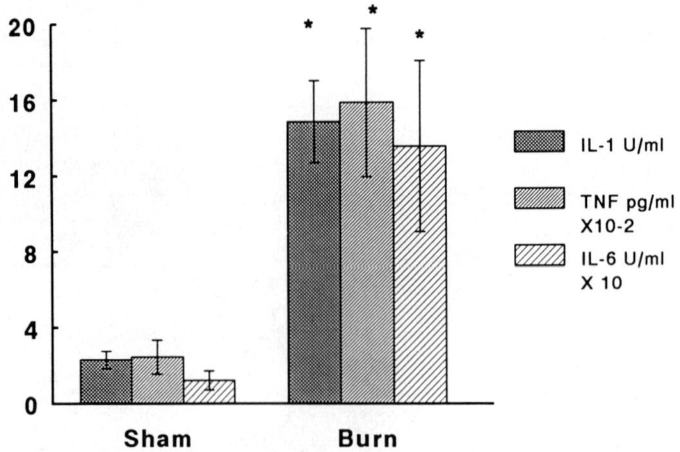

Fig. 7. Effective burn injury on adherent splenocyte secretion of IL-1β, TNF-α, and IL-6 in response to LPS stimulation in culture. IL-1 in u/ml, TNF pg/ml $\times$ 10^{-2}, and IL-6 in u/ml $\times$ 10. Production of all three monokines was significantly increased in cultures from burned animals as compared to those from sham burns. $^*P < 0.01$. (Reprinted with permission of Archives of Surgery)

IL-1β and TNF-α mRNA Expression

Expression of IL-1β and TNF-α mRNA after thermal injury were also examined. IL-1β mRNA expression was increased by 177% and 213% in burned animals at days 4, 7, 10, and 14, respectively. TNF-α mRNA expression was suppressed by 33% on day 4 but increased on days 7, 10, and 14 by 18%, 66%, and 83%, respectively.

Discussion

This study showed impaired in vitro T-cell IL-2 production after burn injury whether the CD3 T-cell receptor complex was directly activated with a mitogenic lectin or whether the early trans-membrane signalling events were bypassed activating cells downstream of these events with the combined use of a phorbal ester and calcium ionophore. These findings suggest that a major defect in T-cell activation occurs beyond the initial membrane-activating events. Although these results do not rule out additional problems in the earlier part of the pathway, the fact that the magnitude of suppression of IL-2 production in PMA/A23187 stimulated cells is very similar to that seen with Con A points toward the principal cellular abnormalities being at or beyond pkC activation and Ca^{2+} mobilization.

We attempted to localize further the perturbation in T cells after thermal injury and in particular, to define the relationship of IL-2 production to IL-2 gene transcription. Whether stimulated by Con A or by PMA/A23187 a significant reduction in IL-2 mRNA expression was seen in burned animals, suggesting that blockage of IL-2 production is pretranscriptional. Although we cannot rule out concomitant post-transcriptional defects, the magnitude of IL-2 mRNA suppression is such that it is unnecessary to hypothesize further distal problems to explain the observed decrease in IL-2 production. Although increased cellular breakdown of IL-2 mRNA is possible, this seems less likely than a defect in regulation of gene transcription.

Other groups have previously addressed the question of IL-2R expression following trauma or thermal injury. Teodorczyk-Injeyan et al. [13] have shown a decrease in the percentage of T lymphocytes expressing IL-2Rα in patients following thermal injury. However, Schluter et al. [14] recently reported increased IL-2Rα expression in severely burned patients. A number of studies have suggested the presence of functional cellular IL-2R by demonstrating a significant proliferative response of lymphocytes from burn victims with the addition of recombinant IL-2 to in vitro cultures [15]. Our results clearly demonstrate normal expression of cell surface IL-2Rα in mitogen-stimulated CD3+ cells following thermal injury. This finding is further strengthened by the demonstration of normal IL-2Rα mRNA expression in this setting. Burn injury in this model was clearly sufficient to induce immunosuppression as demonstrated by reduced lymphocyte proliferation and IL-2 production as noted above.

We further demonstrated in this study that IL-2R function is normal following this degree of thermal injury. Cellular binding of IL-2 was normal early and late and increased on days 10 and 4 after injury, possibly reflecting an increased quantity of cell surface IL-2Rα as demonstrated by Schluter et al. [14]. The addition of human recombinant IL-2 to in vitro cell cultures restored the proliferative response of suppressed lymphocytes to normal, demonstrating the presence of functional IL-2R. Together these studies provide strong evidence that diminished expression or function of the IL-2 receptor does not play a significant role in the immunosuppression seen after thermal injury. These studies further suggest that reduced IL-2 production rather than an abnormality of the IL-2 receptor is the dominant T-cell defect in this setting.

Finally, increased monokine production by macrophages was seen in mice 10 days after burn injury. This time corresponds to the peak mortality from a septic challenge previously shown in this same model [2]. But it is likely that macrophage activation is sustained for many days or weeks after injury. Stimulation of the macrophage may represent an attempt of the injured host to adapt to injury and there are undoubtedly certain advantages gained in doing so [16]. Bacterial phagocytosis may be increased. The cytokines IL-1 and TNF may have beneficial effects [17, 18].

However, the prolonged macrophage activation seen after major burn injury also exerts detrimental effects on the host. The continuing acute phase response leads to inappropriate hypercatabolism with rapid loss of body protein which is ultimately harmful. TNF produced by macrophages may result in the development of the adult respiratory distress syndrome and macrophage activation and increased secretion of pro-inflammatory cytokines has been implicated in the development of multiple system organ failure [19, 20]. Dow-regulation in monokine production, therefore, may not only prevent harmful effects from individual monokines but also the consequences of synergistic toxicity among cytokines. In our studies, increased production of IL-1 and TNF was accompanied by increased expression of mRNA for these cytokines by splenic mononuclear cells and suggests that cytokine production and cytokine gene transcription are coordinated in this model.

Acknowledgements. This work was supported by NIH grant #5R01 GM35633-09, Brigham Surgical Group Foundation and Ainsworth Scholarship, University College, Cork, Ireland.

References

1. Wolfe JH, Wu AV, O'Connor NE et al. (1982) Anergy, immunosuppressive serum, and impaired lymphocyte blastogenesis in burn patients. Arch Surg 117:1266–1271
2. Moss NM, Gough DB, Jordan A, Grbic JT, Rodrick ML, Mannick JA (1988) Temporal correlation of impaired immune response after thermal injury with susceptibility to infection in a murine model. Surgery 104:882–887
3. Teodorczyk-Injeyan JA, Sparkes BG, Mills GB, Peters WJ, Falk RE (1986) Impairment of T cell activation in burn patients: a possible mechanism of thermal injury-induced immunosuppression. Clin Exp Immunol 65:570–581
4. Wood JJ, Rodrick ML, O'Mahoney et al. (1984) Inadequate interleukin 2 production: a fundamental immunological deficiency in patients with major burns. Ann Surg 200:311–320
5. Imboden J, Stobo J (1985) Transmembrane signalling by the T cell antigen receptor: perturbation of the CD3 antigen receptor complex generates inositol phosphates and releases calcium ions from intracellular stores. J Exp Med 161:446–456
6. Kuno M, Gardner P (1987) Ion channels activated by inositol 1,4,5-triphosphate in plasma membranes of human T lymphocytes. Nature 326:301–304
7. Tsudo M, Kozak RW, Goldman CK, Waldmann TA (1987) Contribution of a p75 interleukin-2 binding peptide to a high-affinity interleukin-2 receptor complex. Proc Natl Acad Sci USA 84:4215–4218
8. Szamel M, Kracht M, Krebs B, Hubner U, Resch K (1990) Activation signals in human lymphocytes: interleukin-2 synthesis and expression of high affinity interleukin 2 receptors require differential signalling for the activation of protein kinase C. Cell Immunol 126:117–128
9. Fong Y, Moldawer LL, Shires GT, Lowry SF (1990) The biological characteristics of cytokines and their implications in surgical injury. Surg Gynecol Obstet 170:363–378
10. Takayama TK, Miller C, Szabo G (1990) Elevated tumor necrosis factor alpha production concomitant to elevated prostaglandin E_2 production by trauma patients' monocytes. Arch Surg 125:29–35

11. Sheehan KC, Ruddle NH, Schreiber RD (1989) Generation and characterization of hamster monoclonal antibodies that neutralize murine tumor necrosis factors. J Immunol 142:3884–3893
12. Feinberg AP, Vogelstein B (1983) A technique for radiolabelling DNA restriction endonuclease fragments to a high specific activity. Anal Biochem 132:6–13
13. Teodorczyk-Injeyan JA, McRitchie DI, Peters WJ (1990) Expression and secretion of IL-2 receptor in trauma patients. Ann Surg 212:202–208
14. Schluter B, Wolfgang K, Koller M et al. (1991) Differential regulation of T and B-lymphocyte activation in severely burned patients. J Trauma 31:239–246
15. Grbic JT, Mannick JA, Gough DB, Rodrick ML (1991) The role of prostaglandin E2 in immune suppression following injury. Ann Surg 214:253–263
16. Callery MP, Kamei R, Mangino MJ, Flye MW (1991) Organ interactions in sepsis. Host defense and the hepatic-pulmonary macrophage axis. Arch Surg 126:28–32
17. Silver GM, Gamelli RD, O'Reilly M, Hebert JC (1990) The effect of interleukin-1 alpha on survival in a murine model of burn wound sepsis. Arch Surg 125: 922–925
18. Alexander HR, Langstein HN, Doherty GM, Jensen JC, Norton JA (1990) Human recombinant tumor necrosis factor (hrTNF) protection against endotoxin-induced shock and lethality in the rat. Surg Forum 41:103–105
19. Okusawa S, Gelfand JA, Ikejima T, Connolly RJ, Dinarello CA (1988) Interleukin-1 induces a shock-like effect in rabbits. Synergism with tumor necrosis factor and the effects of cyclooxygenase inhibition. J Clin Invest 81:1162–1172
20. Border JR (1988) Hypothermia, sepsis multiple systems organ failure and the macrophage. Arch Surg 123:285–286

Genomic Fingerprinting for the Evaluation of Epidemic Processes

A. Schwarzkopf, H. Böhm, H. Schmidt, J. Heesemann, and H. Karch

Introduction

Conventional classification of bacteria is based on biochemical features, serology, and chemotaxonomy. Modern taxonomy attempts to separate bacterial species according to their ancestral relationships by molecular methods. Consequently, methods are used which measure genetic relationship by DNA/DNA or DNA/rRNA hybridizations, rRNA gene sequencing, and analysis of restriction fragment-length polymorphism (RFLP). These methods have also revealed applicability for differentiation of pathogens within a single bacterial species. Reliable typing of bacterial isolates from patients is paramount for basic and epidemiological studies of bacterial infections. Typing of clinical isolates also has great potential for hygienic control programs in determining the source of infectious diseases.

Restriction Endonuclease Analysis of Bacterial Genomes

In recent years, restriction endonuclease analysis of bacterial genomes has been shown to be a useful tool for the differentiation of bacteria [1]. In the past the genome fingerprinting was performed with frequently cutting restriction enzymes, yielding a pattern of hundreds of poorly resolved fragments. As shown in Fig. 1A, this procedure could not clearly differentiate between various clinical *E. coli* strains from different patients. This limited the general applicability of genome fingerprinting for epidemiological studies. At present, rare cutting restriction endonucleases are used to digest the bacterial genomes [2]. This procedure yields individual and easy to analyze fragment patterns that are different between unrelated strains. As shown in Fig. 1B, the same genomes of the strains in Fig. 1A were digested with one rare cutting restriction enzyme (*Xba*I), resulting in very distinct fingerprints.

Applicability of Pulsed Field Gel Electrophoresis

Fragments obtained with rare cutting restriction endonucleases are best separated by pulsed field gel electrophoresis (PFGE). An advantage of

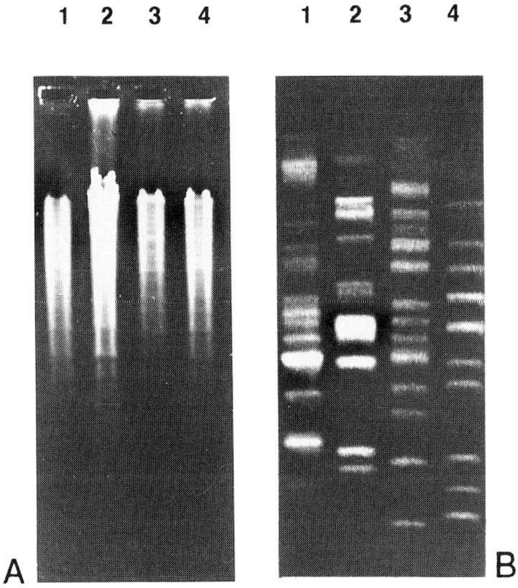

Fig. 1. A Chromosomal DNA of *E. coli* restricted with a frequently cutting restriction enzyme *Eco*RI resulting in hundreds of fragments. Ethidium bromide stained. **B** Chromosomal DNA of the some strains digested with *Xba*I, a rare cutting restriction enzyme

PFGE over conventional gel electrophoresis is its capacity to resolve molecules up to 2000 kb. In the following, the applications of PFGE in the molecular epidemiology of *E. coli* and *S. aureus* infections will be discussed.

The Ability of Restriction Polymorphisms Resolved by PFGE to Distinguish *E. coli* Isolates from Different Patients

Many phenotypic characteristics of different strains of *E. coli* infecting the urinary tract and other extraintestinal sites are often identical. They share virulence properties such as P fimbriae, hemolysin, aerobactin, and the K1 capsule antigen [3]. Since these isolates belong only to a few distinct O-serotypes [4], it is difficult to distinguish these strains by serotyping. However, through analysis with PFGE it is possible to distinguish *E. coli* strains from different patients with urinary tract infection. For any individual isolate, different restriction endonucleases produced distinct RFLP patterns. As shown in Fig. 2, PFGE reveals nine distinct DNA fingerprints from nine isolates from nine different patients.

Comparison of *E. coli* Fingerprinting Between Isolates from Urine and Blood

To determine whether the *E. coli* from primary sources (urinary tract) and secondary sources (blood) are identical, strains from 11 patients with urosepticemia were analyzed. Figure 3 shows the DNA fingerprints of

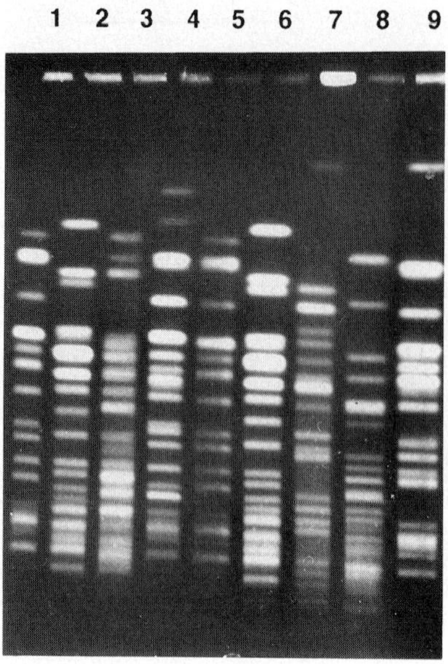

Fig. 2. PFGE agarose gel resolving *Xba*I restriction fragments from nine *E. coli* strains which were isolated from urine cultures of nine different patients

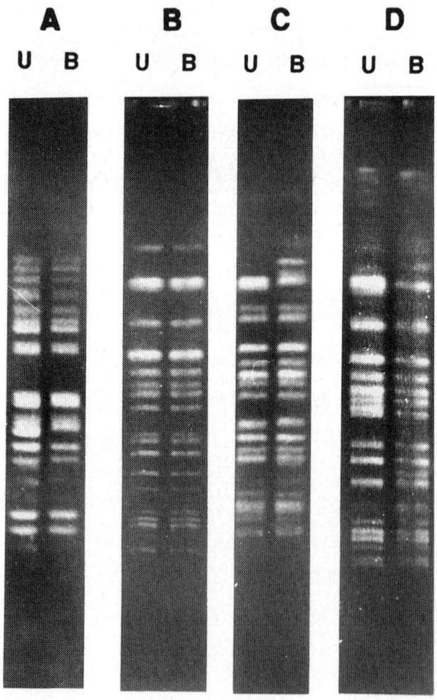

Fig. 3. A comparison of the *E. coli* isolates from four patients (A, B, C, D), obtained from the primary site of infection (urinary tract = *U*) and from blood culture (=*B*)

isolates from four representative patients (blood and urine). Within each patient, the blood and urine isolates were either identical (i.e., patients A, B, D) or very similar (i.e., patient C). However, between patients, the fingerprints of the isolates were noticeably different.

Ability of PFGE to Differentiate Recent Evolutionary Divergence of *E. coli* from Related Lineage

Since 1982, isolates from the *E. coli* serotype 0157:H7 has spread worldwide and are the cause of hemorrhagic diarrhea and hemolytic uremic syndrome [5]. PFGE was used to evaluate whether independent isolates from North America and Germany could be differentiated by DNA fingerprints. PFGE could distinguish most of the isolates between the two countries, and isolates within each country, although the fragment patterns varied only slightly. However, in one case, PFGE revealed that the fingerprints from one strain in North America was identical to those from one in Germany. With this exception, PFGE was found to be able to differentiate not only between epidemiologically independent isolates but also among strains that are evolutionarily highly related. This level of genetic divergence has not been previously shown by other phenotypic or genotypic techniques.

Techniques for Pheno- and Genotyping *S. aureus* Isolates

S. aureus is the most frequent cause of nosocomial infection. After isolating this organism from clinical material, its antimicrobial resistance pattern is routinely analyzed in the clinical laboratory and may provide preliminary evidence of nosocomial infection [6]. Since about 60% of all clinical *S. aureus* strains show identical antibiogram patterns (i.e., most of them are only resistant against penicillins, amino- and acylureidopenicillins), additional methods have been used to phenotype clinical *S. aureus* strains. These other typing methods include: (1) determination of virulence factors (clumping factor, protein A, DNAse, coagulase, (2) capsular polysaccharide serotyping, (3) zymotyping, (4) analysis of cell proteins by SDS-PAGE, and (5) phage typing [7]. How do these methods vary in their validity and reliability to differentiate clincial *S. aureus*? Identification of virulence factors demonstrates that up to 90% are positive for clumping factor, protein A, DNAse, and coagulase. Approximately 10% of *S. aureus* isolates are clumping factor-negative and nosocomial strains are reported in the literature to lack protein A and DNAse [8]. Capsular typing, which is performed with monoclonal antibodies, and SDS-PAGE protein typing also have a low power of discrimination between *S. aureus* strains. Zymotyping performed by esterase polymorphism is also of limited value. Thus, the value of phenotypical methods and their capability to differentiate *S. aureus* increases in the following order: virulence factor typing, capsular serotyping, protein typing by SDS-PAGE, zymotyping and phage typing. Although phage typing has the best capability to distinguish among clinical *S. aureus*, only 80% of clinical isolates will be typable with the international set of phages. Consequently, in addition to phenotyping various genotyping procedures have been developed using plasmid analysis and DNA fingerprinting of chromosomal DNA by ribotyping or PFGE. Plasmid typing is limited to strains which bear plasmids and strains may even change or lose their plasmids in the host or during storage. Ribotyping is usually performed by digestion of chromosomal DNA and subsequent hybridization with probes directed against conserved regions of the RNA genes. When ribotyping was compared with PFGE typing, the results indicated that ribotypes could be further differentiated by PFGE. Moreover, as in *E. coli*, genome typing by PFGE has the highest capacity to distinguish among clinical *S. aureus* strains.

Clonal Structure of Oxacillin-Resistant Clumping Factor-Negative *S. aureus*

A total of 50 oxacillin-resistant *S. aureus* (ORSA) strains were analyzed by PFGE. These strains were clumping factor-negative (CFN) and protein A-negative by latex agglutination and were collected from patients in six different hospitals at different locations in Germany during 1991–1992. All CFN-ORSA strains were isolated between November 1991 and June 1992 from various clinical materials [wound swabs (31 isolates), tracheal secretions (12), blood cultures (4), urine (2), post-mortem swab from ethmoidal cells (1)]. Six CFP-ORSA strains and six *S. epidermidis* strains were used as control strains in the genotyping experiments. It was not known whether there were contacts between patients and medical staff from hospital A and the other clinics (B-F). The reaction for DNAse and coagulase was positive [9]. Biochemical analysis of the isolates resulted in definitive identification (99.9%) of *S. aureus*. Antibiograms, bacteriophage typing, and plasmid analysis were performed. All CFN *S. aureus* strains were resistant to oxacillin (and therefore to all other β-lactam antibiotics and imipenem), gentamicin, clindamycin, erythromycin, ciprofloxacin, and fosfomycin. Susceptibility was found to tetracycline, vancomycin, rifampicin, fusidic acid, and, with one exception, to cotrimoxazole.

All these isolates were nontypable with an international set of phages, an additional experimental phage set indicating phage type 16, 192. Moreover, all isolates possessed a single plasmid of 30 kb, restriction analysis of this plasmid revealing identical patterns. For genotyping these 50 isolates were also analyzed by PFGE. *Sma*I digested chromosomal DNA separated by PFGE was deployed in order to show the interrelationship between the CFN-ORSA strains. The genome type was defined as any fragment pattern varying from another with regard to the number and size of the particular fragment bands concerned. Firstly, we analyzed the outbreak strains from hospital A. They were identical with regard to their fragment number and size. CFP-ORSA stemming from the same hospital revealed a different PFGE pattern. In the next stage we compared the CFN-ORSA strains from hospital A with CFN-ORSA strains from hospitals B, C, D, E, and F. The strain from hospital F, slightly modified in its antibiogram (cotrimoxazole resistant), showed the only exception in fragment patterns. Due to the fact that differences here were minimal, we suggest that we classify such a strain as a genomic subtype [6].

Molecular Typing by Amplification and Restriction Analysis of Virulence Genes

Molecular typing of ORSA strains is of great potential value for basic and epidemiological studies of *S. aureus* infection. In addition to PFGE of chromosomal DNA, which proves cumbersome and time consuming, and therefore less practical for routine investigation, there is a strong tendency nowadays towards molecular typing of *S. aureus* deploying variations in the chromosomal DNA structures. An interesting element in this connection is the coagulase gene, which comprises a region containing several 81-bp tandem repeats, the number differing between *S. aureus* strains. The value of this gene for molecular typing lies in the repeats differing in the presence or absence of *Alu*I restriction sites. Goh et al. [10] recently analyzed 24 methicillin-resistant *S. aureus* isolates recovered from patients and staff members during the investigation of an outbreak. Of these epidemiologically related strains 23 had identical coagulase RFLP profiles, but these profiles were different from those of epidemiologically unrelated *S. aureus* strains. Although we confirmed the essential value of coagulase genotyping when we investigated epidemiologically unrelated CFP-ORSA strains, we were unable to distinguish the CFN-ORSA strains from different hospitals. This probably means that they are even identical in this highly variable gene.

References

1. Grothues D, Tümmler B (1991) New approaches in genome analysis by pulsed-field gel electrophoresis: application to the analysis of *Pseudomonas* species. Mol Microbiol 5:2763–2776
2. McClelland M, Jones R, Patel Y, Nelson M (1987) Restriction endonucleases for pulsed-field mapping of bacterial genomes. Nucleic Acids Res 15:5985–6005
3. Johnson JR (1991) Virulence factors in Escherichia coli urinary tract infections. Clin Microbiol Rev 4:80–128
4. Hacker J, Schrettenbrunner A, Schröter G, Düvel H, Schmidt G, Goebel W (1986) Charaterization of *Escherichia coli* wild-type strains by means of agglutination with antisera raised against cloned P-, S-, and MS-Fimbriae antigens, hemagglutination, serotyping and hemolysin production. Zbl Bakteriol Hyg 261:219–231
5. Böhm H, Karch H (1992) DNA fingerprinting of *Escherichia coli* O157:H7 strains by pulsed-field gel electrophoresis. J Clin Microbiol 30:2169–2172
6. Schwarzkopf A, Karch H, Schmidt H, Lenz W, Heesemann J (1993) Phenotypical and genotypical characterization of epidemic clumping factor-negative, oxacillin-resistant *Staphylococcus aureus*. J Clin Microiol 31:2281–2285

7. Schlichting C, Branger C, Fournier JM, Witte W, Boutonnier A, Wolz C, Goullet P, Döring G (1993) Typing of *Staphylococcus aureus* by pulsed-field gel electrophoresis, zymotyping, capsular typing, and phage typing: resolution of clonal relationships. J Clin Microbiol 31:227–232
8. Neville LO, Billington OJ, Kibbler CC, Gillespie SH (1991) Methicillin resistant *Staphylococcus aureus* without clumping factor, protein A and DNase. Lancet 338:518
9. Schwarzkopf A, Schmidt-Rotte H, Schmidt H, Kunz E, Karch H, Heesemann J (1992) Molecular analysis of nosocomial infection by oxacillin-resistant *Staphylococcus aureus* lacking protein A and clumping factor. Lancet 340:621
10. Goh SH, Byrne SK, Zhang JL, Chow AW (1992) Molecular typing of *Staphylococcus aureus* on the basis of coagulase gene polymorphisms. J Clin Microbiol 30:1642–1645

Interleukin-2 Receptor Expression Is Unaffected by Thermal Injury

D.S. O'Riordain, R.G. Holzheimer, M. Mendez, K. Collins, J.A. Mannick, and M.L. Rodrick

Introduction

Severe traumatic or thermal injury results in depression of cellular immunity, including failure of T-lymphocyte (T-cell) proliferation in response to mitogenic or antigenic stimulation [1, 2]. IL-2, a product of T cells, is the major growth factor for T-lymphocytes and its action on T cells is mediated through binding with IL-2 receptor proteins on the cell surface, with resultant cellular proliferation. This autocrine mechanism is of critical importance to the cell mediated immune response and is obviously dependent both on expression of functional IL-2 receptor on the cell surface and also on normal production and secretion of the IL-2 protein.

Structurally the IL-2 binding complex consists of a number of polypeptide chains, the principal two of which are a 55-kDa, Tac or IL-2Rα chain and the 70- to 75-kDa, IL-2Rβ chain. The β-chain is of intermediate affinity and is expressed on resting cells [3]. The α-chain, on the other hand, is not expressed in the resting state, is of low affinity when expressed alone, but, together with IL-2Rβ, forms a high-affinity IL-2 receptor [4]. Expression of high-affinity IL-2R, and thus cell proliferation, is therefore significantly regulated by IL-2Rα gene expression.

One of the primary immunologic defects in severely burned patients is decreased production of IL-2 [5]. While decreased IL-2 production following thermal injury is undisputed, the status of IL-2R expression and activity in this setting is controversial. Previous studies have variously reported reduced [6] or increased [7] IL-2R p55 expression in severely burned patients. These studies looked only at cell surface expression of the p55 protein, without examining other parameters of IL-2R expression and function. It is clear that we, as yet, do not have a satisfactory answer as to the status of IL-2R in the setting of thermal injury. The following studies were designed to resolve this controversy, through detailed investigation of parameters of both IL-2 receptor expression and function in an established animal model.

Materials and Methods

Under NIH guidelines, a total of 220 8-week-old male A/J mice were anesthetized, subjected to a 20% full thickness scald burn injury or sham burn, sacrificed 4, 7, 10, 14, or 21 days later and splenocytes harvested for in vitro studies. Cells at 1 × 10^6/ml were cultured with concanavalin A (2.5 μg/ml) and/or human recombinant IL-2 (100 U/ml). Lymphocyte proliferation was measured by uptake of tridiated thymidine, and IL-2 production by a CTLL bioassay. Following 48 h stimulation, cells were incubated with both phycoerythrin conjugated anti-IL-2R p55 chain antibody and fluorescein conjugated murine anti-CD3 antibody for assessment of T-cell IL-2R expression or with biotinylated recombinant human IL-2 together with an avidin-fluorescein complex for assessment of IL-2 binding by IL-2R. Samples were processed flow cytometry. Total spleen RNA was isolated by phenol extraction. A Northern blot was prepared and probed sequentially with ^{32}P labelled cDNA for murine IL-2R p55 chain and for β-actin.

Results

Results of in vitro studies are summarized in the Table 1. Mitogen induced lymphocyte proliferation and IL-2 production were both consistently suppressed following burn injury, maximally at day 7. Addition of IL-2 to cultures of cells from burned mice caused a significant increase in the proliferative response on all days following injury (data not shown). IL-2R p55 chain expression in mitogen stimulated CD3+ cells was not changed at any time point. Binding of fluorescein labelled IL-2 was unchanged in burned animals at days 4, 7, and 21 but was increased on days 10 and 14. IL-2R p55 chain mRNA expression in response to in vitro stimulation showed no consistent suppression in thermally injured animals on days 7, 10, or 14.

Discussion

Abnormalities of T-lymphocyte function are central to the immune dysfunction which increases susceptibility to sepsis following thermal or traumatic injury [8, 9]. Our laboratory has previously focused on abnormal lymphocyte proliferation and reduced IL-2 production as being the primary deficiencies in T-cell function in this setting [1, 5]. Expression of functional high-affinity

Table 1. Results of in vitro studies expressed as percentage change in the burned mice compared to the sham burn animals

	Day 4	Day 7	Day 10	Day 14	Day 21
IL-2 production	−22%	−40%*	−36%**	−30%*	+16%
Lymphocyte proliferation (LP)	−25%	−50%*	−37%*	−23%	+12%
IL-2R expression in CD3+ cells	−6%	+9%	+1%	+7%	−5%
Splenocyte IL-2 binding	−3%	+2%	+117%**	+22%	−7%

* $P < 0.05$, ** $P < 0.01$ (Student's t-test)

IL-2 receptors is also critical to the normal lymphocyte response to antigenic or mitogenic stimulation, and is most closely linked to expression of the IL-2Rα (p55) gene and product. Other groups have previously addressed the question of IL-2Rα expression following trauma or thermal injury. Teodorczyk-Injeyan et al. [2, 6] have shown a decrease in the percentage of T lymphocytes expressing IL-2Rα in patients following thermal injury. In these studies marked cellular IL-2Rα suppression was observed in very severe, terminal, burn cases, but in less severely injured patients, IL-2Rα suppression was less severe and transient. There is considerable evidence to dispute depressed cellular IL-2R expression following thermal injury. Schluter et al. [7] recently reported increased IL-2Rα expression in severely burned patients. A number of studies have suggested the presence of functional cellular IL-2R by demonstrating a significant proliferative response in cells from burn victims, with the addition of recombinant IL-2 to in vitro cultures [2, 10]. It is clear that the status of IL-2R following thermal injury has not been satisfactorily determined. The present study addresses these questions in an established, and well controlled, animal model of burn-induced immunosuppression.

Our results clearly demonstrate normal expression of cell surface IL-2Rα in mitogen stimulated, CD3+ cells following thermal injury. These data are further strengthened by the demonstration of normal IL-2R mRNA levels in this setting. That burn injury was sufficiently severe to induce immunosuppression is demonstrated by reduced lymphocyte proliferation and by reduced IL-2 production, and is consistent with our previous reports in the same animal model [1]. Additionally we demonstrate in this study that IL-2R function is normal following this degree of thermal injury. Cellular binding of IL-2 was normal early and late, but actually increased on days 10 and 14, possibly reflecting an increased quantity of cell surface IL-2Rα as demonstrated by Schluter et al. [7]. The addition of human recombinant interleukin-2 to in vitro cell cultures restored the proliferative response of suppressed lymphocytes to normal, demonstrating the presence of functional cellular IL-2R and suggesting that reduced IL-2 production is the principal factor underlying abnormal T-cell responses following burn injury. Additively these morphologic and functional studies provide strong evidence for the notion that suppression of IL-2 receptor does not play a significant role in immunosuppression following moderate thermal trauma. That we can induce abnormal lymphocyte proliferation and abnormal IL-2 production without suppressing IL-2Rα expression or function suggests that reduced IL-2 production, rather than an abnormality of the IL-2 receptor, is the dominant T-cell defect in this clinical setting.

The present studies examine a considerably broader range of parameters of cellular IL-2R expression and function than any previous study in the setting of thermal or traumatic injury and provide strong evidence for normal IL-2R expression and function in the presence of lymphocyte suppression.

References

1. Moss NM, Gough DB, Jordan A, Grbic JT, Rodrick ML, Mannick JA (1988) Temporal correlation of impaired immune response after thermal injury with susceptibility to infection in a murine model. Surgery 104:882–887
2. Teodorczyk-Injeyan JA, Sparkes BG, Mills GB, Peters WJ, Falk RE (1986) Impairment of T cell activation in burn patients: a possible mechanism of thermal injur-induced immunosuppression. Clin Exp Immunol 65:570–581
3. Waldmann TA (1986) The structure function and expression of interleukin-2 receptors on normal and malignant lymphocytes. Science 232:727–732
4. Tsudo M, Kozak RW, Goldmann CK, Waldmann TA (1987) Contribution of a p75 interleukin-2 binding peptide to a high-affinity interleukin-2 receptor complex. Proc Natl Acad Sci USA 84:4215–4218
5. Wood JJ, Rodrick ML, O'Mahony JB et al. (1984) Inadequate interleukin 2 production: a fundamental immunological deficiency in patients with major burns. Ann Surg 200:311
6. Teodorczyk-Injeyan JA, McRitchie DI, Peters WJ (1990) Expression and secretion of IL-2 receptor in trauma patients. Ann Surg 212:202–208
7. Schluter B, Wolfgang K, Koller M et al. (1991) Differential regulation of T and B-lymphocyte activation in severely burned patients. J Trauma 31:239–246
8. Hoyt DB, Ozkan AN, Ninnemann JL, Hansbrough JF, Pinney E, Wormsley S (1988) Trauma peptide induction of lymphocyte changes predictive of sepsis. J Surg Res 45:342–348
9. Wolfe JHN, Wu AV, O'Connor NE et al. (1982) Anergy, immunosuppressive serum and impaired lymphocyte blastogenesis in burn patients. Arch Surg 117: 1266–1271
10. Grbic JT, Mannick JA, Gough DB, Rodrick ML (1991) The role of prostaglandin E2 in immune suppression following injury. Ann Surg 214:253–263

Keratinocytes Express an Intracellular Marker Gene and Regenerate the Epidermis in Porcine Full-Thickness Wounds After Retroviral Gene Transfer

P. Vogt, D. Hatzis, S. Thompson, R. Mulligan, C. Andree, and E. Eriksson

Introduction

Large skin wounds such as in burns lead to significant losses of fluid, electrolytes, and energy and also porvide a portal of entry for infections. Therefore cutaneous wound healing and epithelial coversage is a critical issue in these patients and has led to a number of developments in the field of skin transplantation and skin replacement.

In a new approach to improve epithelial healing it was recently demonstrated that transplanting keratinocytes as single cell suspensions [1] into a cutaneous wound chamber leads to an earlier healing of full thickness skin wounds. This phenomenon was now further studied by tagging the cells with a genetic marker in order to monitor their survival and maturation after autologous transplantation into full thickness skin wounds in pigs.

Material and Methods

Under general inhalational anesthesia split thickness skin grafts were obtained from eight female Yorkshire pigs. Primary keratinocyte cultures were established by dispase and trypsin treatment. At confluence keratinocytes were released from the flasks with 0.01% trypsin and resuspended in normal unbuffered saline (0.9%) containing 100 U/ml penicillin and 100 mg/ml streptomycin at a concentration of 3×10^6 cells/ml.

We injected 1.2 ml of this suspension into full thickness wounds (15×15 mm, 9 mm deep) created on the pig dorsum. Keratinocytes resuspended in saline were found to be more than 95% viable as confirmed by trypan blue uptake and reculturing of the content of individual syringes in culture flasks.

For retroviral gene transfer experiments 60%–70% confluent keratinocyte cultures were incubated on three consecutive days with a murine Moloney leukemia vector *MFG-acZ* containing the β-galactosidase gene. Keratinocytes expressing this gene turn blue when stained with X-Gal (5-bromo-4-chloro-3-indolyl-*b*-D-galactoside).

Full thickness wounds (1.5×1.5 cm, 0.9 cm deep) were created surgically within tattooed margins, down to the panniculus carnosus muscle and covered by a liquid tight vinyl chamber. The chamber (P.A. Medical Corp., Columbia, Tenn.) consists of a flexible transparent vinyl top bonded to an adhesive base. The base has a central opening compatible with the created wound margin. Keratinocyte suspensions were injected through the chamber onto the bottom of the wound. Chambers were filled with 1.2 ml of either normal saline 0.9% with 100 IU penicillin + 100 μg streptomycin/ml (n = 33), or normal saline containing unmodified autologous keratinocytes (3×10^6 cells/ml, n = 37), or normal saline containing transduced autologous keratinocytes (expressing the *lacZ* gene; 3×10^6 cells/m, n = 32).

Chambers were exchanged daily and refilled. Wound fluid collected daily from individual wounds were centrifuged at 1000 rpm for 10 min and then filtered through a 0.45-mm filter (Millipore, Inc.). Endogenous protein as a noninvasive marker of restoration of the epithelial barrier function was measured with a turbidimetric assay (Stanbio CSF, Stanbio Laboratory Inc., San Antonio) as described previously [2]. Wounds were biopsied and stained with X-Gal and hematoxylin and eosin.

Results

Wounds receiving either normal keratinocytes or keratinocytes expressing the *lacZ* gene reepithelialized significantly faster than controls (12 days vs 16 days; $P < 0.01$).

Wounds receiving keratinocytes also developed a significantly earlier barrier function to endogenous protein than wounds treated with saline alone (12 dyas vs 15 days; $P < 0.001$).

Keratinocyte expressing the *lacZ* gene as well as normal kertinocytes first appeared on day 4 biopsies as cellular clusters on the bottom of the wound and later (days 8–12) in all layers of the newly regenerated epidermis. *LacZ* expression was observed in all biopsies of wounds that had received keratinocytes transduced with the *lacZ* gene. Biopsies at 19–27 days showed *lacZ* expression in the stratum corneum, but no longer in basal cells.

Discussion

Restoration of the epithelial barrier is a critical issue for the treatment of patients with large skin defects. In animal experiments Billingham and Reynolds [3] have first demonstrated in a rabbit model and later Worst et al. in a mouse model [4–6] that suspensions of keratinocytes injected into wounds are reorganized in vivo to an epithelium showing all the characteristic features of a stratified epidermis. More recently hair growth could be induced after injecting hair follicles into full thickness wounds in mice [7].

Morgan et al. [8] showed first that human keratinocytes can be genetically engineered in vitro by retroviral gene transfer and secrete human growth hormone after transplantation into nude mice. In addition plasmids have been used as vectors for successful transfection of keratinocytes [9].

Enclosing wounds in a wet closed chamber system creates a liquid environment favorable for the healing of skin wounds [2] and this system also provides a useful system for transplantation of cells, by serving as an in vivo culturing system [1].

In this study we have transplanted suspensions of autologous keratinocytes in a porcine model into full thickness wounds and tracked the transplanted cells after marking them with a genetic marker: *lacZ*. The results suggest that keratinocytes transplanted as single cell suspensions survive and regenerate the epithelium. The pattern of expression indicates that transduced keratinocytes reconstitute the new epidermis and undergo terminal differentiation. This technique of regenerating skin epidermis with naive and genetically engineered transplantable keratinocytes provides new possibilities for introduction and expression of therapeutic proteins in skin disease, skin replacement, and wound healing.

References

1. Eriksson E, Liu PY, Zeckel Y, Binder T, Breuing K, Miller DR (1991) In vivo cell culture accelerates reepithelialization. Surg Forum 41:670–673
2. Breuing K, Eriksson E, Liu PY, Miller DR (1992) Healing of partial thickness porcine skin wounds in a liquid environment. J Surg Res 52:50–58
3. Billingham RE, Reynolds J (1952) Transplantation studies on sheets of pure epidermal epithelium and on epidermal cell suspensions. Br J Plast Surg 5:25–36
4. Mackenzie IC, Fusenig NE (1983) Regeneration of organized epithelial structure. J Invest Dermatol 81(1):189s–194s
5. Worst PKM, Valentine EA, Fusenig NE (1974) Formation of epidermis after reimplantation of pure primary epidermal cell cultures from perinatal mouse skin. JNCI 53(4):1061–1064
6. Worst PKM, Mackenzie IC, Fusenig NE (1982) Reformation of organized epidermal structure by transplantation of suspensions and cultures of epidermal and dermal cells. Cell Tissue Res 225
7. Weinberg WC, Goodman LV, George C, Morgan DL, Ledbetter S, Yuspa SH, Lichti U (1993) Reconstitution of hair follicle development in vivo: determination of follicle formation, hair growth and hair quality by dermal cells. J Invest Dermatol 100:229–236
8. Morgan JF, Barrandon Y, Green H, Mulligan RC (1987) Expression of an exogenous growth hormone gene by transplantable human epidermal cells. Science 237:1476–1479
9. Teumer J, Lindahl A, Green H (1990) Human growth hormone in the blood of athymic mice grafted with cultures of growth hormone-secreting human keratinocytes. FASEB J 4:3245–3250

The Influence of Non-specific Inflammatory and Immunological Reactions on the Expression of Major Histocompatibility Complex and Activation Antigens After Murine Hepatic Transplantation

H.-J. GASSEL, R. ENGEMANN, W. TIMMERMANN, A.M. GASSEL, and A. THIEDE

The orthotopic replacement of the liver is a well-established means of treating end-stage liver diseases. Since the technical problems have mostly been solved, it is immunological questions that still challenge both clinicians and scientists.

The model of orthotopic rat liver transplantation is a well-developed standard technique for the study of various pathomechanisms after hepatic transplantation. Standard technique can include arterialization [1–3] of the graft, serving as a physiological transplantation model. Previous studies in genetically defined inbred rat strains have shown that non-specific inflammatory responses occur if arterialization is omitted [4, 5] in a syngeneic LEW-LEW (RT11) combination.

Using an allogeneic major histocompatibility complex (MHC) and non-MHC disparate DA (RT1a)-LEW combination, a strong rejection reaction is induced [6].

MHC antigens are known to play an important role in the induction of immune responses. Whereas class I antigens are expressed on most nucleid cells, class II antigens show a more restricted distribution. It is known that class II antigen expression is inducible under various pathological situations. MHC antigens may act as targets for an anti-allograft response. In addition, the expression of activation antigens such as the interleukin-2 (IL-2) receptor is accepted as a signal of immunological activation.

The purpose of this study was to evaluate the influence of the transplantation technique and the effect of an alloresponse on the expression of MHC class II and activation antigens on various hepatic cellular components.

In order to study the influence of the technically related inflammatory reaction on antigen expression, the two different transplantation techniques in the syngeneic combination were compared. The model of allogeneic arterialized liver transplantation served for the study of the influence of an immunological alloresponse.

Materials and Methods

Orthotopic rat liver transplantation was performed according to the methods previously described [1, 7] in the LEW-LEW and DA-LEW combination.

Two groups were formed in the LEW-LEW combination (a) with or (b) without reconstruction of the arterial blood supply of the graft. At days 3, 5, 10, 15, 20, 30 and 100 postoperatively (p.op.) biopsies were taken and routinely processed for haematoxylin-eosin staining. In addition, immunoperoxidase staining was performed with monoclonal antibodies directed against MHC class II antigen only (MRC-Ox6), rat Kupffer cells (KI-M2R) and the IL-2 receptor (MRC-Ox39). The number and distribution of positive cells was determined by light microscopic evaluation.

Results

The Influence of a Non-specific Inflammatory Reaction: LEW-LEW Combination

After syngeneic orthotopic rat liver transplantation without arterialization ($n = 38$), 67% of the recipients went on to long-term survival as defined by survival for more than 100 days p.op. (Fig. 1). By contrast, re-arterialization of the graft increases the survival rate to more than 90%.

Histologically, non-arterialized rat liver grafts showed a strong mononuclear cell infiltrate between day +5 and day +20 p.op. In many cases, bile duct proliferation occurred and in severe cases complete liver fibrosis was seen (Fig. 2a). By contrast, the liver architecture was preserved when the

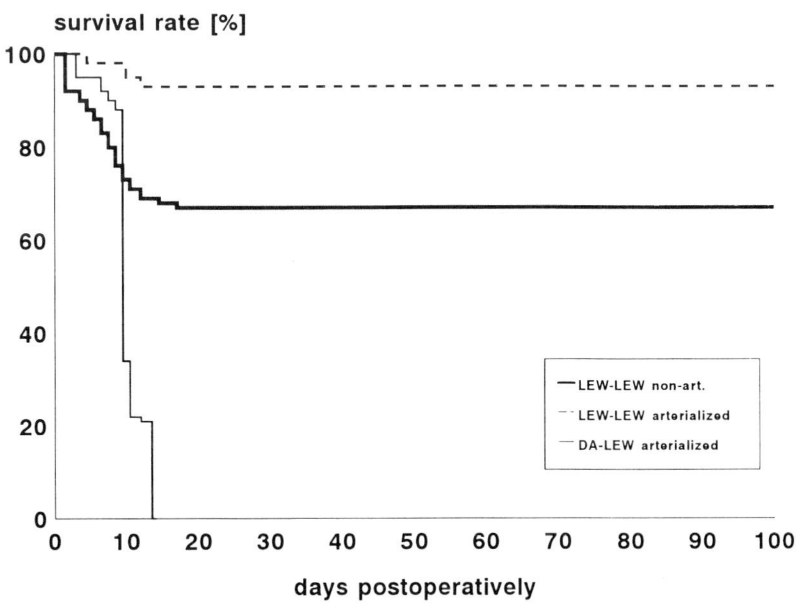

Fig. 1. Survival rates after orthotopic rat liver transplantation

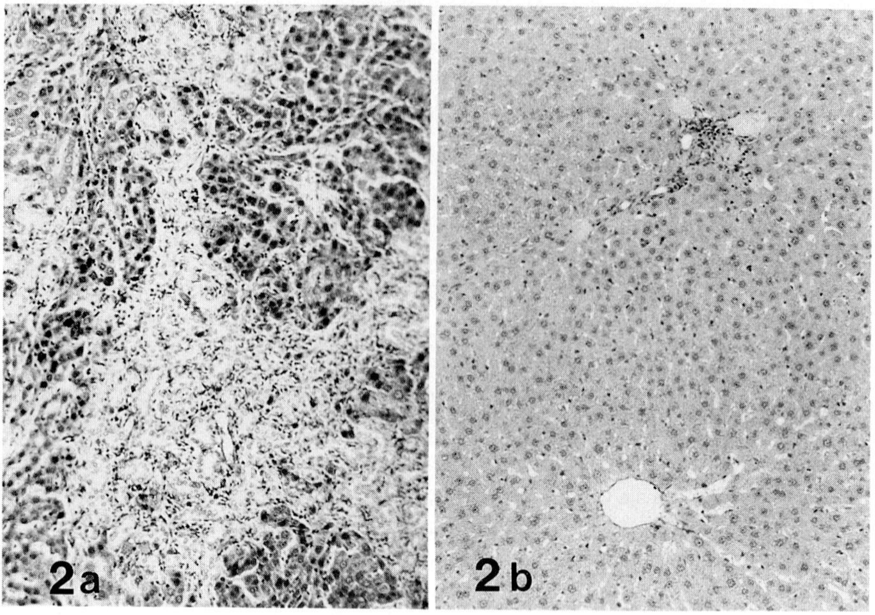

Fig. 2. a Syngeneic non-arterialized liver graft 30 days p.op. HE stain. **b** Syngeneic liver graft, arterialized, 100 days p.op. HE stain

graft was arterialized (Fig. 2b). Occasionally, mononuclear cells were seen in the early p.op. period (day +5 p.op. until day +20 p.op.) in the portal tracts. These cells diminished in the later stages. Particularly, no bile duct disturbances occurred after arterialized rat liver transplantation.

The immunohistological staining for rat Kupffer cells was performed with KI-M2-R (Fig. 3). The Kupffer cells were distributed regularly throughout the parenchyma. No KI-M2-R staining was seen in the portal tracts. Staining for MHC class II antigen with the monoclonal antibody MRC Ox-6 revealed that Kupffer cells were MHC class II negative in the normal rat liver. Only a few mononuclear and dendritic cells stained Ox-6 positive in the portal tracts of the normal liver. A very similar picture was seen after syngeneic transplantation with rearterialization of the graft (Fig. 4a). No MHC class II expression was found on Kupffer cells, hepatocytes or bile duct and endothelial cells.

By contrast, in non-arterialized liver grafts, MHC class II antigen expression was induced on Kupffer cells, but not parenchymal cells, bile duct cells and endothelial cells. This expression was seen from day 10 p.op. until the late stage after transplantation, as long as the inflammatory process was going on (Fig. 4b). The analysis of activation antigen expression was performed by the use of MRC Ox-39 antibody. The monoclonal antibody, directed against the 55-kDa protein (β-chain) of the rat IL-2 receptor stained with Kupffer cells in non-arterialized isografts. The expression was

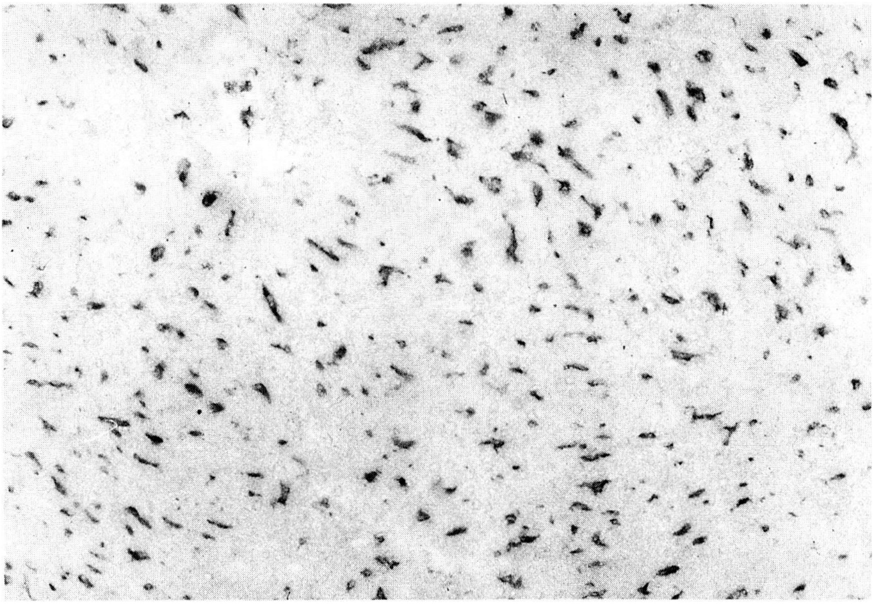

Fig. 3. Naive LEW rat liver. Stained cells represent Kupffer cells. Immunoperoxidase stain with monoclonal antibody KI-M2R

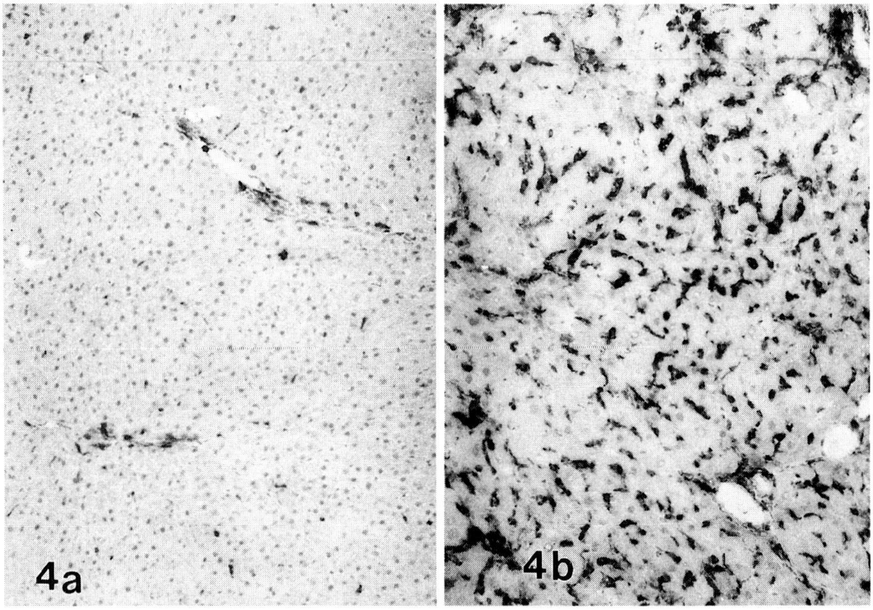

Fig. 4. **a** Syngeneic arterialized liver graft, day 20 p.op. Parenchymal cells mostly not stained. Immunoperoxidase stain with monoclonal antibody MRC Ox-6. **b** Syngeneic non-arterialized liver graft on day 30 p.op. Immunoperoxidase stain with monoclonal antibody MRC Ox-6. Mostly positive parenchymal cells

mild to moderate and strictly restricted to Kupffer cells. By contrast, arterialized syngeneic grafts did not express any IL-2 receptor on either Kupffer cells or parenchymal cells.

The Effect of the Immunological Alloresponse: DA-LEW Combination

In the fully allogeneic DA-LEW combination, rat liver transplantation was performed with arterialization throughout. Thus, non-specific inflammatory reactions could be excluded by the transplantation technique. All LEW recipients of a DA liver died within 14 days after transplantation if no immunosuppression was administered.

A strong rejection reaction occurred after allogeneic liver transplantation (Fig. 5) if no immunosuppression was administered. A dense mononuclear cell infiltrate in the portal tracts as well as in the liver parenchyma was seen. Confluent necroses of hepatocytes and destruction of bile ducts led to total necrosis of the whole organ. Consequently, the recipients died within the first 14 days after transplantation (Fig. 1). During this rejection crisis MHC class II antigens were strongly induced on Kupffer cells of the graft. The induction of MHC class II antigen preceded the rejection and was seen on day +5 p.op. By contrast, parenchymal cells and bile duct cells remained class II negative throughout.

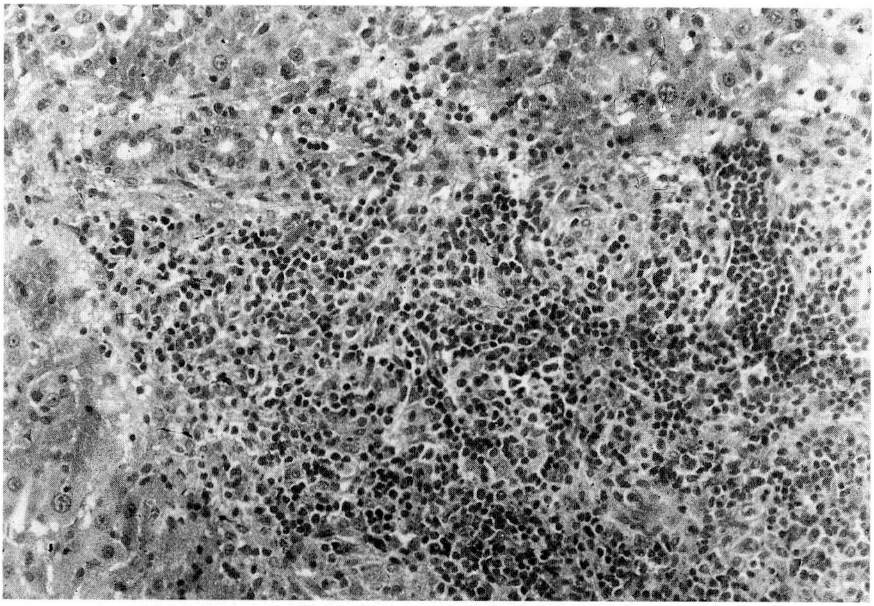

Fig. 5. Allogeneic DA liver graft, day +10 p.op. Strong rejection response with mononuclear cell infiltrate and liver destruction. HE stain

No expression of IL-2 receptors on allograft liver cells was seen within the first 3 p.op. days (Fig. 6a). However, from day 3 onwards, the expression of IL-2 receptors on rat Kupffer cells was constantly increasing (Fig. 6b). Hepatocytes, bile duct cells and endothelial cells remained negative throughout the rejection.

Discussion

The influence of the transplantation technique on the survival rates after liver transplantation is clearly demonstrated. Reconstruction of the arterial blood supply provides a physiological transplantation model with a consequent increase in the long-term survival rate of the recipients from 67% to more than 90%. The main cause of death in the non-arterialized group is bile duct complications leading to liver fibrosis. This is due to the lack of perfusion of the donor bile duct in the early p.op. period. The blood supply to the donor bile duct is achieved through the donor hepatic artery exclusively in the first 14 postoperative days. If the artery is ligated, reperfusion via capillaries from the omentum majus occurs within weeks. Thus, the majority of the more recently published transplantation techniques involve re-arterialization

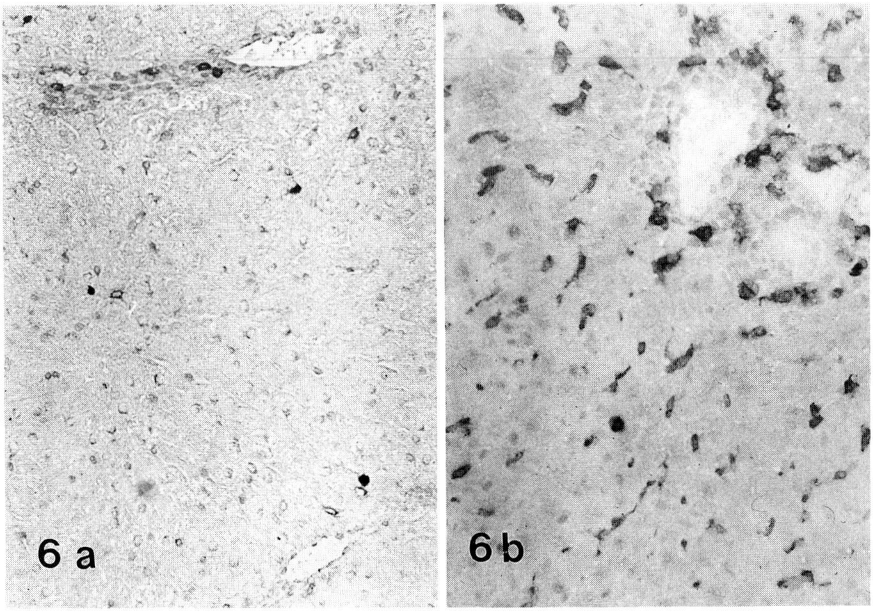

Fig. 6. a DA liver allograft, day 3 p.op. No expression on parenchymal cells. Immunoperoxidase stain with monoclonal antibody MRC Ox-39. **b** DA liver allograft, day 5 p.op. Expression of the IL-2 receptor on both infiltrating cells and Kupffer cells. Immunoperoxidase stain with monoclonal antibody MRC Ox-39

of the graft by different means [2, 8]. The influence of arterialization of a liver graft on MHC class II and IL-2 receptor expression is demonstrated. Whereas in naive rat livers MHC class II antigen and IL-2 receptors are expressed not at all or very rarely, the non-specific inflammatory reaction caused by omitting the arterialization of the graft leads to a strong induction of MHC class II and IL-2 receptor antigens on Kupffer cells. This induction correlates with severe histological changes and may have important implications for the immune response after liver transplantation: The Kupffer cell of the liver is thought to be able to function as an antigen-presenting cell and it is immunogenic as it can induce T-cell proliferation [9]. Thus, a Kupffer cell presenting MHC class II and activation antigens on its surface could serve as a target for specific autoreactive T-cell responses. Whether the antigen induction is due to this specifically activated autoreactive T cells or whether it is regulated by cytokines and mediators (e.g. γ-interferon) [10] released from inflammatory mononuclear cells remains unsolved at this point. The role of other class II inducible factors needs to be discussed. The expression of MHC class II antigens in the rat is restricted to certain cells, such as dendritic cells, macrophages and B cells. They play an important role in the induction and regulation of the immune response and they are recognized by mainly CD4-positive T cells. Therefore, a non-specific inflammatory reaction resulting in the induction of MHC and activation antigens could trigger a rejection reaction of an allograft similar to a viral infection. As it is well known in clinical liver transplantation that viral infections can cause expression of class II antigens on liver cells [11] and consequently trigger a rejection response, the technically related antigen induction on rat Kupffer cells may be responsible for the impaired outcome of liver allografts which are not arterialized in comparison to liver allografts arterialized in inbred rat strain combinations, as previously published [6].

The rejection response to an allograft itself induces a strong expression of MHC class II antigens on cells that do not constitutively express these antigens. Similarly, the IL-2 receptor expression is induced by the rejection response. In this study, all these experiments were done using the arterialized technique in order to exclude technically related problems. Hence, at every autopsy, the patency of the arterial anastomosis was checked.

In conclusion, this study demonstrates that the MHC class II and IL-2 receptor expression on rat Kupffer cells is inducible by both inflammatory and specific immunological factors. Therefore, in the rat, the arterialized model should be used for immunological studies throughout.

Whether the sequential analysis of the expression of activation markers could be a useful tool in the early diagnosis of a rejection has not yet been clarified. Regarding the expression of MHC class II antigens, it is commonly accepted that the induction of the MHC class II expression on liver cells (mostly hepatocytes in the clinical situation) is a relatively non-specific phenomenon which can be due to viral infections, cholestasis, ischaemia or toxic reactions as well as graft rejections. However, there might be a role for the routine analysis of activation antigen expression.

The role of the induction of activation and MHC antigens by technically related factors needs to be kept in mind when an alloresponse is considered.

References

1. Engemann R (1985) Technique for orthotopic rat liver transplantation. In: Thiede A, Deltz E, Engemann R, Hamelmann H (eds) Microsurgical models in rats for transplantation research. Springer Berlin Heidelberg New York, pp 69–75
2. Steffen R, Ferguson DM, Kron RA (1989) A new method for orthotopic rat liver transplantation with arterial cuff anastomosis to the recipient common hepatic artery. Transplantation 48:166–169
3. Gao W, Lemasters JJ, Thurman RG (1993) Development of a new method for hepatic rearterialization in rat orthotopic liver transplantation. Reduction of liver injury and improvement of surgical outcome by arterialization. Transplantation 56:19–24
4. Kamada N, Calne RY (1979) Orthotopic liver transplantation in the rat. Transplantation 28:47–50
5. Gassel HJ, Engemann R, Hamelmann H (1987) Major histocompatibility complex class II antigen expression on Kupffer cells after orthotopic rat liver transplantation: a consequence of non-specific inflammation or allograft rejection? Transplant Proc 19:3017–3018
6. Engemann R, Ulrichs K, Thiede A, Müller-Ruchholtz W, Hamelmann H (1985) Graft tolerance after orthotopic liver transplantation in a primarily nontolerant strain combination following temporary ciclosporin A treatment. In: Thiede A, Deltz E, Engemann R, Hamelmann H (eds) Microsurgical models in rats for transplantation research. Springer, Berlin Heidelberg New York, pp 247–254
7. Gassel HJ, Engemann R, Thiede A, Hamelmann H (1986) Orthotopic rat liver transplantation: the influence of rearterialization of the graft on liver morphology and antigen expression. A new, simplified model. Eur Surg Res 18 [Suppl 1]: 181–182
8. Marzi J, Knee J, Menger MD, Harbauer C, Duhren V (1991) Hepatic microcirculatory disturbances due to portal vein clamping in the orthotopic rat liver transplantation model. Transplantation 52:432–436
9. Rubinstein D, Rosta AK, Lipsky P (1985) The role of the Kupffer cells in antigen activation process. Gastroenterology 88:1688–1696
10. Franco A, Barnaba V, Natali P, Balsano C, Musca A, Balsano F (1988) Expression of class I and class II major histocompatibility complex antigens on human hepatocytes. Hepatology 8:449–454
11. Lautenschlager J, Höckerstedt K, Salmela K (1990) Fine-needle aspiration biopsy in the monitoring of liver allografts. Different cellular findings during rejection and cytomegalovirus infection. Transplantation 50:798–803

Cellular Activation (1)

Cellular Endothelial Interaction and the Activation of Plasma Cascade Systems in Sepsis

A.O. Aasen and L. Buø

Release of proteases and mediators from circulating cells occurs during the early stages of sepsis [1]. These phenomena, being a part of cellular activation, have wide-ranging effects of importance for the pathophysiology of this disease. In experimental animals exposed to endotoxin, accumulation of leukocytes in various organs such as the lung and the liver is a prominent feature. As a part of these morphological changes, damage to endothelial cells is regularly seen. This process leads to exposure of the subendothelial basement membrane. The basement membrane is known for its capacity to activate the contact system of plasma.

Mediator Release and Endothelial Activation

When endotoxin is given intravenously to experimental animals or to human volunteers, release of cytokines is seen within minutes after the start of the infusion. Peak values are reached within the first few hours. Recent studies have shown that these mediators play a key role in the activation of the vascular endothelium [2]. During this process, surface molecules are expressed on the endothelium, leading to adhesion of circulating leukocytes. Such adhesion molecules are found both in the selectin family (E-selectin and P-selectin) and in the immunoglobulin gene super family (ICAM-1, ICAM-2, and VCAM-1). Leukocytes express counter-receptors for these molecules of the vascular endothelium which also promote adherence of leukocytes to the endothelial cells [3].

These processes of leukocyte endothelial interaction lead to injuries of the vascular endothelium and exposure of the subendothelial basement membrane.

The Contact System

As a consequence of exposure of proteins belonging to the plasma cascade systems to the subendothelium, the contact system is activated [4]. Contact activation represents a common mechanism for the initiation of several body defences against injury, such as intrinsic blood coagulation, fibrinolysis, the plasma kallikrein-kinin system, and complement activation. In the cascade reactions of contact activation the zymogens FXII, FXI, and prekallikrein (PKK) are converted to active serine proteases by limited proteolysis. High-molecular-weight kininogen (HK) is a nonenzymatic cofactor in these conversions. Binding of the zymogen FXII to a negatively charged surface (subendothelium) where autoactivation of FXII occurs, initiates activation of the contact system. Contact activation initiates the intrinsic coagulation cascade through activation of FXII and FXI (Fig. 1). FXI and PKK circulate as noncovalently associated bimolecular complexes with HK. When these complexes are bound to the negative surface adjacent to activated FXII, active serine proteases are generated from the bound zymogens. The zymogens can bind directly to the surface, but activation only occurs in the presence of HK. Surface-bound FXIIa cleaves PKK to kallikrein and FXI to FXIa. Kallikrein generates additional FXIIa from FXII. FXIa remains bound to HKa on the surface, while kallikrein is released into the fluid phase. Kallikrein can diffuse and hydrolyze its substrate HK to HKa composed of a heavy and a light chain linked by disulfide bonds. The coagulation activity resides in the light chain, which contains both the surface-binding regions and the domain responsible for complex formation with PKK and FXI. FXII in plasma is converted to FXIIa and to FXII fragments (FXIIf) which retain the active site of FXIIa but not the surface-binding domain.

The contact activation system is closely regulated by plasma protease inhibitors [5], C1-inh and α_2-M being the most important natural inhibitors. C1-inh is the major inhibitor of FXIIa and is also a major inhibitor of kallikrein (Fig. 1). Kallikrein is also inhibited by α_2-M. The predominant inhibitor of FXI is α1-PI. Kallikrein and FXIa complexed with HK are protected against inactivation.

The plasma kallikrein-kinin system is initiated by contact activation (Fig. 1). Kallikrein can cleave its natural substrate HK, releasing the very potent vasodilator bradykinin [6]. Kinins are responsible for several physiological effects such as increase in vascular permeability, induction of hypotension, smooth muscle contraction, stimulation of cellular glucose uptake, provocation of pain, and tissue plasminogen activator (t-PA) release. C1-inh and α_2-M control the release of kinins from HK, while kininases control the plasma level of kinins by inactivation. Recently, the kininogens were demonstrated to be potent inhibitors of cystein proteases such as cathepsins, papain, and calpain.

Thus kininogens are multifunctional proteins which (a) serve as substrates for kallikrein and release kinins, (b) bind and assemble coagulation zymogens on activating surfaces, allowing contact activation to occur, and (c) inhibit cysteine proteases [7]. The plasma kallikrein-kinin system, furthermore, has a role in the activation of coagulation and fibrinolysis, and participates in healing of wounds and defence against infections (phagocytosis).

Bradykinin probably stimulates the release of t-PA from the vascular endothelial cells. This kinin action provides a link between the kallikrein-

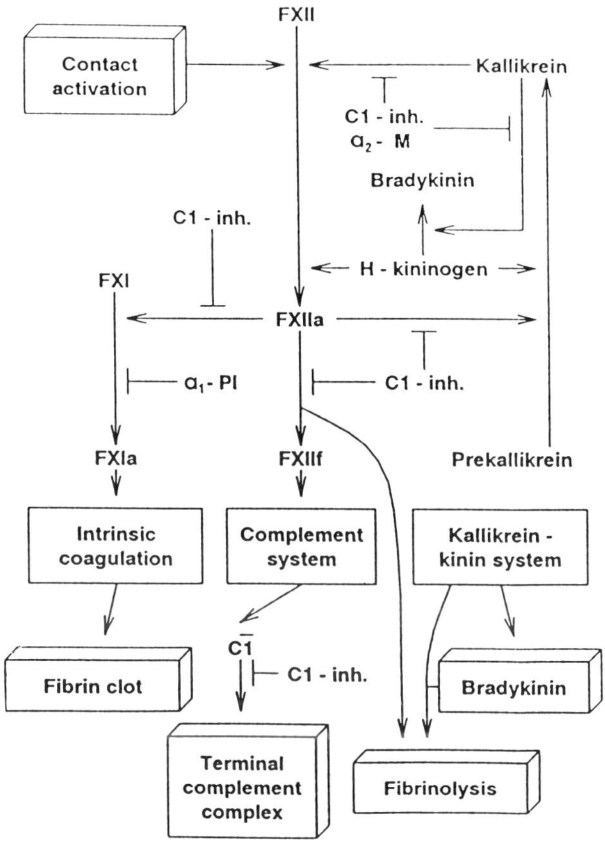

Fig. 1. Interactions between the plasma cascade systems induced by contact activation

kinin system and the extrinsic pathway of fibrinolysis. Kallikrein and FXIIa are believed to contribute to the generation of urokinase plasminogen activator (u-PA) from its precursor pro-u-PA, thereby interlinking the contact and kallikrein-kinin systems with the intrinsic pathway of fibrinolysis. The physiologic significance of kallikrein and FXIIa as directly acting plasminogen activators (FXII-dependent PA) is unclear and weak compared to u-PA. Plasmin is thought to participate in the activation of FXII and to release BK from its precursor HK, providing connections between the fibrinolytic system, contact activation, and the kallikrein-kinin system.

The complement system is activated and controlled as a consequence of contact activation. FXIIf, a cleavage product of FXII, activates the first component (C1) in the classical pathway of complement (Fig. 1), in a manner analogous to the activation by antigen-antibody complexes. Plasmin has also been shown to be capable of activating C1, while plasma kallikrein has been shown to inactivate it. C1-inhibitor, the major inhibitor of activated C1, also inhibits the activities of FXIIa, FXIIf, kallikrein, and plasmin. A wide variety of mediator substances, like peptides having pronounced effects on the vasculature, are formed during complement activation.

Thus activation of the contact system initiates several interacting proteolytic cascades and is thereby responsible for a wide variety of physiologic effects. The proteolytic cascades initiated and amplified by the proteins of the contact system are of importance in several host defence reactions.

Experimental Studies

On injecting rats with purified human FXII fragments, decreases in blood pressure of about 20% were seen immediately after injection of the compound [8]. After depleting the animals of circulating PKK by the administration of dextran sulfate, the decreases in blood pressure following FXII fragment injections were, however, prevented. Furthermore, recent experiments performed in our laboratory showed that small quantities of purified plasma kallikrein with activities corresponding to values found in humans with sepsis promptly reduced peripheral vascular resistance and left ventricular stroke work [9]. Additional support for a role of the plasma kallikrein-kinin system in sepsis was provided by Andreasson and co-workers using a lung-lymph fistula model in septic sheep. In these experiments, marked decreases in functional plasma kallikrein inhibition were found in the lymph at 4 h after the start of endotoxin infusion [10].

Clinical Studies

During the last two decades, several clinical studies have emphasized that the plasma kallikrein-kinin system might be of importance in the pathophysiology of sepsis. Using functional assays, our group demonstrated that patients with sepsis have marked reductions in plasma PKK and functional plasma kallikrein inhibition activities [11, 12]. Kalter et al. [13] observed a significant correlation between functional plasma kallikrein inhibition and the C1-inhibitor antigen values. Studies by Lämmle and the groups of Fritz, Colman, and Hack have also underlined the importance of plasma kallikrein in patients with sepsis [14–17].

References

1. Schlag G, Redl H (1993) Pathophysiology of shock, sepsis and organ failure. Springer, Berlin Heidelberg New York
2. Prober JS, Cotran RS (1990) The role of endothelial cells in inflammation. Transplantation 50:537–544
3. Bevilacqua MP (1993) Endothelial-leukocyte adhesion molecules. Annual Rev Immunol 11:767–804

4. Colman RW (1984) Surface-mediated defense reactions. The plasma contact activation system. J Clin Invest 73:1249–1253
5. Schapira M (1987) Major inhibitors of the contact phase coagulation factors. Semin Thromb Hemost 13:69–78
6. Erdös EG (1976) Commentary. The kinins. A status report. Biochem Pharmacol 25:1563–1569
7. Müller-Esterl W, Iwanaga S, Nakanishi S (1986) Kininogens revisited. TIBS 11:336–339
8. Waeber G, Schapira M, Waeber B, Aubert JF, Nussbergen J, Brunner HR (1988) Hypotensive effect of the active fragment derived from factor XII is mediated by an activation of the plasma kallikrein-kinin system. Circ Shock 26:375–382
9. Naess F, Waage A, Roeise O, Stadaas JO, Aasen AO (1992) Hemodynamic and proteolytic effects of intravenous injection of purified human plasma kallikrein. Am J Physiol 263:4405–4409
10. Andreasson S, Smith L, Aasen AO, Saldeen T, Risberg B (1988) Local pulmonary activation of proteolytic enzymes after Escherichia-coli-induced lung injury in sheep. Eur Surg Res 20:289–297
11. Aasen AO, Smith-Erichsen N, Amundsen E (1983) Plasma kallikrein-kinin system in septicemia. Arch Surg 118:343–346
12. Smith-Erichsen N, Aasen AO (1984) Evaluation of severity and prognosis in early stages of septicemia by means of chromogenic peptide substrate assays. Eur Surg Res 2:140–146
13. Kalter ES, Timmermanns A, Bouma BN (1982) The kinin generating system during sepsis and bacterial shock. Agents Actions 9:638–644
14. Lämmle B, Tran TH, Ritz R, Duckert F (1984) Plasma prekallikrein, factor XII, antithrombin III, C1(−)-inhibitor and alpha 2-macroglobulin in critically ill patients with suspected disseminated intravascular coagulation (DIC). Am J Clin Pathol 82:396–404
15. Jochum M, Duswald K-H, Neumann S, Witte J, Fritz H (1984) Proteinases and their inhibitors in septicemia – basic concepts and clinical implications. Adv Exp Med Biol 167:391–404
16. Pixley RA, De La Cadena R, Page JD, Kaufman N, Wyshock EG, Chang A, Taylor FB, Colman RW (1993) The contact system contributes to hypotension but not disseminated intravascular coagulation in lethal bacteremia. J Clin Invest 91:61–68
17. Nuijens JH, Huijbregts CCM, Eerenberg AJM, Abbink JJ, Strac van Schijndel RJM, Felt-Bersma RJF, Thijs LG, Hack CE (1988) Quantification of plasma factor XIIa-C1(−)-inhibitor and kallikrein-C1(−)-inhibitor complexes in sepsis. Blood 72:1841–1848

The Role of the Macrophage in Early Post-traumatic Immunosuppression

C.C. Baker

Introduction

The macrophage has achieved an area of preeminence over the last 10 years in sharp contradistinction to its previous image as a relatively inert phagocyte. This chapter will attempt to give some background on the reasons why the macrophage is important in trauma and multiple organ failure, some specific studies relating to post-traumatic immunosuppression, and some thoughts about future directions.

Clinical correlates of immunosuppression following injury have been known for some time. In mechanical trauma, sepsis causes 78% of late deaths when the neurologic deaths (50% of total deaths) are eliminated [1]. Conversely, when inhalation injury deaths are eliminated, sepsis causes 75% of deaths following thermal injury. Studies on the sepsis syndrome has been extensive over the last 10 years. Sepsis can be defined as a pathophysiologic state due to disruption of homeostasis from infection, the toxic products of microbes, and/or the action of inflammatory mediators. It is this last area that has captured the interest of surgeons and basic scientists alike and I will spend some of my time referring to studies in this area.

The disruption of homeostasis that occurs following major injury or operative intervention is a complex process. The balance between premorbid disease, the nutritional state, host resistance, and the insults of shock, soft tissue injury, and malnutrition, result in disruptions in homeostasis leading to sepsis. There are a number of factors that play into this balance, including immune factors, coagulation factors, toxic factors, gas exchange, energy metabolism, wound healing, and clinical errors of omission and commission. Many of these are beyond the scope of this paper, which will concentrate on the specific immune abnormalities that have been studied. When development of sepsis cannot be traced to a treatable cause, mortality is usually proportional to the number of organs that fail.

Macrophage Function

Macrophage function is at the center of the specific immune cell interactive network that is critical for host resistance. It is now known that the macrophage is the main cell responsible for antigen recognition and antigen processing. In the normal setting this leads to production of interleukin-1 (IL-1) and IL-1 receptors leading to T-cell elaboration interleukin-2 (IL-2) receptors, T-cell replication, and T-cell production of IL-2. This leads to B-cell activation and antibody production. All of these steps, together with complement lead to opsonization of bacteria, phagocytosis and killing by neutrophils. Macrophages have been found to be a very complex set of cells. A simplistic way to characterize macrophages is to divide them into facilitatory and inhibitory macrophages. Facilitatory macrophages carry immune response (IR) genes on their surface, interact with T-helper cells, produce IL-1, and are inhibited by prostaglandin E_2, steroids and T-suppressor cells. Inhibitory macrophages lack an IR gene, interact with T-suppressor cells, are stimulated by prostaglandin E_2 and T-suppressor cells, and are resistant to steroids. Macrophages have a host of functions, including the following: complement synthesis; interaction with the coagulation system (plasminogen activator and tissue thromboplastin factor synthesis); antigen recognition; monokine production; and immune regulation. This set of functions was very carefully described by Ron Maier in his treatise describing the angry macrophage [2]. An adaptation of these functions is shown in Table 1. The main thing to remember is that the macrophage is a cell that occupies a critical position relative to a number of inflammatory systems, and it causes a large number of interactions through a host of inflammatory mediators.

Table 1. Macrophage-derived inflammatory mediators

Chemoattractants
C5a
Leukotriene B_4 (LTB_4)
Interleukin-8
Vasoactive agents
C3a
Prostacycline
Leukotrienes (LTC_4, LTD_4)
Thrombotic factors
Thromboxane A_2
Procoagulant activity
Plasminogen activator inhibitor
"Metabolic" agents
Interleukin-1
Interleukin-6
Pathophysiologic agents
Tumor necrosis factor
Platelet activating factor
Immunosuppressors
Prostaglandin E_2
Interferon-γ depressed

Macrophage and Multiple Organ Failure (MOF)

There are several possible roles for the macrophage in MOF. Bacterial translocation of antigen across the gut is one area that has received a great deal of interest. The macrophage has been clearly shown by Carol Wells to be responsible for trafficking of antigen from the gut lumen to the mesenteric lymph node [3]. Another possible area involves the alteration in the antigen recognition processing and presentation, which may lead to macrophage dysfunction [4]. One of the possible etiologic theories in this regard is that disruption of soft tissues, altered bone or altered brain, act as altered self antigen, which causes down regulation in order to avoid an autoimmune response. Another area where significant attention has been addressed is the paracrine interactions in the liver (between the hepatocyte and the Kupffer cell) and in the lung (between the alveolar macrophage and the endothelial cell). In both of these areas, substances produced by the macrophage, such as interleukin-6 in the liver, lead to stimulation of a nearby cell (e.g., hepatocyte). These interactions are not well understood but clearly have a role in multiple organ failure. Nitric oxide is attaining a substantial amount of interest in this area [5].

Studies of Macrophage Function Following Injury

A number of years ago we studied splenectomy patients and found that their response to phytohemagglutinin (PHA) was decreased to negligible levels at about 15 days following injury. Although PHA is a T-cell mitogen, it requires macrophage cooperation for optimal function. Therefore we chose to study the effect of macrophage depletion on these results. Human mononuclear cells were depleted of macrophage by passage over a Sephadex G-10 column. When depleted cells were tested they had normal mitogen responses, whereas unfiltered cells continue to show only 20% mitogen response at 15 days [6]. This was presumptive evidence that inhibitory macrophages, previously cleared by the spleen, were elaborated in larger amounts around 2 weeks following injury. There is no evidence, however, that this abnormality has anything to do with overwhelming postsplenectomy sepsis. Faist et al. [7] have continued studies on trauma patients in my laboratory and in Germany showing decreases in total T cells and particularly T-helper cells in the first three weeks following injury. Conversely the patients had a monocytosis and were found to have increased production of prostaglandin E_2 at 7–10 days [8]. Depressions in IL-2 synthesis and IL-2 receptor elaboration were shown in the same 7–10 day period. Interestingly, addition of indomethacin to the cultures significantly increased the production of IL-2. Although the IL-2 levels were not restored to normal, this is suggestive evidence of inhibitory macrophage function early following injury.

The hypotheses that came from these studies are as follows:

1. Major trauma is immunosuppressive.
2. Alterations in self antigens may trigger macrophage dysfunction following injury.
3. Macrophage release of mediators may potentiate post-traumatic immunosuppression.

To test these hypotheses we chose to study antigen presentation in a model of sepsis using cecal ligation and puncture (CLP). This model provides polymicrobial sepsis which is parallels human sepsis. The model was originally described in a rat [9] and later adapted to the mouse [10]. We studied two strains of mice that are congenic except for the one abnormality in their macrophage response to endotoxin. The mice from the C_3H/HEJ strain are resistant to endotoxin, whereas mice from the C_3H/HEN strain are sensitive to endotoxin. Mortality rates for these two strains of mice for cecal ligation and puncture and femur fracture are shown in Table 2. Antigen recognition was studied in these animals using a T-cell clone, D10 G4.1 developed by Kaye et al. [11]. This system allows assessment of antigen recognition and IL-1 production. Briefly, C_3H/HEJ animals were seen to have profound increases in antigen presentation with a 14-fold increase in 8 h and a 4 1/2-fold increase at 4 days, compared to C_3H/HEN animals, which nearly had normal responses throughout the time period studied [12]. With respect to IL-1 production, the C_3H/HEJ animals had a 28-fold increase at 4 h which dropped to a 20-fold increase at 1 day and a fourfold increase at 6 days. The C_3H/HEN animals were able to mount a fourfold increase at 6 days, but this was rather a late response. Our conclusion from these studies was that the C_3H/HEJ mice had markedly increased antigen presentation and IL-1 production by macrophages after CLP compared to endotoxin sensitive C_3H/HEN mice. The differences in mortality in these two strains of mice may relate to the supernormal response of the C_3H/HEJ mice or to an inadequate response of the macrophages from the C_3H/HEN mice in this model.

We then went on evaluate the interaction between femur fracture as a trauma model and CLP as a sepsis model. Basically, the same two strains of mice were used and CLP was performed at 1, 3, 5, and 7 days following femur fracture. C_3H/HEN mice had significantly enhanced mortality and essentially all mice died when CLP was performed with a 25-gauge needle, 7

Table 2. Mortality after CLP and femur fractures

Strain	CLP (25 gauge)	CLP (19 gauge)	Femur fracture
C_3H/HEJ	0	25%	10%
C_3H/HEN	45%[a]	100%[a]	10%

[a] Increased versus C_3H/HeJ ($P < 0.05$, χ^2)

days following femur fracture. Interestingly, the C_3H/HEJ mice, which normally have minimal mortality after CLP with a 25-gauge needle, or with femur fracture, had 35% mortality when CLP followed femur fracture by 1 day and 45% mortality when CLP followed femur fracture by 3 days [13]. At 5 days there was no excessive mortality and at 7 days there was no mortality at all. These data would suggest that, even in the endotoxin-resistant C_3H/HEJ mice, there is a macrophage abnormality occurring early after injury that leaves the animals at increased risk for mortality from sepsis. If we could better understand this early macrophage defect, we might be able to intervene and alter the outcome.

More recently, we have followed studies from Schirmer et al. [14] and studied open and closed femur fracture in AKR mice. We hypothesized that the closed femur fracture with its crush injury might involve more immunosuppression and more alterations in gut permeability than the open femur fracture. The open femur fracture group did not demonstrate any reduction in mitogenic response or a change in gut permeability. The closed femur fracture group was associated with increases in B- and T-cell responses and gut permeability early after injury. Significant immunosuppression occurred 96 h after closed femur fracture (L. Napolitano, unpublished data). These data suggest that the magnitude of the injury and the type of injury may well determine the degree of immunosuppression.

The Future

With all the studies looking at immune regulation and macrophage function following injury, a number of studies are bound to be performed looking at immunomodulation. Some of the possible therapeutic strategies are listed in Table 3. As we look at immunomodulation in this area, we must remember several things. First of all, detection of cytokines in the serum does not necessarily relate to what is going on at the cell membrane level. In addition,

Table 3. Immunomodulation strategies

Problem	Strategy
Endotoxin	Monoclonal antibodies (HA-IA, J-5)
	Neutralize (polymyxin)
Prostaglandin E_2	Indomethacin
	Ibuprofen
TNF	Monoclonal antibodies
Oxygen radicals	Scavengers
	WBC endothelial CD14 blockade
	Allopurinol
Nitric oxide	Arginine
	n-Monomethyl arginine

we must learn to recognize the difference between endocrine, autocrine, and paracrine roles for a number of these inflammatory mediators. In order to optimize immunomodulatory therapy, we must stratify patients at risk, maximize standard therapy, and limit immunomodulator therapy to those patients with a favorable risk-benefit ratio. Because these therapies are often expensive and do have risks, we must be very careful in using them. Finally, one must realize that by altering the immune system in another direction, we may be upsetting the delicate balance of the immune system. All therapies must be carefully considered and scrupulously tested before being put into widespread use.

Conclusion

A great deal of information has accrued over the last 10–15 years regarding immunosuppression following injury. Substantial insights have been obtaind about the central role of the macrophage in this process. Nonetheless, our understanding is still limited. This chapter has attempted to describe some of the studies regarding the role of the macrophage in post traumatic immunosuppression. Our understanding is still incomplete in this area, but it appears that the macrophage tends to exert some of its dysfunctional effects early after injury. Before we consider invasive efforts at immunomodulation, we must understand these processes further and recognize that efforts at immunomodulation may upset the delicate balance of the immune system in the opposite direction.

References

1. Baker CC, Openheimer L, Stephens B, Lewis FR, Trunkey DD (1980) The epidemiology of trauma deaths. Am J Surg 140:144–150
2. Maier RV (1993) The angry macrophage and its impact on host response mechanisms. In: Faist E, Merakins J, Schildberg R (eds) Host defense dysfunction in trauma, shock, and sepsis. Springer, Berlin Heidelberg New York, pp 191–197
3. Wells CL, Jechorek RP, Gillingham KJ (1991) Relative contributions of host and microbial factors in bacterial translocation. Acta Med Scand 126:247–252
4. Baker CC, Yamada A, Faist E, Kupper TS (1987) Interleukin-1 and T cell function following injury. J Burn Care Rehabil 8:503–508
5. Lancaster JR Jr (1992) Nitric oxide in cells. Am Sci 80:248–259
6. Baker CC, Miller CL, Trunkey DD (1979) Identity of mononuclear cells which compromise trauma patients' resistance. J Surg Res 26:478–487
7. Faist E, Kupper TS, Baker CC, Chaudry IH, Dwyer J, Baue AE (1986) Depression of cellular immunity after major injury: its association with posttraumatic complications and its restoration with immunomodulating agents. Arch Surg 121:100–105
8. Faist E, Mewes A, Baker CC, Strasser T, Alkan SS, Reiber P, Heberer G (1987) Prostaglandin E_2 (PGE_2)-dependent suppression of IL-2 production in patients with major trauma. J Trauma 27:837–848

9. Wichterman KA, Baue AE, Chaudry IH (1980) Sepsis and septic shock – a review of laboratory models and a proposal. J Surg Res 29:189–201
10. Baker CC, Chaudry IH, Gaines HO, Baue AE (1983) Evaluation of factors affecting mortality rate after sepsis in a murine +cecal ligation and puncture model. Surgery 94(2):331–335
11. Kaye J, Gillis S, Mizel SB et al. (1984) Growth of a cloned T cell line induced by monoclonal antibody specific for antigen receptor: interleukin-1 is required for the expression of receptors to interleukin-2. J Immunol 133:1339–1345
12. Baker CC, Niven-Fairchild AS, Yamada A, Caragnano CL, Kupper TS (1991) Macrophage antigen presentation and interleukin-1 production after cecal ligation and puncture in C_3H/HeN and C_3H/HeJ mice. Arch Surg 126:253–258
13. Baker CC, Niven-Fairchild T, Caragnano C, Kupper TS (1991) Outcome following femur fracture and subsequent cecal ligation and puncture in endotoxin-sensitive (C_3H/HeN) and Endotoxin-resistant (C_3H/HeJ) mice. J Surg Res 50: 170–174
14. Schirmer WJ, Schirmer JM, Townsend MC, Fry DE (1988) Femur fracture with associated soft-tissue injury produces hepatic ischemia. Arch Surg 231:412–415

Role and Measurement of Endotoxin in Septic Shock

R. URBASCHEK, K.-P. BECKER, R.S. MCCUSKEY, and B. URBASCHEK

The development of severe septicemia is a major complication in patients after multiple trauma, burn trauma, or abdominal surgery. In spite of modern surgical procedures, constant improvement in intensive care medicine, and new antimicrobial agents, the incidence and lethality rate of patients developing gram-negative sepsis remain high.

Numerous clinical and experimental studies have been performed with the aim of identifying a parameter for use as an initial index for the development of sepsis. In regard to sepsis induced by gram-negative bacteria, the measurement of circulating endotoxin – the lipopolysaccharides from the outer membrane of the gram-negative bacterial cell wall – would be a plausible early candidate, particularly since the isolation of circulating bacteria is relatively rare and time-consuming.

Measurement of Endotoxin

In pg amounts, endotoxins are capable of specifically activating an enzymatic cascade present in the lysate of amebocytes of the horseshoe crab *Limulus polyphemus* (LAL, limulus amebocyte lysate) [1]. This reaction results in the formation of a clot that also can be evaluated by measuring an increase in optical density, or the intensity of color when additional chromogenic substrates are used.

Difficulties in measuring endotoxin in plasma is due to factors present in protein-containing substances that interfere with the LAL-endotoxin reaction. It was found that dilution and heating of the samples, reduces these difficulties. In our laboratory, an automated, kinetic turbidimetric, LAL-microtiter assay was developed that takes into account plasma-related interferences by performing an individual internal standardization in each sample [2, 3]. This method avoids the procedure widely used of reading the reaction of the sample on a standard curve in a plasma pool from normal plasma, a procedure widely used. The course of the endotoxin-LAL reaction of plasma samples in regard to the endogenous and spiked endotoxins concentrations may vary intra- and interindividually. In Fig. 1. an example is demonstrated indicating possible errors in the detection of endotoxin levels in plasma when a standard curve in pooled normal plasma is used.

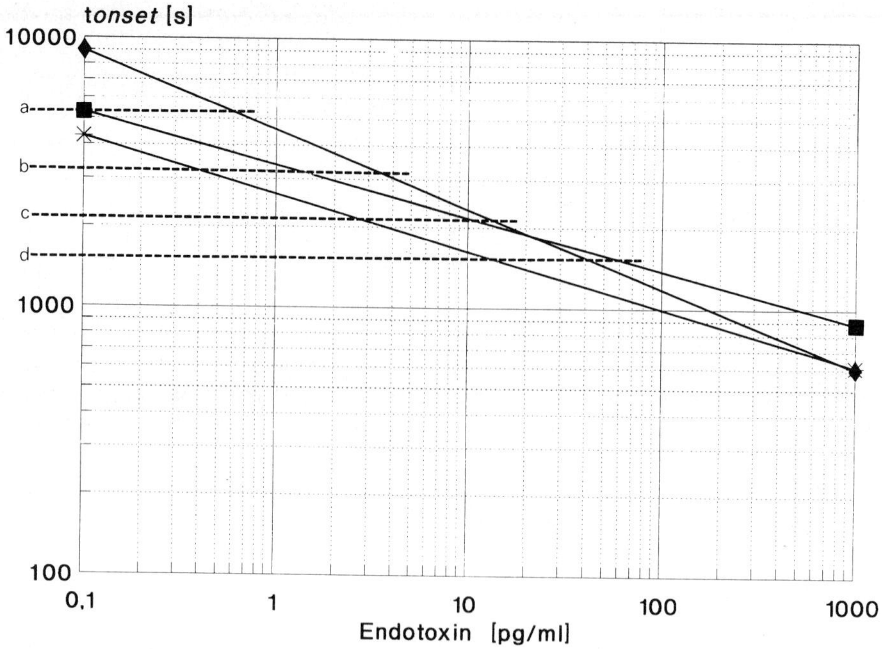

Fig. 1. Reading of plasma samples of patients at three different plasma pool reference curves (reference 1 [◆]; reference 2 [■]; reference 3 [*]). The t_{onset} at 40 mAbs of the kinetics (reading for 100 min at 30-s intervals at 405 nm and 37°C) is shown versus the endotoxin concentrations added. *a* to *d* indicate the endotoxin values in plasma samples of four different patients. As an example in plasma *b* 4, 12, or 33 pg/ml of endotoxin would be measured when reading at reference [1], reference [2], or reference [3] respectively

In general, further disadvantages of LAL methods are: (a) that they are not widely available in hospitals; and (b) that no comparison of the results between laboratories is possible, since these depend on the kind of method used – end-point, kinetic, turbidimetric, or colorimetric – for the pretreatment of the plasma, the volumes of the reagents, the lysate, and the standard endotoxins used.

Interpretation of Results

Humans are the most sensitive species to endotoxic effects, so that extremely low concentrations of endotoxin (for instance 10 pg/ml plasma) can indicate the development of a severe gram-negative sepsis. This implies that the test procedure has to be extremely sensitive. Although the biological LAL test systems currently are the most sensitive procedures for the detection of endotoxins, only a positive result is helpful in indicating development, course, or prognosis of gram-negative sepsis. An individual negative result does not exclude that endotoxins and their mediators are already active locally in their microenvironment, without detectable amounts of circulating endotoxin. This is mainly due to the facts that endotoxin clearance is extremely effectful and rapid, and that factors are present in the circulation that are capable of neutralizing endotoxin [4, 5]. In this context, it also should be mentioned that endotoxin-induced cytokines are capable of inducing other cytokines and that these may act synergistically. In addition, endotoxins per se elicit synergistic effects with a number of cytokines. Very often, even in severely ill patients, only a transient increase in endotoxin level is detectable. In regard to the onset of detrimental endotoxin-induced pathophysiological mechanisms, only the tip of the iceberg is detectable, which also applies to the results of measuring cytokines in patients with sepsis [6]. Moreover, endotoxins have potentiating effects on endotoxin-induced permeability, increasing substances such as the vasoactive amines, histamine, and serotonin [7].

The Status of Response to Endotoxin

The detrimental effects involved in the development of sepsis, septic shock, and death reflect the consequences of the release of large amounts of endotoxins that – also depending on the status of the major target cell, the macrophage – result in overstimulation, dysregulation, and failure of the organisms to regulate and counteract their activities. It is well known that minute amounts of endotoxins are capable of inducing beneficial effects, such as enhanced nonspecific resistance to microbial infections, tolerance to its own effects, stimulation of hematopoiesis, radioprotection, and tumor regression [8]. It has been shown that also small amounts of endotoxin-induced mediators, such as TNF, IL-1, IL-6, or TGF-β, can transfer such beneficial effects [8–12]. Several mechanisms are involved, primarily the role of the functional state of macrophages, the major target cells of endotoxic effects. In addition, an increase in clearance of endotoxin, increased detoxification, lack of production of toxic mediators, downregulation of receptors, and a decrease in the number of receptors have been discussed. Thus, the state of reactivity to endotoxin is involved in the manifestation of their effects in the host. This implies that an absolute value of circulating endotoxin cannot be indicative of the severity of the clinical situation.

The Effect of Immunoglobulins

In regard to the specificity of the results obtained using LAL detection methods, a report and our own experiences indicating that IV-immunoglobulin (IVIG) preparations may result in false-positive endotoxin levels [13, 14] are of interest. In conventional lysates, besides the endotoxin-specific C-factor pathway of activation, a second factor of the coagulation cascade – factor G – is present that can be activated by substances other than endotoxin, for instance by (1-3)-β-D-glucans or fungal polysaccharides [15]. Such nonspecific reactions have been described in plasma from patients suffering from infections with *Candida albicans*. IV preparations obviously contain nonendotoxic *Limulus*-reactive material that also can activate the described nonspecific pathway. Evidence was obtained by using endotoxin-specific G-factor-free lysates that did not react with IVIGs. Our experiments, comparing eight immunoglobulin preparations in saline or human plasma with six different lysates, revealed that lysate-dependent false-positive reactions are measurable. Experimentally, an increase in LAL activity in plasma of mice was observed 6 h after treatment with homologous IG which was given at the time when a polymicrobial intra-abdominal infection was induced by cecal ligation and puncture (McCuskay et al., submitted). In vital microscopic studies of the microcirculature of the liver revealed that this treatment drastically improved the hepatic microcirculation by minimizing the numbers of leukocytes that normally plug the sinusoids in septic mice after

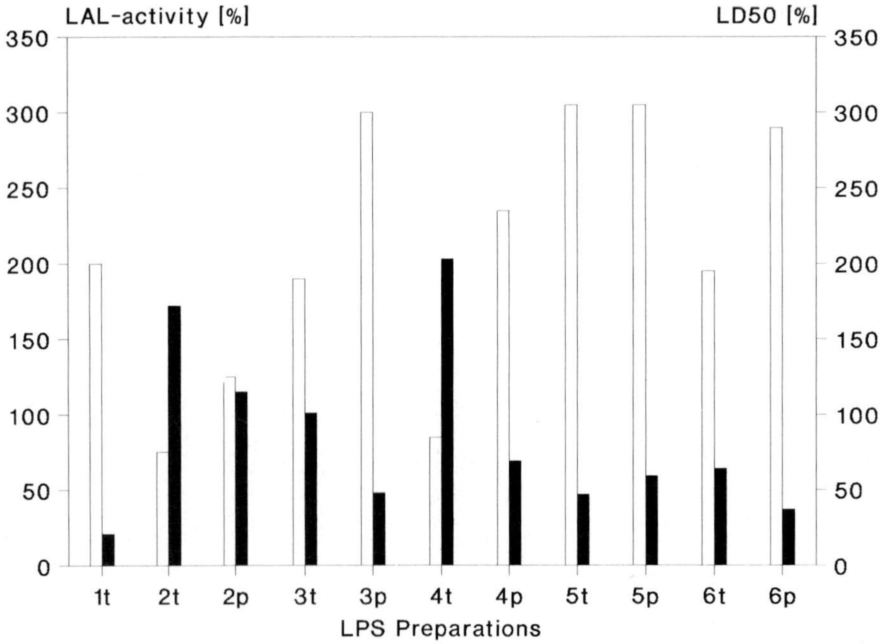

Fig. 2. LAL activity [□] versus toxicity (LD_{50}) [■] in mice of different LPS preparations, related to Novo Pyrexal (*Salmonella abortus equi*, the standard endotoxin used in the LAL assay) as 100%. *t*, Trichloroacetic acid; *p*, phenol water extraction. *1*, *E. coli O111:B4* (extracted in our laboratory); *2*, *E. coli O111:B4*; *3*, *E. coli O55:B5*; *4*, *S. enteritidis*; *5*, *S. typhosa* and *6*, *S. typhimurium* (2–6 Difco Laboratories)

cecal ligation and puncture. These studies clearly indicate that IgG reduced hepatic microvascular inflammatory responses to invading bacteria and endotoxin but that an LAL-positive reaction remained.

The Activiey of Different LPS Preparations

Different gram-negative bacteria have different amounts of endotoxins, and endotoxins derived from different gram-negative bacteria have varying LAL activity that does not correlate to their biological activity. This further implies that the absolute level of endotoxin measured does not necessarily reflect the severity of the underlying disease. Figure 2 illustrates the missing correlation between LAL activity with the LD_{50} of the different LPS preparations in mice.

Summary

In spite of the limitations described in the detection of endotoxin in plasma samples, the LAL test remains a valuable tool as a diagnostic and prognostic means for the evaluation of gram-negative sepsis and for monitoring the effect of therapeutic means used. The limitations involved, however, should be realized by both the clinician and the laboratory.

References

1. Levin J, Bang FB (1964) Bull Johns Hopkins Hosp 115:265–274
2. Ditter B, Becker K-P, Urbaschek R, Urbaschek B (1983) Arzneimittelforschung 33:681–687
3. Becker K-P (1993) Zum Endotoxinnachweis mit *Limulus* Amöbozyten Lysat. Dissertation, University of Heidelberg
4. Urbaschek B, Becker KP, Ditter B, Urbaschek R (1985) In: Leive L (ed) Microbiology-1985. American Society of Microbiology, Washington, pp 39–43
5. Prior RB (ed) Clinical applications of the limulus amoebocyte lysate test. CRC, Boca Raton
6. Cavaillon J-M, Munoz C, Fitting C, Misset B, Carlet J (1992) Circ Shock 38:145–152
7. Urbaschek B, Versteyl R (1965) Nature 207:763–764
8. Nowotny A (ed) (1983) Beneficial effects of endotoxins. Plenum, New York
9. Urbaschek R, Urbaschek B (1987) Rev Infect Dis 9:607–615
10. McCuskey RS, Urbaschek R, McCuskey PA, Urbaschek B (1987) Rev Infect Dis 9:616–619
11. Liu Z, Simpson RJ, Cheers C (1992) Infect Immun 60:4402–4406
12. Urbaschek R (1993) Prog Med Microbiol 4:1–11
13. Ikemura K, Ikegami K, Shimazu T, Yoshioka T, Sugimoto T (1989) J Clin Microbiol 27:1965–1968
14. Urbaschek R, Becker K-P (1993) Infusionsther Transfusionsmed 20:16–20
15. Obayashi T, Tamara S, Tanaka S (1985) Clin Chim Acta 149:55–65

Normal Human Immune Peritoneal Cells: Predominance of Memory Lymphocytes

U. KUBICKA, W.L. OLSZEWSKI, W. TARNOWSKI, K. BIELECKI, and A. ZIOLKOWSKA

Introduction

The peritoneal cavity contains immune cells derived from the blood circulation. These cells, macrophages, lymphocytes, and granulocytes, play a crucial role in the local immune responsiveness. Clinically, they maintain the sterility of the peritoneal cavity and protect against the development of intraperitoneal infections.

Intraabdominal infections and subsequent peritonitis in man remain a basic surgical problem. Despite progress in immunology, little is known about the kinetics of the immune response in human peritonitis.

We found in our previous studies that the human peritoneal cavity contains populations of free cells different from those in peripheral blood; this suggests a nonrandom accumulation of immune cells in the peritoneal cavity. More than 50% of these cells were lymphocytes, mostly of cytotoxic phenotype (CD4/CD8 ratio 0.4) [1]. The peritoneal cells (PCs) responded to standard mitogens such as PHA or ConA, although more weakly than the peripheral blood mononuclear cells (PBMCs).

The fact that PCs can be rapidly recruited in the peritoneal cavity indicates that these cells should belong to the memory cell population. This process is regulated by adhesion molecules. The question arises as to which adhesion molecules are expressed on PCs.

Our experiments were designed to investigate whether peritoneal lymphocytes represent a memory cell population and to identify adhesion molecules on PCs.

Material and Methods

Subjects

The study population comprised 16 patients of both sexes (age range: 32–71 years) undergoing elective cholecystectomy; informed consent was obtained from all patients. The patients had normal peripheral blood leukocyte counts, no symptoms of infection, and were not under any form of treatment with steroids or cytostatics.

Collection and Isolation of Peritoneal and Peripheral Blood Cells

Peritoneal cells were obtained intraoperatively, by means of peritoneal lavage, before any intraperitoneal manipulations were done. One thousand ml of 37°C prewarmed normal saline was infused slowly into the peritoneal cavity through a Trocath peritoneal dialysis catheter (Lab. Don Baxter, Italy). After 5 min the fluid was removed by gentle suction. Erythrocyte-contaminated fluid (hematocrit > 1) was eliminated from further studies. Collected fluid was centrifuged (10 min, 1200 rpm), then washed and resuspended in proper cell density in wash medium RPMI 1640 (Gibco, UK) supplemented with 10% decomplemented fetal calf serum (DFCS) (Gibco) and 100 U/ml penicillin/streptomycin solution (Gibco).

Before surgery 10 ml of peripheral blood was drawn from the cubital vein. PBMCs were isolated on a Lymphoprep gradient (Nyagard, Norway) according to the method of Boyum [2].

Cell Identification

Cell viability was determined by the trypan blue exclusion method. For immunocytochemical identification cytospins were stained with monoclonal antibodies (moAb) against CD11b (Mac-1) (Dako, Dania), CD14 (monocyte/macrophage) (Becton-Dickinson, USA), CD49d (VLA-4) (Immunotech), and CD54 (ICAM-1) (Becton-Dickinson) by the immuno-alkaline phosphatase anti-alkaline phosphatase (APAAP) staining technique according to the Dakopatts working procedure.

Flow Cytometric Analysis

PCs or PBMCs ($2–5 \times 10^6$) in 100 μl 0.01 M PBS were stained with 10 μl of Dako fluorochrome-conjugated primary antibody against CD2 and CD3 (pan T cells), CD4 (T helper cells), CD8 (T cytotoxic/suppressor cells), CD11a (LFA-1), CD11b (Mac-1), CD11c (p 150.95), CD18 (β_2 integrins), and CD45RO (UCHL1; memory cells). The cells were then analyzed with a fluorescence activated cell sorter (FACStar, Becton-Dickinson, USA) equipped with an argon ion laser. The green, red, and two-color fluorescence was measured. In each sample a total of 10 000 cells were analyzed. Data were presented as isometric displays of dot plots or single histograms. Results were expressed as a median percentage of positive cells.

Statistical Evaluation

The results were expresed as median values with the range of data. Comparisons were done using a nonparametric paired Wilcoxon test.

Results

The applied peritoneal lavage procedure allowed us to collect from 0.5 to 4.3×10^6 cells (M = 1.3×10^6). Their mean viability was 90.0%, and in no case below 80.0%.

The results of flow cytometric analysis of peritoneal and blood mononuclear cell subpopulations are shown in Figs. 1–3. They are expressed as a median percentage of the total mononuclear cell population. We found 61.7% (33.1%–71.4%) CD2, 51.0% (43.7%–58.3%) CD3, 93.9% (92.2%–95.5%) CD18, 96.4% (88.1%–96.4%) CD11a, 27.2% (12.0%–48.2%) CD11b, and 20.4% (18.8%–35.5%) CD11c positive cells in the entire PC population. The CD4/CD8 ratio was 0.9. For comparison, the respective values in the PBMC population were as follows: 75.5% (63.1% –88.2%) CD2, 62.0% (59.0%–66.4%) CD3, 97.8% (96.7%–99.0%) CD18, 97.7% (97.2%–98.7%) CD11a, 47.4% (36.5%–59.9%) CD11b, and 22.2% (13.3%–22.7%) CD11c; the CD4/CD8 ratio was 1.2.

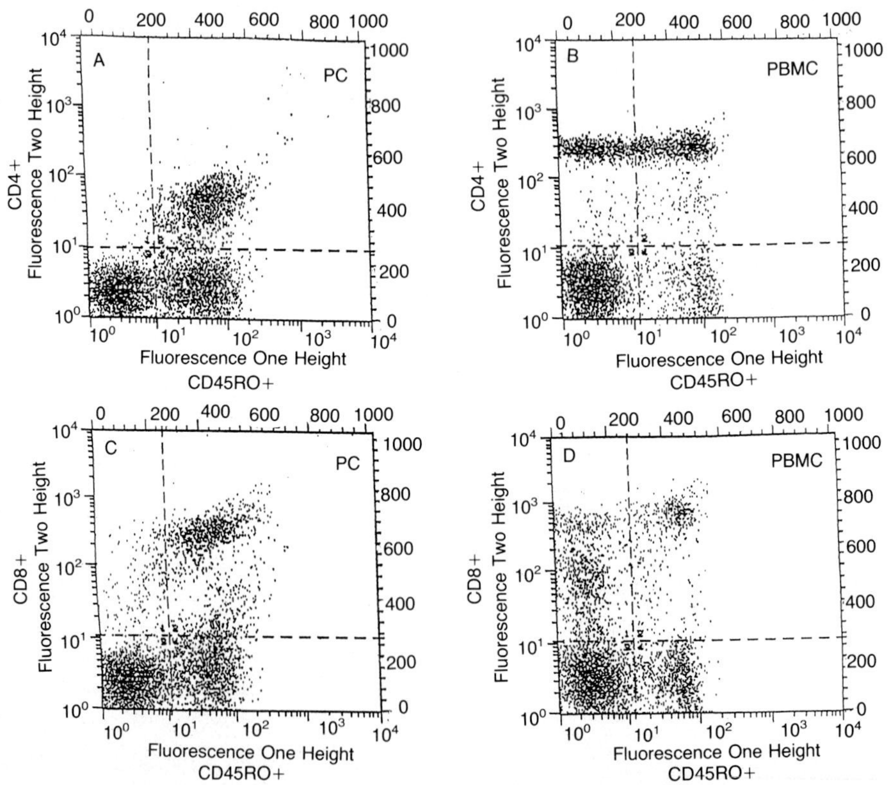

Fig. 1. Dot plot displays of the two-color analysis of peritoneal (*PC*) and peripheral blood mononuclear cells (*PBMC*) stained with anti-CD4 (**A**, **B**) or anti-CD8 (**C**, **D**) and anti-CD45RO (UCHL1) monoclonal antibodies

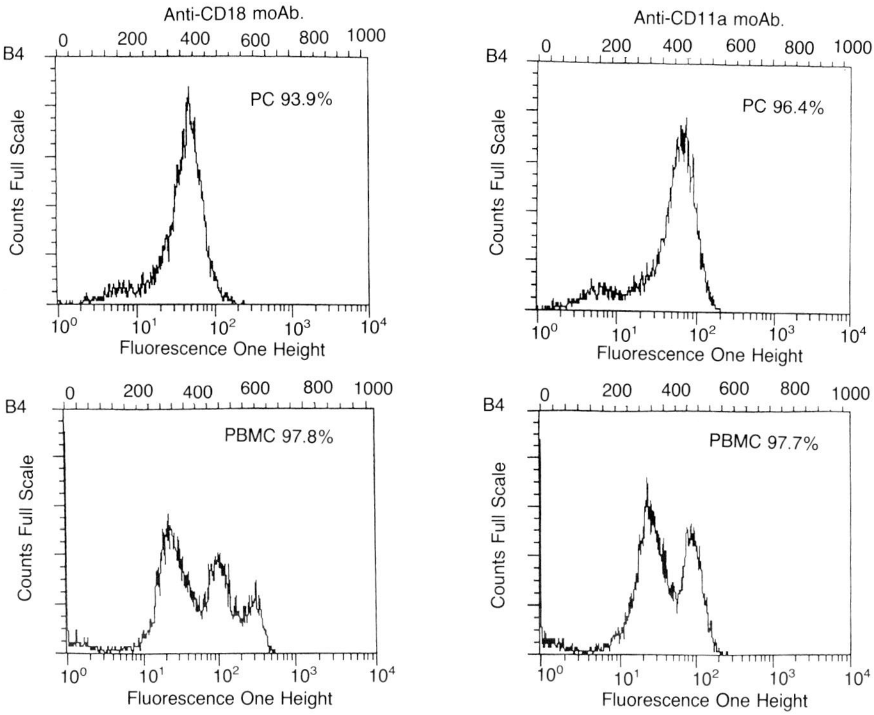

Fig. 2. Histograms of peritoneal (*PC*) and peripheral blood mononuclear cell (*PBMC*) populations stained with anti-CD18 and anti-CD11a monoclonal antibodies

Increased expression of CD2 molecule by peritoneal lymphocytes was detected in all patients, with the mean fluorescence intensity increasing from 457 (377–479, $n = 5$) on blood lymphocytes to 488 (405–522, $n = 6$) on peritoneal lymphocytes. The expression of CD3 was reduced in the peritoneal lymphocyte population compared with peripheral blood [474 (387–492, $n = 6$) and 514 (422–622, $n = 6$), respectively].

Memory Cell Identification

We found a significant difference in expression of the CD45RO (UCHL1) molecule on peritoneal and peripheral blood lymphocytes. Two-color analysis of PCs with a-CD4 (PE in FL2) and a-CD45RO (FITC in FL1), and with a-CD8 (PE) and a-CD45RO (FITC) are presented in Fig. 1A,C. The corresponding cell display patterns of PBMCs are shown in Fig. 1B,D. It revealed that a majority of CD4 and CD8 positive peritoneal lymphocytes were simultaneously UCHL1 positive, representing a memory/effector cell population (92.4% and 73.1%, respectively). In contrast, 50.2% CD4+ and

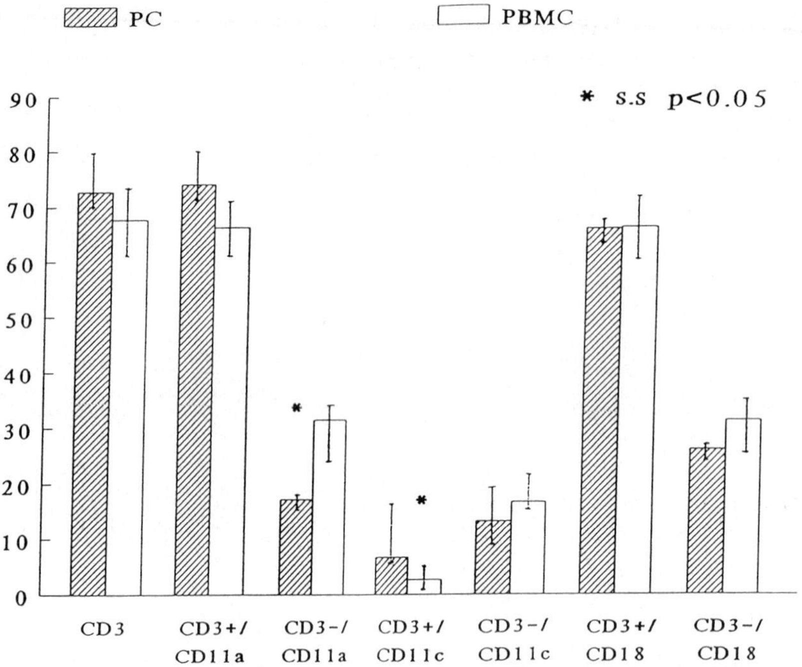

Fig. 3. The presence of adhesion molecules on CD3+ and CD3-peritoneal (*PC*) and peripheral blood mononuclear cells (*PBMC*) (median, $n = 3$, FACS)

30.1% CD8+ cells among PBMCs were UCHL1 positive; thus PBMCs contained more naive immune cells.

Adhesion Molecule Identification

Flow Cytometry. In contrast to significant differences in CD11b+ (Mac1+) cell frequency in peritoneal cavity and peripheral blood, we did not observe any differences in the percentages of CD18, CD11a, and CD11c positive cells in total peritoneal and blood cell populations. However, we found homogeneous CD18 (β_2 integrin chain) and CD11a (α-chain, LFA1) expression in PCs compared with bright and dim CD18+ and CD11a+ cells in peripheral blood (Fig. 2). In addition to an observed right shift in the mean fluorescence intensity of CD2, there were increases in CD11a [from 490 (414–510) in PBMCs to 503 (461–549) in PCs] and CD11c [from 320 (296–444) in PBMCs to 372 (368–433) in PCs] expression in the peritoneal CD3+ lymphocyte population. Moreover, we found more CD3+/CD11c+ lymphocytes in the peritoneal than in the blood cell population (6.7% and 2.7%, respectively) (Fig. 3). There were significantly less CD3−/CD11a+ cells among PCs than PBMCs (17.2% and 31.4%, respectively).

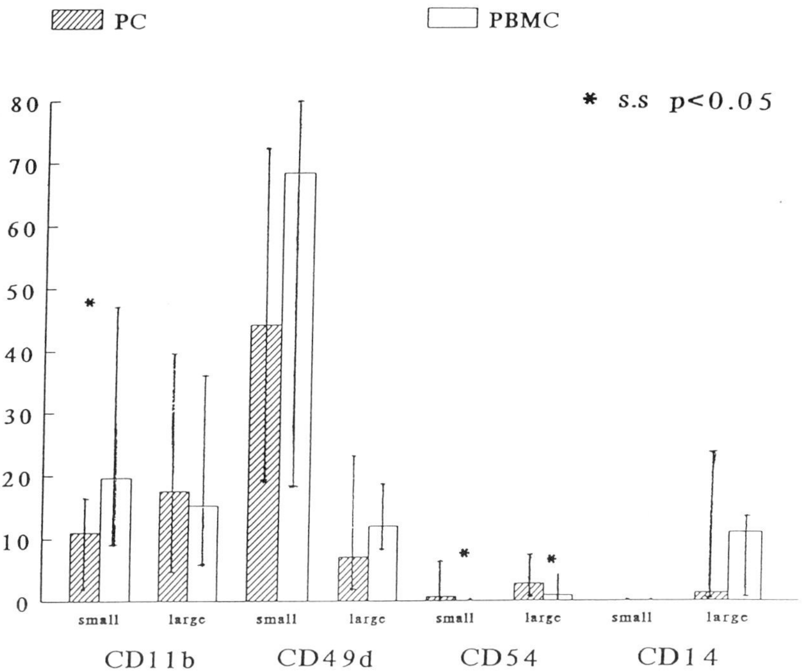

Fig. 4. The presence of adhesion molecules on peritoneal (*PC*) and peripheral blood mononuclear cells (*PBMC*) (median, $n = 6$, immunocytochemistry)

Immunocytochemistry. Immunocytochemical staining confirmed the results obtained in FACS, that there are significantly less cells expressing the CD11b (Mac1) adhesion molecule in the peritoneal cavity than in peripheral blood. This difference was seen in a cell-population morphologically resembling small lymphocytes (11.0% and 19.7%, respectively) (Fig. 4). Using the immunocytochemical method we found 44.2% (18.7%–70.0%) CD49d (VLA-4) positive cells in peritoneal and 68.3% (17.7%–76.9%) in the peripheral blood small, lymphocyte-like cell population. Because of the wide range of data the difference was not statistically significant. Moreover, we observed only 1.3% (0.3%–23.0%) CD14+ PCs and 10.9% (5.1% –13.0%) CD14+ PBMCs. A mean of 3.5% of PCs and 0.9% of PBMCs were CD54+ (ICAM1+).

Discussion

Evidence from the studies presented here, in which we characterized human PCs obtained intraoperatively by means of peritoneal lavage from patients undergoing elective cholecystectomy, indicates that the human peritoneal cavity contains a cell population rich in T lymphocytes, mainly T cytotoxic/

suppressor cells. The majority of CD4 and CD8 peritoneal lymphocytes belong to the memory/effector (UCHL1+) cell population. There is a high percentage of CD2, CD11a, CD11c positive lymphocytes and CD54+ cells in the whole PC population. In contrast, the percentage of CD11b+, CD49d+, CD14+ cells in the total peritoneal population, and of CD3-/CD11a+ cells, is low.

Cichocki et al. [3] and Davies et al. [4], using flow cytometry, demonstrated that in the majority of their patients treated with continuous ambulatory peritoneal dialysis, lymphocytes accounted for at least 50% of PCs. From our previous immunocytochemical studies it appeared that the PC population contains 45% CD68+ monocytes/macrophages, 42% CD2+ T lymphocytes, and 2% CD22+ B lymphocytes [1]. The present flow cytometric analysis confirmed the results and revealed that the percentage of T lymphocytes in the peritoneal cavity was even higher, with 61.7% CD2+ cells and 51.0% CD3+ cells, and an absence of CD19+ B lymphocytes (from 0% to 2.3%, data not shown). T4/T8 ratio was less than 1, which may suggest a preferential accumulation of the cytotoxic or suppressor lymphocytes in the peritoneal cavity.

It is known that resting T cells comprise two distinct subpopulations: CD45RA+/CD45RO− naive/virgin T cells and CD45RA−/CD45RO+ memory/effector T cells [5–8]. T lymphocytes lose CD45RA and gain CD45RO molecules during priming [6]. These cell subpopulations differ with respect to their activation requirements and responsiveness to mitogen [7–9]. We analyzed the normal human PC population by two-color flow cytometry to evaluate proportions of memory and naive cells in the peritoneal compartment. We found that the majority (92.4%) of CD4+ PCs, but only half (50.2%) of the CD4+ PBMCs were CD45RO+. Moreover, 73.1% of CD8+ PCs, but only 30.1% of CD8+ PBMCs, were CD45RO+. The presence of a significant proportion of CD45RO+ T lymphocytes in normal subjects may be a consequence of natural immunization to environmental antigens. Such a phenomenon was also found in normal human skin [10]. The predominance of the memory cell population in the peritoneum may explain the observation by us of lower responsiveness of peritoneal lymphocytes, compared with peripheral blood lymphocytes, to standard mitogens [11].

Immune specificity of the peritoneum strongly suggests that cell distribution in the peritoneal cavity is not a random process. It raises the question of which molecular factors and/or structures are responsible for such a cellular composition. There is little information about adhesion molecule expression on normal human PCs. Using a rat model it was shown that peritoneal exudate lymphocytes express the VLA-4 molecule and specifically migrate to the inflamed skin. This migration was blocked by moAb a-VLA-4 [12]. An increase in VLA-4 adhesion molecule on the surface of PCs in CAPD patients was observed [13]. We were not able to demonstrate an elevated percentage of CD49d (VLA-4)-positive cells in the peritoneal cavity, in comparison to the peripheral blood of the same patients. The frequency of VLA-4+ cells, like that of CD11b+, CD14+, and CD3−/CD11a+ cells, was even lower in peritoneal fluid than in blood.

It is known that macrophages and neutrophils express less CD11a and more CD11b and CD11c as α-chain β_2 integrins [14, 15]. Our observation in relation to nonlymphocytic CD11a+ PCs is in agreement withthis. We found less CD11b+ cells, no difference in CD11c+ cells and no more intense expression of these adhesion molecules in the entire PC population as compared with peripheral blood. The low values of CD14+ cells (1.3%) that we observed in the peritoneum were unexpected. We demonstrated that monocytes/macrophages stained with moAb against CD68 comprised approximately 40% of the entire PC population (data not shown, and [1]). It seems probable that molecules engaged in adhesion and migration of monocytes through endothelium and mesothelium, namely CD14, CD11b, and CD11c [16], and of lymphocytes (CD49d) [12, 13] into the peritoneum, are subsequently internalized or shed. Another possibility is that these surface receptors are occupied by their natural ligands and are not available for specific monoclonal antibody.

Slightly higher expression of CD2, CD11a, and CD11c on peritoneal than on peripheral blood lymphocytes and a higher percentage of CD54 positive cells in the PC than in the PBMC population may reflect a natural immune activation occurring in the peritoneal cavity.

In conclusion, the predominance of memory lymphocytes (CD45RO+) and lymphocytes with more intense CD2, CD11a, and CD11c molecule expression, as well as a higher frequency of CD54+ cells in the peritoneal population, compared to peripheral blood, suggests a permanent immune alert in the peritoneal cavity.

References

1. Kubicka U, Olszewski WL, Maldyk J, Wierzbicki Z, Orkiszewska A (1989) Normal human immune peritoneal cells: phenotypic characteristcs. Immunobiology 180:80
2. Boyum A (1976) Isolation of lymphocytes, granulocytes and macrophages. Scand J Immunol 5:9
3. Cichocki T, Hanicki Z, Sulowicz W, Smolenski O, Kopec J, Zembala M (1983) Output of peritoneal cells into peritoneal dialysate. Cytochemical and functional studies. Nephron 35:175
4. Davies SJ, Suassuna J, Ogg CS, Cameron JC (1989) Activation of immunocompetent cells in the peritoneum of patients treated with CAPD. Kidney Int 36:661
5. Smith SH, Brown MH, Rowe D et al. (1986) Functional subsets of human helper-inducer T cells defined by a new monoclonal antibody, UCHL1. Immunology 58:63
6. Akbar AN, Terry L, Timms A et al. (1988) Loss of CD45R and a gain of UCHL1 reactivity is a feature of primed T cells. J Immunol 140:2171

7. Byrne JA, Butler JL, Cooper MD (1988) Differential activation requirements for virgin and memory T cells. J Immunol 141:3249
8. Mackay CR (1992) Migration pathways and immunologic memory among T lymphocytes. Semin Immunol 4:51
9. Morimoto C, Letvin NL, Boyd AW et al. (1985) The isolation and characterization of the human helper inducer T cell subset. J Immunol 134:3762
10. Bos JD, Hagenaars C, Das PK et al. (1989) Predominance of "memory" T cells (CD4+, CDw29+) over "naive" T cells (CD4+, CD45R+) in both normal and diseased human skin. Arch Dermatol Res 281:24
11. Kubicka U, Maldyk J, Wierzbicki Z, Orkiszewska A, Rowinski W, Olszewski WL (1987) Immunological characteristics of human peritoneal cells. Eur Surg Res 19/S1:42
12. Issekutz TB, Wykretowicz A (1991) J Immunol 147:109
13. Van Dinther-Janssen ACHM, Horst E, Koopman G, Newmann W, Scheper RJ, Meijer CJLM, Pals ST (1991) The VLA-4/VCAM-1 pathway is involved in lymphocyte adhesion to endothelium in rheumatoid synovium. J Immunol 147: 4207
14. Tamatani T et al. (1991) Eur J Immunol 21:627
15. Morisaki T, Torisu M (1991) Enhanced adherence activity of OK-432-induced peritoneal neutrophils to tumor cells correlates to their increased expression of CD11b/CD18. Clin Immunol Immunopathol 59:474
16. Beekhuizen H, Blokland I, van Furth R (1993) Cross-linking of CD14 molecules on monocytes results in a CD11/CD18- and ICAM-1-dependent adherence to cytokine-stimulated human endothelial cells. J Immunol 150:950

Supplementation of Postoperative Enteral Nutrition with Arginine, RNA, and Omega-3 Fatty Acids Increases the Activity of Blood Monocytes in Cancer Patients

M. SENKAL, M. KEMEN, H.-H. HOMANN, T. HARINGS, J. BAIER, and V. ZUMTOBEL

Introduction

Early postoperative enteral feeding helps to ameliorate weight loss and to decrease the nitrogen losses in catabolic states after extensive surgical procedures [6]. Supplementation of enteral diets with arginine, omega-3 fatty acids, and RNA has been described to improve clinical outcome after major surgery [4] and to overcome postoperative immune dysfunction [8]. Since the activity of monocytes is a major part of the immune system we investigated in a prospective randomized trial the effect of an arginine, RNA, and omega-3 fatty acids supplemented enteral diet on the monocyte activity. This includes the ability of peripheral blood monocytes to express the human leukocyte antigen DR (HLA-DR) and the percentage of antigen-presenting monocytes. The percentage of peripheral blood monocytes that express HLA-DR antigen appears to be an accurate marker of both the infection and disease associated with immunodepression [3].

Patients and Methods

Forty-two adult patients with upper gastrointestinal malignancies who were to undergo major abdominal surgery were entered into the study. Exclusion criteria were the presence of insulin-dependent diabetes mellitus, pregnancy, or the use of steroids or anti-immune medication before study entry, as well as renal failure. All patients underwent surgical procedures as indicated by their primary site and stage of disease. Intraoperatively, a needle catheter jejunostomy (NCJ) was placed in the proximal jejunum. Enteral feeding started 12 h after surgery via this NCJ with 20 ml/h and progressed to the optimal goal of 80 ml/h by the fifth postoperative day (1 ml = 1 kcal). Patients were fed 10 days postoperatively with the study diet.

After surgery patients were randomly assigned to receive either an arginine, omega-3 fatty acids, and RNA enriched diet or an isocaloric and isonitrogenous placebo diet. Both diets were whole protein formulas in liquid form. The supplemented diet was fortified with 125 mg/dl arginine, 12.3 mg/dl RNA, and 292 mg/dl omega-3 fatty acids. The oral intake was allowed when clinically indicated between the 5th and 7th postoperative day and started with clear liquids. All patients received intravenous fluids and electrolytes as needed. When complications occurred they were treated adequately with either antibiotics or surgical revision.

Determination of Monocyte HLA-DR Antigen Expression. All cell samples were analyzed on a FAC-Scan flow cytometer (Beckton Dickinson). Briefly, the expression of HLA-DR antigen on monocytes was determined using fluorescent-labeled dual monoclonal antibody staining and flow microfluorometric analysis. A 100-μl aliquot of whole blood was stained with antihuman fluorescein isothiocyanate-coupled monoclonal antibody, which specifically stains monocytes, and with phycoerythrin-coupled antihuman HLA-DR. Samples were analyzed on a flow cytometer (Beckton Dickinson). The results are described as the percentage of total sample monocytes (monoclonal antibody-staining cells) that expressed HLA-DR antigen as well as the mean fluorescent intensity, a measure of antigen density. All antibodies were purchased from Beckton Dickinson.

Results

Forty-two patients were studied. There were 21 patients in the supplemented diet group and 21 patients in the placebo diet group. The preoperative diagnoses and operative procedures were similar between the two groups. At entrance into the study, there were no significant differences in nutritional status or type of surgical pathology; the age ranges were similar in both groups. There were no significant differences between groups in mean percent usual body weight, mean operative duration, or number of patients who received transfusions during the surgical procedure or postoperatively. The most common operative procedure was total gastrectomy, which was performed in nine patients who received the supplemented diet and seven patients who received placebo.

Gastrointestinal tolerance of both formula diets was excellent and no difference occured between the groups. No dropouts occurred due to intolerance.

The percentage of activated monocytes was similar preoperatively and on the first three postoperative days in both diet groups (Fig. 1). In the placebo diet group activated monocytes increased from 77% ± 2.1% on the 7th postoperative day to 81.6% ± 2.1% and 80% ± 2.6% on the 10th and 16th postoperative days compared to the group with supplemented diet, in which the percentage of activated monocytes varied from 86.7% ± 2.2% on the 7th postoperative day to 86.8% ± 2.1% and 91% ± 2.5% on the 10th and 16th postoperative days respectively. On postoperative days 7 and 16 the statistical difference between the two groups was significant ($P < 0.05$), whereas on postoperative day 10 the percentage of activated monocytes was only suggestively higher in the supplemented diet group.

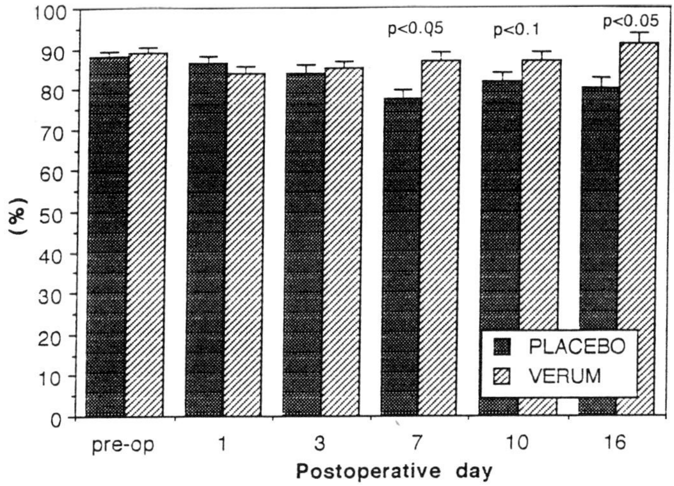

Fig. 1. Percentage of HLA-DR antigen-expressing monocytes in patients postoperatively fed either with an arginine-, omega-3 fatty acids-, and RNA-supplemented enteral diet (verum) or an isonitrogenous and isocaloric placebo diet. On postoperative days 7 and 16 HLA-DR expression in monocytes was significantly higher in the supplemented diet group ($P < 0.05$)

Preoperative values of HLA-DR expression of the individual monocyte decreased postoperatively in both diet groups (Fig. 2). HLA-DR expression levels did not show any significant difference between the two diet groups until the 7th postoperative day, when the fluorescence intensity, i.e., HLA-DR expression, was suggestively higher in the supplemented diet group. In this group HLA-DR expression of the monocyte increased from 160 ± 12 on the 7th postoperative day to 188 ± 15 and 194 ± 14 on the 10th and 16th postoperative days respectively. In contrast, the placebo diet group showed HLA-DR antigen expression levels of 119 ± 17, 166 ± 18, and 158 ± 19 during the same period.

Discussion

The ability of peripheral blood monocytes to express HLA-DR and the capacity of serum to support neutrophil phagocytosis correlates with the development of infection and late death after major trauma. Moreover, these values seem to be predictive for patient outcome both in development and recovery from major infection and in death from such infection [7, 9]. Persistence of a septic state is associated with a continued low expression of HLA-DR antigen and low levels of interferon-γ.

Certain nutrients such as the semiessential amino acid arginine, RNA, and omega-3 fatty acids may act pharmacologically on the immune system.

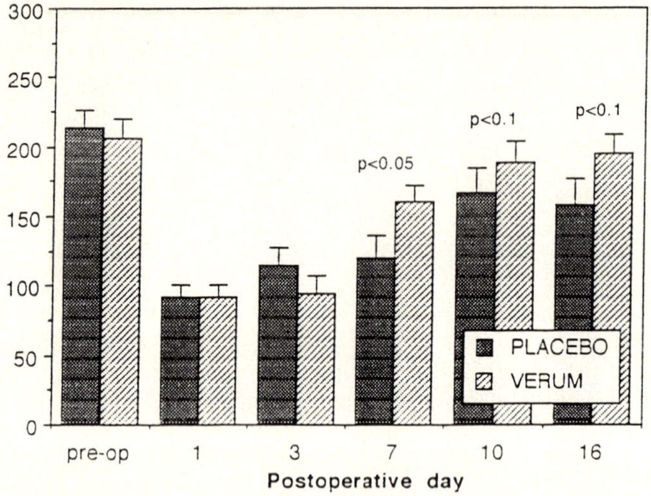

Fig. 2. The phagocytosis capacity of each monocyte, i.e., antigen density of the individual monocyte, was significantly higher on postoperative day 7 in the supplemeneted diet group ($P < 0.05$). On postoperative days 10 and 16 the antigen density (fluorescence intensity) was suggestively higher in the group with the arginine, RNA and omega-3 fatty acids enriched diet

It has been suggested that these nutrients may improve host immune defenses. The specific nutrient substrates seem to act via different mechanisms.

In different clinical trials the effect of dietary supplementation with arginine, omega-3 fatty acids, and RNA on immune defenses in surgical patients has been compared with a standard commercially availible enteral diet [1, 2, 4]. The purpose of this study was to evaluate the immunologic state of patients who underwent operations for upper gastrointestinal cancer and were fed postoperatively either with an arginine-, omega-3 fatty acids-, and RNA-supplemented enteral diet or with an isonitrogenous and isocaloric placebo diet.

There was a significant difference in the immunologic responses between the supplemented and the placebo diet group. Analysis of variance with repeated measures (ANOVA) showed significant differences ($P < 0.05$) between the two diet groups for the percentage of activated monocytes and the expression of the monoctyte antigen HLA-DR.

Cheadle et al. [3] found lower mean percentage of monocytes that expressed HLA-DR antigen and a lower mean fluorescence intensity in patients with postoperative infection and in those with severe sepsis. Furthermore, a delayed return to normal values in patients after general anesthesia and laparotomy has been described [5].

Our data show a significantly higher percentage of activated monocytes and expression of the HLA-DR antigen within the second postoperative week in patients who were postoperatively fed with an arginine, omega-3 fatty acids, and RNA supplemented enteral diet. Since a low percentage of activated monocytes and a low HLA-DR expression level correlate with immune dysfunction and are predictive of patient outcome [9] for infections and sepsis, our data show that application of an arginine, RNA, and omega-3 fatty acids supplemented diet is likely to reduce the occurrence of post-operative infections and sepsis. This would support the results of Daly et al., who described a better clinical outcome and an amelioration of the post-operative immune deficiency in patients who received this supplemented enteral diet [4].

In conclusion, supplementation of enteral nutrition with arginine, RNA, and omega-3 fatty acids improves recovery from postsurgical immune depression. This improved postsurgical immune response may be accountable, at least in part for the improved clinical outcome in surgical patients fed postoperatively with supplemented enteral nutrition [4].

References

1. Bower RH (1992) A modified enteral formula reduces hospital length of stay in patients in intensive care units. Clin Nutr 11 (Suppl):305
2. Cerra FB, Lehman S, Kostantinides N, Kostantinides F, Shronts EP, Holman R (1990) Effect of enteral nutrient on in vitro tests of immune function in ICU patients: a preliminary report. Nutrition 6:84–87
3. Cheadle WG, Hershman MJ, Wellhausen SR, Polk HC (1991) HLA-DR antigen expression on peripheral blood monocytes correlates with surgical infection. Am J Surg 161:639–645
4. Daly JM, Lieberman MD, Goldfine J et al. (1992) Enteral nutrition with supplemental arginine, RNA, and omega-3 fatty acids in patients after operation: immunologic, metabolic, and clinical outcome. Surgery 112:56–67
5. Faist E, Mewes A, Strasser T et al. (1988) Alteration of monocyte function following major injury. Arch Surg 123:287–292
6. Fletcher JP, Little JM (1986) A comparison of parenteral nutrition and early postoperative enteral feeding on the nitrogen balance after major surgery. Surgery 100:21–24
7. Hershman MJ, Cheadle WG, Kuftinec D, Polk HC Jr, George CD (1988) An outcome predictive score for sepsis and death following trauma. Injury 19: 263–266
8. Liebermann MD, Shou J, Torres AS et al. (1990) Effects of nutrient substrates on immune function. Nutrition 6:88–91
9. Polk HC J, George CD, Wellhausen SR et al. (1986) A systematic study of host defense processes in badly injured patients Ann Surg 204:282–299

Mild Surgery-Induced Changes in Human Peripheral Blood Lymphocytes

E. Bresciano, D. Mancino, M.L. Vuotto, P. Gazzerro, M.T. Ielpo, V. Mazzoccoli, M. Mosti, and A. Barbarisi

Surgery, though purposeful, induces a stress that greatly affects organism homeostasis. This in turn induces an impairment of immune specific and nonspecific mechanisms of defense that, despite advances in patient care, still are very often responsible for death [1]. A great deal of research is therefore directed toward monitoring surgical subjects [2–5].

Surgery-induced immune modifications have been studied for some time. It is common knowledge that surgery is immunosuppressive, but findings are partially conflicting, chiefly because of the variability of parameters under study [6]. In fact, together with the nonsurgical workup, such as immunological profile, postoperative monitoring times, and different study approaches, one must take into account those parameters strictly linked to surgery: duration, anesthesia, antibiotic prophylaxis, transfusions, and, above all, degree. Our field of research is mild elective surgery. In other investigations we analyzed, both in vivo and in vitro, cell-mediated immunity through phenotypic and functional changes of the T compartment in a limited sample of patients. We found transitory immunodepression in the postoperative period.

Here we confirm the previous data, comparing them with findings from a larger sample of patients. We also studied possible phenotypic changes in B cells under the same experimental conditions. Our aim was to gather information that may be useful for surgical planning and follow-up.

Materials and Methods

Population

Forty-five surgical patients (mean age 43 years) constitute the sample of the present work. Subjects with proven immunodepression, recent blood transfusions, or use of steroids, cyclo-oxygenase inhibitors, or immunomodulating drugs and narcotics in the 6 months prior to the study were not included. Splenectomy, jaundice, recurrent or local infections, malnutrition, diabetes mellitus, neoplasia, and liver, renal, and endocrine diseases constituted further reasons for exclusion. All subjects were also screened for anti-HIV antibodies. Each patient underwent elective clean or clean-contaminated surgery without rising above an ASA index of 2. Mild surgery, performed by the same team, using standardized mix balanced general anesthesia lasted no more than 120 min. Blood loss was held below 500 ml. None of the patients were transfused and all were placed on the same antibiotic prophylaxis regimen.

PBMC Phenotype Analysis

Heparinized whole blood samples were drawn before surgery (PreO) and on the second (PO2) and seventh (PO7) postoperative days. A complete blood count was taken. The samples were labeled for 15 min at room temperature with monoclonal antibodies (Becton Dickinson, Mountain View, Calif., USA) recognizing specific markers on T (CD3, CD4, CD8, HLA-Dr, CD25, CD71) and B (CD19) lymphocytes. Erythrocytes were then lysed by incubation in the presence of a commercial FACS lysing solution. The labeled cells were assayed by flow cytofluorimetry (FACScan, Becton Dickinson).

Statistical analysis

Student's *t* test was used for statistical analysis of results.

Results

Pre O blood counts were within the reference range. On PO2 they indicated transitory leukocytosis coupled with lymphopenia. All values tended to return to normal on PO7.

Flow cytometric analysis revealed a significant impairment in the percentage of classic T-cell phenotypic markers (CD3, CD4, CD8) expressing lymphocytes on PO2. On PO7 the values fell back to baseline. The B-lymphocyte compartment showed no significant phenotypic changes during the whole test period (Fig. 1).

The number of activation markers (HLA-Dr, CD25, CD71) expressing lymphocytes did not change remarkably on PO2. All increased on PO7, but the change was significant only in the case of CD71 (Fig. 2).

Conclusions

These results confirm previous findings where we suggested that, under our experimental conditions, there is a selective involvement of the T-compartment. Phenotypic changes seem to predominate over functional ones that, in addition, appear later. The B-compartment does not seem to be involved.

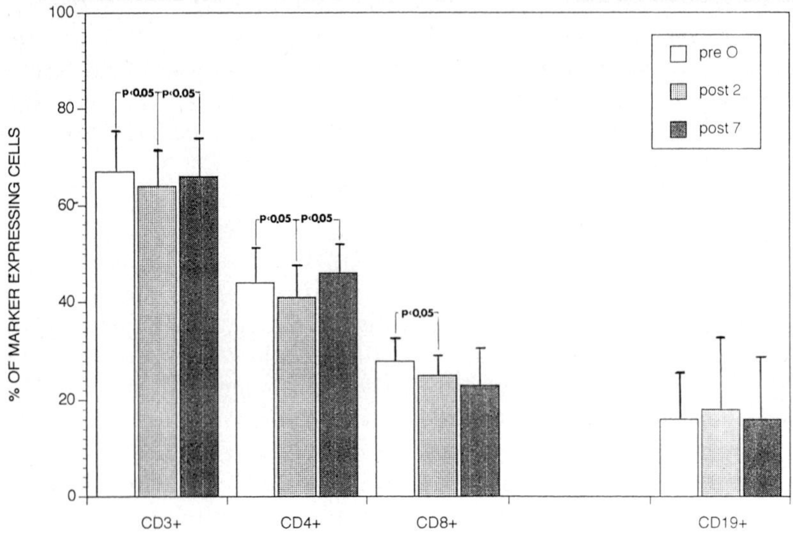

Fig. 1. Percentages of peripheral blood lymphocyte phenotypic markers in elective mild surgery-managed patients before surgery and on the 2nd and 7th postoperative days

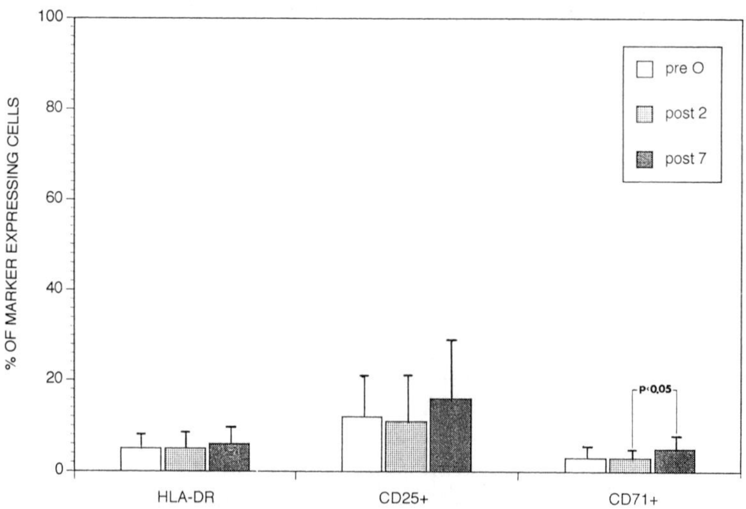

Fig. 2. Percentages of peripheral blood lymphocyte activation markers in elective mild surgery-managed patients before surgery and on the 2nd and 7th postoperative days

The degree of surgery can influence postoperative immune behavior. After elective mild surgery, in fact, there is a rapid recovery of immunocompetence, as demonstrated by the 7-day follow-up. This could be linked to a favorable postoperative outcome and constitutes an important diagnostic parameter in postsurgical care. The clinical evolution of our patients who failed to show signs of sepsis supports this.

References

1. Mannick JA (1993) Trauma, sepsis, and immune defects. In: Faist E, Meakins JL, Schildberg FW (eds) Host defense dysfunction in trauma, shock and sepsis. Springer, Berlin Heidelberg New York
2. Baue AE (1993) Progress in trauma care through understanding the cell biology of injury. In: Faist E, Meakins JL, Schildberg FW (eds) Host defense dysfunction in trauma, shock and sepsis. Springer, Berlin Heidelberg New York
3. Maldonado MD, Venturoli A, Franco A, Nunez-Roldan A (1991) Specific changes in peripheral blood lymphocyte phenotype from burn patients. Probable origin of the thermal injury-related lymphocytopenia. Burns 17(3):188–192
4. Spagnoli GC, Heberer M, Vogelbach P, Rosso R, Jorgensen J, Harder F (1993) Phenotypic and functional characteristics of peripheral blood lymphocytes in a defined group of polytrauma patients. In: Faist E, Meakins JL, Schildberg FW (eds) Host defense dysfunction in trauma, shock and sepsis. Springer, Berlin Heidelberg New York
5. Volk HD, Thieme M, Ruppe U, Heym S, Docke D, Manger D, Zuckermann S, Golosubow A, Nieter B, Klug H, van Baehr R (1993) Alterations in function and phenotype of monocytes from patients with septic disease: predictive value and new therapeutic strategies. In: Faist E, Meakins JL, Schildberg FW (eds) Host defense dysfunction in trauma, shock and sepsis. Springer, Berlin Heidelberg New York
6. Meakins JL (1993) Clinical factors influencing host defense integrity. In: Faist E, Meakins JL, Schildberg FW (eds) Host defense dysfunction in trauma, shock and sepsis. Springer, Berlin Heidelberg New York

Cell Activation (2)

Tissue Perfusion and Oxygenation Related to Wound Healing and Resistance to Infection

F. Gottrup

Perioperative mortality has not changed significantly in the last 20–30 years in spite of advances in the observation and treatment of patients in intensive care units [1]. Among patients undergoing different types of surgery, the overall mortality has been reported to be three times higher than normal in patients treated in intensive care units postoperatively [2]. Sixty percent of these patients died from sepsis with multiple organ failure. Although different types of advanced monitoring systems have been introduced, the overall mortality remains unchanged. One of the fundamental reasons for this is that available methods of hemodynamic monitoring all assess the central hemodynamic situation, whereas little is known of the extent to which requirements of peripheral cells are fulfilled. In order to improve morbidity and mortality, both central and peripheral perfusion and oxygenation are necessary, being essential to the optimal function of both central and peripheral cells.

The fundamental change after tissue injury is destruction of the nutritional supply to tissue and development of local hypoxia [3–6]. Inadequate tissue perfusion and oxygenation has been found to be the most important determinant of wound healing and resistance to infection following injury. Tissue oxygenation is vital for the metabolic processes of the cells, because 95% of the body energy is generalized by aerobic processes. An anaerobic metabolism is much less economic and can maintain cell function for only a short period. Thc delivery of an adequate volume of oxygen at a sufficient partial pressure for cell metabolism therefore is critical for the normal function of cells and tissues. Oxygen tension in tissue affects both wound healing and resistance to infection [7].

Collagen accumulation in healing wounds has been found to be a direct function of arterial oxygen tension over a certain physiological range [8]. Oxygen tension of approximately 20 mmHg has been shown to be a crucial level beneath which accumulation of collagen is definitely impaired [9, 10]. This is primarily based on the function of enzymes important for wound healing and development of infection. Collagen synthesis is dependent on the enzyme propyl hydroxylase with a K_m (concentration of substrate at which the rate of reaction is 50% of maximum) of approximately 20 mmHg O_2 [11] and a W_{max} (maximum rate or velocity of reaction) of 50–100 mmHg O_2. More recently these figures have been suggested to be even higher [12].

Other enzymes important for cross-linking and development of strength of the wound have similar K_m's for oxygen at more than 20 mmHg, and if oxygen tension in tissues falls below 40 mmHg the maximal function rate starts to fall. Furthermore the synthesis of collagen seems to be limited if collagen-producing fibroblasts exist in an extracellular environment in which oxygen tension is less than 50 mmHg but clinically this will probably not be seen before the range of 20–30 mmHg [13]. Above this level of tissue oxygen tension there will be sufficient deposition and cross-linking of collagen, this process being directly related to the development of biomechanical strength of all surgical wounds [14].

Adequate tissue perfusion and oxygenation is also the most important determinant of *resistance to infection* following tissue injury such as that due to surgery. This is obvious from our knowledge of healing of wounds of the face and anus. In spite of massive contamination of the latter, both types of wounds nearly always heal without infection if the patient has normal function of the immune system. The difference between these types of wound and other wounds is not due to improved local immunity but rather to an increased perfusion and oxygenation. The improved resistance to infection with increased oxygen tension is provided through an improved leukocyte function. When leukocytes ingest bacteria, an oxidase in the phagosomal membrane is activated and converts dissolved molecular oxygen to superoxide radicals [15, 16]. Together with other radicals, superoxides account for about half the capacity of granulocytes to kill *Staphylococcus aureus*. The rate of superoxide production in leukocytes depends on oxygen tension, and bactericidal activity of human leukocytes begins to fail as oxygen tension falls below about 30–40 mmHg. This has been demonstrated in experimental studies in flaps after injection of bacteria [6, 17, 18]. Invasive infections were only found in flap areas in which the oxygen tension was less than 40 mmHg. With raised oxygen tension in inspired gas the infection rate decreased and correlated with the tissue oxygen tension but not with the oxygen-carrying capacity.

Perfusion and Oxygenation in Tissues

The metabolic needs of the cell, especially related to oxygen, depend on peripheral tissue perfusion, which again is influenced by the function of the lungs and cardiovascular regulatory mechanisms. The oxygen delivery depends on the amount of oxygen delivered and exchanged in the lungs, the flow of blood to and in the tissue, and the capacity of blood to carry oxygen. The second important factor for tissue oxygenation is the oxygen diffusion capacity in the tissue itself. Finally, the rate of oxygen consumption in tissue is important for optimal cell function. A sensitive control system and external factors influence this system. In response to hemorrhage this system maintains blood flow to vital organs such as the heart and brain while most other tissues have a decrease in blood flow [7].

Exchange between the microcirculation and interstitial fluid occurs by *diffusion and filtration* across the microvascular walls. Respiratory gasses (O_2-CO_2) move between the systemic capillary blood and their cells by diffusion. Oxygen diffuses from a higher concentration in the bloodstream into the interstitial fluid while carbon-dioxide has the opposite concentration relation and diffuses from cell environments to blood, but about 20 times faster than oxygen through tissue. For this reason elimination of carbon-dioxide is much less of a problem than oxygen delivery. As oxygen diffuses away from the capillary it is consumed by the tissue and the oxygen tension falls. Diffusion distances vary therefore directly with the oxygen tension along the length of the capillary. In the venous end of the capillary minor changes in blood oxygen tension may provide an anoxic region in the intercapillary area, and the oxygen partial pressure may be as low as 1–2 mmHg in cerebral cortex [19]. Hyperbaric treatment of 3 atmospheres absolute pressure (ata) will increase the diffusion distance by twofold at the venous and by fourfold at the arterial end of the capillary. This increase in oxygen diffusion distance may be especially important in tissues compromised by infection or local injury. With regard to direct evaluation of tissue oxygenation, measurements of tissue oxygen tension in a representative area of peripheral tissue have been shown to be a valuable measure of the status of oxygenation in peripheral tissue.

The distribution of blood flow in the presence of a pathological condition may be altered between different types of organs. Local metabolism will change the distribution of blood according to the metabolic needs of the different types of tissues. Some tissues, e.g., muscle, have the capacity to increase the number of active capillaries while others, e.g., subcutis and the gastrointestinal tract, do not. Their perfusion is primarily regulated by autonomic nerve reflexes. In the gastrointestinal tract the mucosa, furthermore, has been found to be one of the most sensitive areas in the gut during impaired tissue perfusion in the critically ill [20]. The tissue pH is constant related to oxygen delivery until a critical point where oxygen delivery equals oxygen requirement. Below this point the pH in the mucosa falls in parallel with the further decrease in oxygen delivery and the corresponding fall in oxygen consumption. Thus it seems reasonable to direct monitoring systems toward the subcutis and the mucosa of the gastrointestinal tract because they may give an early warning of tissue hyperperfusion and hypoxia.

Clinical Relevance of Tissue Perfusion and Oxygenation

After tissue injury such as that caused by surgery, local hypoxia due to vascular damage develops rapidly, and in this relative absence of oxygen the wound repair process and resistance to infection may be impaired. For this reason detection of poor tissue perfusion, and especially tissue oxygenation, is crucial in postoperative care. Monitoring systems evaluating the adequacy of central hemodynamics are routinely used. Prevention of tissue ischemia secondary to flow-limited oxygen delivery has been the rationale for hemodynamic monitoring in the intensive care unit [21]. Routine measurements of hemodynamic variables such as systemic blood pressure, heart rate, pulmonary artery pressure, cardiac output, and mixed venous blood oxygenation have been used. To make the measurements, both noninvasive and invasive devices have been used. These measurements, however, assess the central hemodynamic situation and little is known of the extent to which the peripheral tissue oxygenation fulfils the demand for oxygen in the peripheral tissue, which may be of particular importance in surgery. Evaluation of perfusion has, for most surgeons, primarily been based on assessment of parameters such as skin temperature, urine output, blood pressure, and pulse. Assurance of sufficient tissue perfusion is, however, a far more complex process which has been shown to be weakly related to the aforementioned parameters. In the case of nonoptimally functioning hemostatic mechanisms the surgical patient therefore may be underperfused postoperatively and have decreased tissue oxygenation in the area of wounded tissue. Consequently, healing and resistance to infection may be impaired.

The term *tissue perfusion* has been likened to blood flow, oxygen delivery, or a combined concept of flow and nutritional supply including oxygen. It has been used with reference to the functional and circulatory status of the tissue but no clear definition has been proposed. If the patient was "well perfused," tissue function has generally been accepted as good and undisturbed. It would therefore be useful to have a parameter that would permit monitoring of both tissue perfusion and tissue oxygenation as a "mirror" of sufficient nutrition in order to provide optimal cell function. Such a concept could be called *tissue oxygen perfusion* [7]. This concept would be a measure of the ability of the central cardiovascular mechanisms to deliver a volume of oxygen to the peripheral tissue that is adequate to meet metabolic demands. This general concept combines oxygen delivery, tissue oxygen transport, and tissular oxygen consumption (Table 1). The concept has to be defined for each type of pathological condition but allows us to evaluate the applicability of the presently used monitoring systems for tissue oxygenation. This concept could be a useful tool for clinicians to describe the general oxygenation of tissues or organs.

The best means of assessing the adequacy of tissue oxygenation and perfusion is to evaluate the situation at the *local tissue level*. Simultaneous monitoring of tissue perfusion and oxygenation in all organ systems would be ideal, because not all organs or even all parts of the same organ are similarly oxygenated at the same time. It can then be a question of whether one single measurement in one single tissue can give an idea of the situation in all tissues of the body. If information on general tissue perfusion and

Table 1. Main determinants of tissue oxygen perfusion

I. *Oxygen delivery to tissue*
Oxygen in arterial blood
Delivery of arterial blood to tissues
Microcirculation
Oxygen from blood to tissue
II. *Oxygen transport in tissue*
Diffusion distance
Oxygen partial pressure
III. *Oxygen consumption of tissue*
Activation status of cells
Hormones
Temperature of tissue
Drugs

oxygenation is, however, wanted, we need to find at least an "essential" tissue in which perfusion is the first to be sacrificed during change in oxygen delivery and consumption and the last to be restored. At the same time these tissues should be easily available for monitoring. This means a "surface" would be preferable. Subcutis and mucosa in the gastrointestinal tract are, as earlier described, such tissues. Both types of tissue have been shown to be among the first to be affected in different types of shock and provide an indirect measure of the adequacy of tissue perfusion and oxygenation in the whole body. Many different monitoring systems are presently available (Table 2). However, only two of these allow assessment of the tissue oxygen perfusion and fulfil the criteria of the ideal monitoring system. These two monitoring systems are measurements of the tissue oxygen tension and of intramural pH in the gastrointestinal tract.

Monitoring of Tissue Perfusion and Oxygenation

The cell has a *critical oxygen partial pressure* below which the enzymes in the cell do not function optimally. In order to judge oxygen supply to an organ tissue the cellular oxygen partial pressure is important [19]. As the cell wall has no diffusion barrier against oxygen, the interstitial fluid close to the cell has a partial pressure similar to that inside the cell. Measuring tissue oxygen tension in the interstitial fluid therefore is the most important parameter for evaluating oxygen perfusion in the tissue. Measuring tissue oxygen tension in subcutaneous tissue has been found to be a mirror of perfusion in other peripheral tissues [16]. Changes in blood flow of bone, skin, spleen, pancreas, and bowel parallel changes in the tissue oxygen tension in subcutis during hemorrhage. Oxygen tension in subcutis has been reported to be dependent on both cardiac output and tissue perfusion in normovolemia and hypovolemia, and from a physiological point of view, oxygen delivery/

Table 2. Techniques presently available for evaluation of tissue oxygen perfusion

1. Laser Doppler velocimetry
2. Postcapillary venous pressure measurements
3. Skin temperature measurements
4. Vital capillary microscopy
5. Pulse oximetry
6. Intramural pH measurements in stomach and colon
7. Tissue oxygen tension measurements
8. Other methods (nuclear magnetic spectroscopy, infrared techniques for measuring the functional status of cytochrome a_3)

oxygen consumption has been found to be of greater clinical interest than cardiac output alone [22]. Recent work has shown that oxygen tension measurements in subcutaneous tissue are an important parameter for observation of tissue perfusion experimentally as well as in surgical patients [7, 18, 23–28]. During cardiovascular surgery and extracorporeal circulation, oxygen tension in subcutis falls and stays low for 3–4 h, and a distinction between supply/demand ratio and tissue oxygen tension seems to occur [25, 29]. A relationship between oxygen tension in subcutis and infectious and lethal complications after colorectal surgery has been suggested in recent work [30, 31]. These studies show that tissue oxygen tension measurements represent a measure of tissue oxygen perfusion. The measurements provide clinician with an early warning of a decrease in oxygen delivery to the tissue, probably before tissue acidosis and tissue damage have developed. The usability of this parameter, however, in critically ill patients with multiple organ failure remains to be investigated.

Measurements of tissue oxygen tension can be performed using different types of monitoring systems [32]. Such measurements have not yet become routine because of methodological problems which have prevented the technique from being used daily at the bedside. Recent developments have, however, made the method almost atraumatic, reliable, and constant. Continuous measurement of peripheral tissue oxygen tension may therefore be employed routinely in the near future. Single device sensors as shown in Fig. 1A are presently being developed specifically for measurements directly in the tissue. A sensor for peroperative trans-serosal measurements is shown in Fig. 1B. Further information can be found in surveys on this topic [7, 32].

A measuring system for evaluating *pH in the gastrointestinal mucosa* during splanchnic ischemia and multiorgan failure has recently been described [20, 33]. Underlying this monitoring system is the finding that the splanchnic circulation seems to be very consistently affected by endogenous vasoconstrictors when they are released during hemorrhage, cardiac failure, or sepsis. This vasoconstriction cause visual ischemia and inadequate mu-

A

B

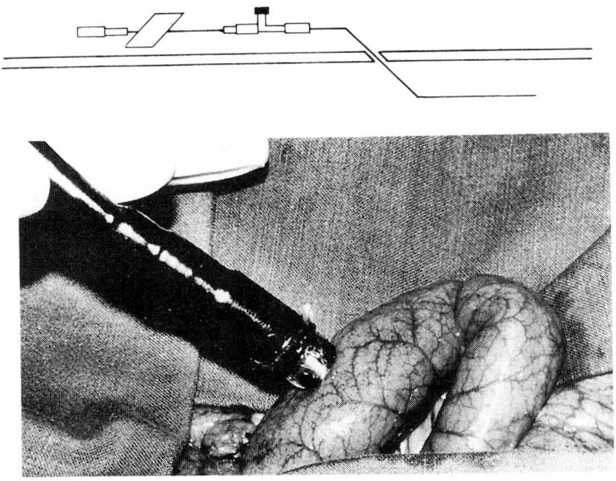

Fig. 1A,B. Tissue oxygen tension measurements. **A** Schematic drawing of a single device oxygen sensor placed directly in the tissue (e.g., subcutaneous tissue). The principles for clinically used sensors are most often based on polarographic or optical fluorescence techniques. The diameter of the sensor is 0.5–0.7 mm. **B** Sensor for surface measurements in the abdominal cavity during surgery (e.g., trans-serosal measurement of the bowel). (Modified from [7])

cosal oxygenation, leading to acidoses in the tissue and a falling pH. Recording a normal pH in mucosa indicates that oxygenation exceeds the critical values associated with tissue hypoxia. Low values can be caused by reduction of oxygen delivery and/or utilization in relation to need. The gut is selectively impaired in shock and one of the first organs to be affected in compensated shock. Recent studies have indicated that measurement of mucosal pH (pHi) may be a guide during resuscitation and help to improve outcome by allowing prevention of splanchnic organ hypoxia and development of systemic oxygen deficit and tissue acidosis [34]. Presently pHi is measured in the stomach or in the bowel using a catheter with a gas-permeable balloon (Fig. 2). The advantage of this method is that it is noninvasive, relatively simple, and reliable when correctly applied. The disadvantage of the method is that it does not provide continuous assessment and changes in pHi may take time to develop. This implies that the technique cannot be used for constant monitoring of rapid changes which may follow hemorrhage, for example. Furthermore, this method has been reported to be less sensitive for evaluation of non-critically ill elective surgical patients [35]. This monitoring system is, however, the only practical method available for monitoring visceral perfusion in clinical practice and fulfils the requirement of measurements of both tissue perfusion and oxygenation.

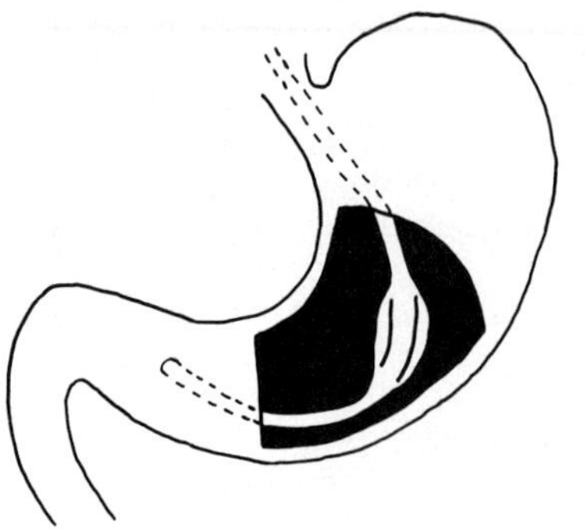

Fig. 2. PH measurements in gastrointestinal mucosa. Schematic drawing of pH measurement in gastric mucosa using a gas-permeable balloon. (Modified from [7])

Conclusion

Assuring the delivery of adequate oxygen to meet the metabolic demands for wound healing and resistance to infection requires monitoring systems to assess both perfusion and oxygenation in the tissue. Measurements of *tissue oxygen tension* provide the clinician with a continuous measure of changes in oxygen delivery and tissue perfusion, while measurements of the *mucosal pH* provide an intermittent evaluation of the total metabolic situation in the patient. Combinations of these types of measurements presently seem to be the best monitoring systems for the evaluation of tissue perfusion and oxygenation. These methods are complementary because measurements of oxygen tension in subcutis will give an early warning of a decrease in oxygen delivery to the tissue while pH measurements in the gastrointestinal mucosa will provide the clinician with the metabolic end point. This allows treatment which can improve the outcome in critically ill patients, in particular. Monitoring of tissue oxygen tension and intermucosal pH may in the future be of fundamental value in predicting wound healing and development of wound infection after tissue injury.

References

1. Ahnefeld FW, Heinrich H (1983) Hat sich in der Routine des Anästhesisten die Berücksichtigung von Risikofaktoren bewährt? Langenbecks Arch Chir 361:263–267
2. Mayr O, Hannemann L (1989) Preoperative assessment and monitoring of high-risk patients: In: Reinhart K, Eyrich R (eds) Clinical aspects of O_2 transport and tissue oxygenation. Springer, Berlin Heidelberg New York, pp 151–161
3. Hunt TK, Twomey P, Zederfeldt B (1967) Respiratory gas tensions in healing wounds. Am J Surg 114:302–307
4. Silver IA (1969) The measurement of oxygen tension in healing tissue. 3:124–135
5. Niinikoski J, Heughan C, Hunt TK (1972) Oxygen tension in human wounds. J Surg Res 12:77–82

6. Gottrup F, Firmin R, Hunt TK, Mathes S (1984) The dynamic properties of tissue oxygen in healing flaps. Surgery 95:527–537
7. Gottrup F (1992) Measurement and evaluation of tissue perfusion in surgery (to optimize wound healing and resistance to infection. In: Leaper DJL, Branicki FJ (eds) International surgical practice. Oxford University Press, Oxford, pp 15–39
8. Hunt TK, Pai MP (1972) Effect of varying ambient oxygen tensions on wound metabolism and collagen synthesis. Surg Gynecol Obstet 135:561–567
9. Silver IA (1980) The physiology of wound healing. In: Hunt TK (ed) Wound healing and wound infection: theory and surgical practice. Appleton-Century-Crofts, New York, pp 11–31
10. Niinikoski J (1980) The effect of blood and oxygen supply on the biochemistry of repair. In: Hunt TK (ed) Wound healing and wound infection: theory and surgical practice. Appleton-Century-Crofts, New York, pp. 56–71
11. Myllyla R, Tuderman L, Kivirikko KI (1977) Mechanism of the prolyl hydroxylase reaction. II. Kinetic analyses of the reaction sequence. Eur J Biochem 80:349–357
12. De Jong L, Kemp A (1984) Stoichiometry and kinetics of the prolyl 4-hydoxylase partial resection. Biochim Biophys Acta 787:105–111
13. Niinikoski J, Gottrup F, Hunt TK (1991) The role of oxygen in wound repair. In: Janssen H, Rooman R, Robertson JIS (eds) Wound healing. Wrightson, Petersfield, pp 165–174
14. Viidik A, Gottrup F (1986) Mechanics of healing soft tissue wounds. In: Schmid-Schönbein GW, Woo SLY, Zweifach BW (eds) Frontiers in biomechanics. Springer, Berlin Heidelberg New York, pp 263–279
15. Hunt TK, Rabkin J, Jensen JA, Jonsson K, Goodson WH (1987) Tissue oximetry: an interim report. World J Surg 11:126–132
16. Hunt TK, Halliday BJ, Hopf HW, Scheuenstuhl H (1991) Measurement and control of tissue oxygen tension in surgical patients. In: Gutierrez G, Vincent JL (eds) Tissue oxygen utilization. Springer, Berlin Heidelberg New York, pp 337–349 (Update in intensive care and emergency medicine, vol 12)
17. Gottrup F, Orredsson S, Price DC, Mathes SJ, Hohn DC (1984) A comparative study of skin blood flow in musculocutaneous and random pattern flaps. J Surg Res 37:443–447
18. Jonsson K, Hunt TK, Mathes SJ (1988) Oxygen as an isolated variable influences resistance to infection. Ann Surg 208:783–787
19. Grote J (1989) Tissue respiration. In: Smidt RF, Thews G (eds) Human physiology. Springer, Berlin Heidelberg New York, pp 598–612
20. Fiddian-Green RG (1989) Studics in splanchnic ischemia and multiple organ failure. In: Marston A, Bulkley GB, Fiddian-Green RP, Haglund U (eds) Splanchnic ischemia and multiple organ failure. Arnold, London, pp 349–363
21. Fink MP (1989) Clinical care in the ICU: hemodynamic considerations in the management of the critically ill. In: Marston A, Bulkley GB, Fiddian-Green RG, Haglund U (eds) Splancnic ischemia and multiple organ failure. Arnold, London, pp 365–375
22. Reinhart K (1989) Monitoring O_2 transport and tissue oxygenation in critically ill patients. In: Reinhart K, Eyrich K (eds) Clinical aspects of O_2 transport and tissue oxygenation. Springer, Berlin Heidelberg New York, pp. 195–211
23. Chang N, Goodson WH, Gottrup F, Hunt TK (1983) Direct measurement of wound and tissue oxygen tension in postoperative patients. Ann Surg 197: 470–478
24. Gottrup F, Firmin F, Rabkin J, Halliday BJ, Hunt TK (1987) Directly measured tissue oxygen tension and arterial tension assess tissue perfusion. Crit Care Med 15:1030–1036

25. Kuttila K (1989) Tissue perfusion and oxygenation in cardiac surgery. Scand J Thorac Cardiovasc Surg Suppl 38
26. Hjortdal VE, Awwad A, Gottrup F, Kirkegaard L, Gellett S (1990) Tissue oxygen tension measurement for monitoring musculocutaneous and cutaneous flaps. Scand J Plast Reconstr Hand Surg 24:27–30
27. Hartmann M (1992) Tissue perfusion and oxygenation in relation to wound healing. Experimental and clinical studies. Thesis, University of Lund
28. Kallehave F, Hovendal CPH, Gottrup F (1992) Surface tissue oxygen tension in assessment of local perfusion in colonic interposition in infants. Surg Res Commun 13:239–243
29. Gellett S, Asmussen J, Gottrup F (1990) Measurement of oxygen in patients during extra-corporeal circulation. J Int Care Med 16 Suppl 1:98
30. Göte H, Raahave D, Bæch J (1989) Tissue oximetry as a possible predictor of lethal complications after emergency intestinal surgery. Surg Res Commun 7:243–249
31. Gys T, Van Esbroeck G, Hubens A (1991) Assessment of the perfusion in peripheral tissue beds by subcutaneous oximetry and gastric intramucosal pH-metry in elective colorectal surgery. J Int Care Med 17:78–82
32. Gottrup F (1991) Tissue oxygen tension monitoring: relation to hemodynamic and oxygen transport variables. In: Gutierrez G, Vincent JL (eds) Tissue oxygen utilization. Springer, Berlin Heidelberg New York, pp 322–336 (Update in intensive care and emergency medicine, vol 12)
33. Montgomery A (1991) Intramucosal pH of the gut. A measure of splanchnic ischemia. Thesis, University of Lund
34. Fiddian-Green RG (1993) Intramucosal pH: what, how, whom, when and where? In: Vincent J-L (ed) Yearbook of intensive care and emergency medicine. Springer, Berlin Heidelberg New York, pp 258–269
35. Van Esbroeck G, Gys T, Hubens A (1992) Evaluation of tissue oximetry in perioperative monitoring of colorectal surgery. Br J Surg 79:584–587

Cell Cycle Progression and Signal Transduction in Normal and IgM Transgenic B Cells

U. CHEN, D. THORPE, H. MOK, M. KUHN, and R.G. ROEDER

The questions we have been trying to address are really very simple: Do resting B cells respond to antireceptor antibodies? Do such antibodies mimic the antigens that would normally stimulate these cells? Although there is no reason to believe that different antireceptor antibodies behave differently, the one we actually use is almost always anti-μ heavy chain.

Two-Parameter Cell Cycle Assay

To study the cell cycle after stimulation, we need an assay. In the past few years, we have adopted a two-parameter and a three-parameter assay to study the B cell cycle in normal [1–4] as well as IgM-transgenic (Chen, submitted) mice. The two-parameter assay involves labelling cells with BrdU in culture for certain lengths of time, harvesting, treating the cells with NP-40 to permit the entrance of dyes, labelling the nuclei with two fluorescence dyes, and then analyzing them with flow cytometry.

Both dyes stain DNA. Hoechst 33258 binds to thymidine. Whenever thymidine is replaced by BrdU during DNA synthesis, the Hoechst fluorescence is quenched. So the more BrdU incorporation, the less Hoechst fluorescence. This is shown on the x-axis. Ethidium bromide fluoresce is *not* quenched by BrdU. Thus, the intensity of fluorescence, plotted on the y-axis, reflects the DNA content, which varies regularly throughout the cell cycle.

Combining these two fluorescence parameters, we can trace cells in any specific compartment: the G_0/G_1, S, G_2 of the first cycle; then, G_1, S, G_1 of the second cycle, and then, G_1, S, G_2 of the third cycle. We can even trace cells into the fourth cycle. With the help of a computer program written by Peter Rabinovitch, we can calculate how many cells are in each compartment at any time [1, 2, 4].

While the measurement of cell cycle pattern was an established technique, we had to define tissue culture conditions for incorporation of BrdU into primary mouse B cells. This took a long time. We shall not present the details of development of the methods here; rather we shall describe some results with primary mouse B cells [1–4].

Activation of Normal B Cells Via Receptors

When small, dense, resting B cells are freshly isolated from animals, they give a pattern like the one shown in Fig. 1A. The cells are in the resting stage, the so-called G_0/G compartment. Note that essentially all of the cells are in this cluster – that is, they are synchronized. When these B cells are

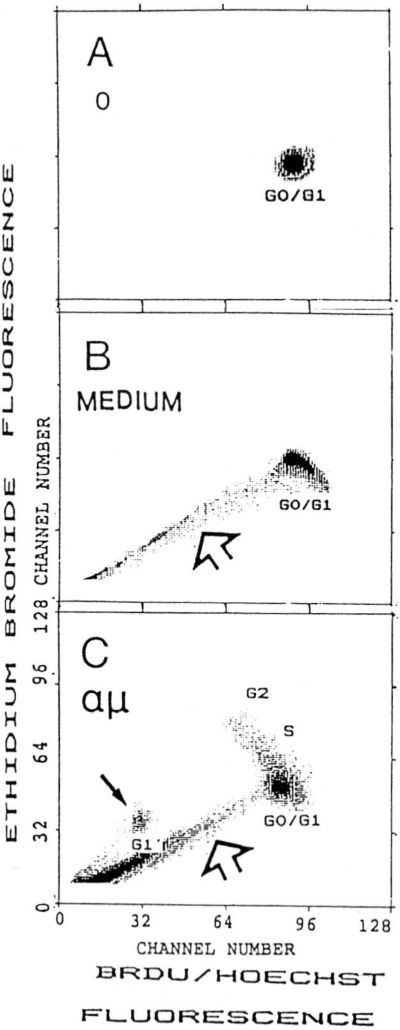

Fig. 1A–C. BrdU/Hoechst 33258 fluorescence (*abscissa*) and ethidium bromide fluorescence (*ordinate*) of small, resting B cells from normal *nu/nu* mice analyzed at 60 h after stimulation. Each scale is linear and arbitrary (channel numbers). G_1', S', G_2' are the G_1, S, G_2 compartments of the second cycle. **A** No stimulation, measured at 0 h; **B** medium, **C** aμ, anti-μ; *open arrow* denotes apoptotic cells kept in "medium" for a few days, many of them never leave G_0/G_1. But some of them go into the "nuclear degradation" compartment, which most immunologists like to call "apoptosis" (open arrow in Fig. 1B). We can stimulate B cells with various reagents. Anti-μ (Fig. 1C) stimulates 30%–40% of the cells through the cycle, that is, through S and G_2 of the first cycle, and some reach the G_1 of the second cycle (solid arrow in Fig. 1C). No cells move further than G_1 of the second cycle during the time they are cultured. Note that the cycling B cells are no longer synchronized. Again, many cells are in the apoptotic compartment (open arrow in Fig. 1C).

Activation of Transgenic B Cells Via Receptors

Stimulated, transgenic B cells can also remain in the G_0/G_1, enter the apoptosis compartment, or enter the cycling compartments. Anti-μ stimulates a small percentage of the transgenic B cells to enter the cell cycle (6.1%, Fig. 2C); they go through S and G_2 of the first cycle and are arrested at G_1 of the second cycle. Antigen stimulates even fewer transgenic B cells to enter the cell cycle (2.7%, Fig. 2D): Some go through S and G_2 of the first cycle, and are arrested at G_1 of the second cycle, just like the anti-μ stimulated cells, but some go through S and G_2 of the second cycle and reach G_1 of the third cycle. Note that many IgM-transgenic B cells remain at G_0/G_1 although they are neither dead nor degraded.

Figure 3 summarizes the data discussed so far. When small, dense, resting, B cells are activated by either anti-μ or antigen, they can remain unaffected (G_0/G_1), they can die by apoptosis, or they can enter the cell cycle. There are, however, clear differences between anti-μ and antigen stimulation. Upon anti-μ stimulation, B cells cycle once and give rise to two daughter cells. This is the same for normal B cells and transgenic B cells. Upon antigen stimulation, transgenic B cells cycle twice and give rise to four granddaughter cells. It is impossible to stimulate normal B cells with antigen due to the extremely low frequency of antigen-specific normal B cells.

Other Differences Between Normal and Transgenic B Cells

There are several other differences between normal and transgenic B cells of which we shall mention only one. When normal B cells are stimulated by anti-μ+LPS, 90%–95% of B cells enter the cycle. This is synergy; that is, the effect of the two together is more than the sum of each [1]. Transgenic B cells respond very differently. When transgenic B cells are stimulated by anti-μ+LPS, anti-μ actually *inhibits* the proliferative action of LPS (Chen, submitted).

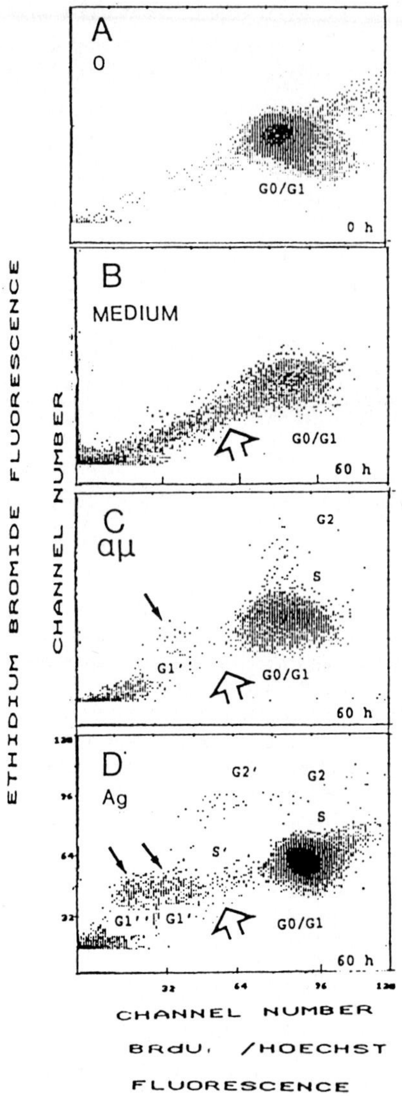

Fig. 2A–D. BrdU/Hoechst 33258 fluorescence (*abscissa*, linear scale) and ethidium bromide fluorescence (*ordinate*, linear scale) of small, resting B cells from PC-specific transgenic mice, analyzed at 60 h after stimulation. Each scale is linear and arbitrary (channel numbers). *Solid arrows* point to cells in the G_1 phase of the second (*G1'*) and third (*G1''*) cell cycle. **A** No stimulation, measured at 0 h; **B** no stimulation, after 60 h of culture in medium; **C** anti-μ; **D** antigen. *Open arrow* denotes apoptotic cells

Calcium Influx Assay and PI Assay

We have also studied calcium influx after stimulation with anti-μ and antigen. While normal B cells respond to anti-μ with an influx of calcium (Fig. 4A), this is not the case with all the other reagents tested so far, including LPS and NIP-Ficoll (Fig. 4B,C). Transgenic B cells respond similarly. There is a calcium influx *only* when they are stimulated with anti-μ (Fig. 4D,G).

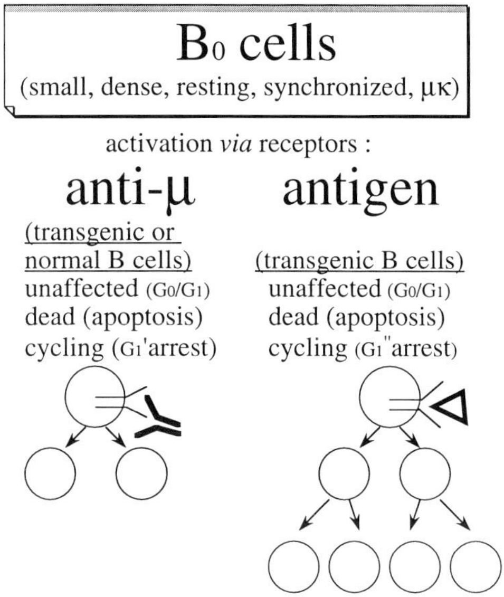

Fig. 3. The interpretation of the data from Figs. 1 and 2. Small, dense, resting, synchronized B cells from either normal C57B16 *nu/nu* mice or anti-PC *μ*k transgenic mice are activated via receptors. The stimulation with antireceptor activators leads normal as well as transgenic B cells to three states: no touch (remain at G_0/G_1), death (apoptosis), or cycling. With anti-*μ* (thick fork-like symbol) stimulation, cells divide once and arrest at the G_1 phase (G_1') of the first cycle for both normal and transgenic B cells, while antigen (*thick triangle*) breaks this arrest. Some transgenic B cells divide twice and reach the G_1 phase of second cycle (G_1'')

The surprise is that when antigen was used, it did not stimulate a calcium influx. This observation was made with anti-PC-transgenic B cells from Storb et al. [5] (Fig. 4E,F) and NIP-transgenic B cells from David Baltimore (data not shown). With TNP-transgenic B cells from George Köhler [6], the results were ambiguous. TNP-OVA (Fig. 4H) did not cause a calcium influx, while TNP-Ficoll (FIg. 4I) had some effect.

Kenny et al. measured the PI rather than calcium influx with anti-PC-transgenic B cells [7] (personal communication). They found that although anti-*μ* and LPS are capable of stimulating B cells in this assay, antigen has no effect at all. As we have seen, antigen does stimulate cells into cycle, but the pattern is very different from that after anti-*μ* stimulation.

What is the meaning of the fact that the effect of anti-*μ* is different from that of antigen? In fact it is easier to say what it does not mean. We usually assume that B cells in IgM-transgenic mice are basically the same as B cells from normal mice, except that most of them express a surface receptor for a known, cognate antigen. Our data presented here are not consistent with this concept, at least not for B cells from the IgM-transgenic mice that we

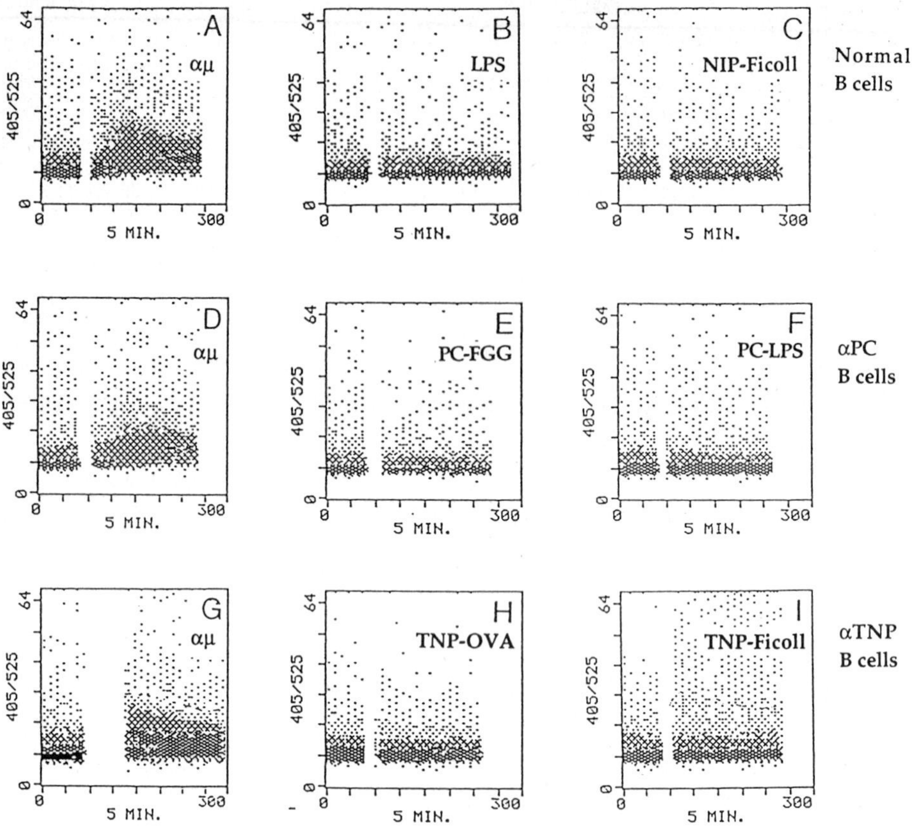

Fig. 4. The calcium response of small dense B cells from C57B6 *nu/nu* mice and IgM transgenic mice. *Row 1*: *nu/nu* fice; *row 2*: PC-μk transgenic mice; *row 3*: TNP-μ transgenic mice. Cells were loaded with Indo-1 for 45 min at 37°C. B cells were identified by gating out T cells, i.e., by labelling cells with biotinated anti-T24 and PE-streptavidin for 30 min on ice after Indo-1 loading **A**, **D**, and **G** Anti-μ 10 μg/ml; **B** LPS; **C** NIP-Ficoll; **E** $PC_{3.6}$-FGG 20 μg/ml; **F** PC_{12}-LPS 20 μgml; **H** TNP-OVA 10 μg/ml; **I** TNP-Ficoll 10 μg/ml. **C** shows the response of normal B cells of *nu/nu* mice stimulated with NIP-Ficoll, and served as the negative control. The emission ratio on the y-axis is plotted (405/525 nm, 0–64) versus time on the x-axis (5 min, 0–300 s)

used. We have also learned that anti-μ does not necessarily mimic antigen in activating B cells (Chen, submitted).

The Effect of Anti-μ+ Factor on Normal B Cells

As discussed above, we found that anti-μ induce normal resting B cells to divide once. We have also studied the effect of anti-μ + lymphokines such as

Table 1. Anti-μ acts differently from antigen on B cells

Assay	Normal B cells			Transgenic B cells		
	Anti-μ	Ag	LPS	Anti-μ	Ag	LPS
Ca^{2+} influx	+	ND	–	+	–	–
PI[a]	+	ND	(+)	+	–	+
Cell cycle	+	ND	+	+	++	+

[a] Kenny et al. 1992, and personal communication

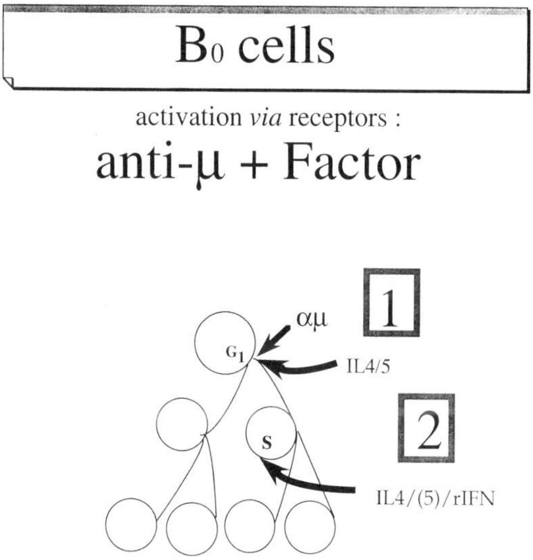

Fig. 5. A model of normal mouse B cell cycle after anti-μ and lymphokine stimulation. Upon activation of small resting B cells with anti-μ alone, or anti-μ plus lymphokines, B cells exit from the G_0/G_1 phase. In the presence of anti-μ alone, small B cells have completed the first cycle and arrested at the G_1 compartment. IL4 acts as a costimulator of anti-μ, exits the majority of B cells from G_0/G_1 phase, and progresses through three cycles. IL-4 alone is also a cell cycle-progressing factor. IL-5 acts mainly on B cells as a co-competence factor of anti-μ. It has no effect in exciting resting B cells; it has some S phase progression effect on activated B cells. Anti-μ activation is shown by *black straight arrows*, lymphokines as co-competence factors by the *curved arrow*, and IL-4/(5)/γ-IFN (*rIFN*) as S phase progression factor by *curved arrows*. Two restriction points are marked in black, and framed as *1* and *2* in the *boxes*

IL2, IL4, IL5, and γ-interferon (Fig. 5). IL4, IL5, and γ-interferon all stimulate cells to enter the cell cycle, while IL2 has no effect [1–4]. Every lymphokine is different, and we can assign a role to each lymphokine. For example, IL4 and IL5 are costimulators of anti-μ. In addition, IL4 is an S-

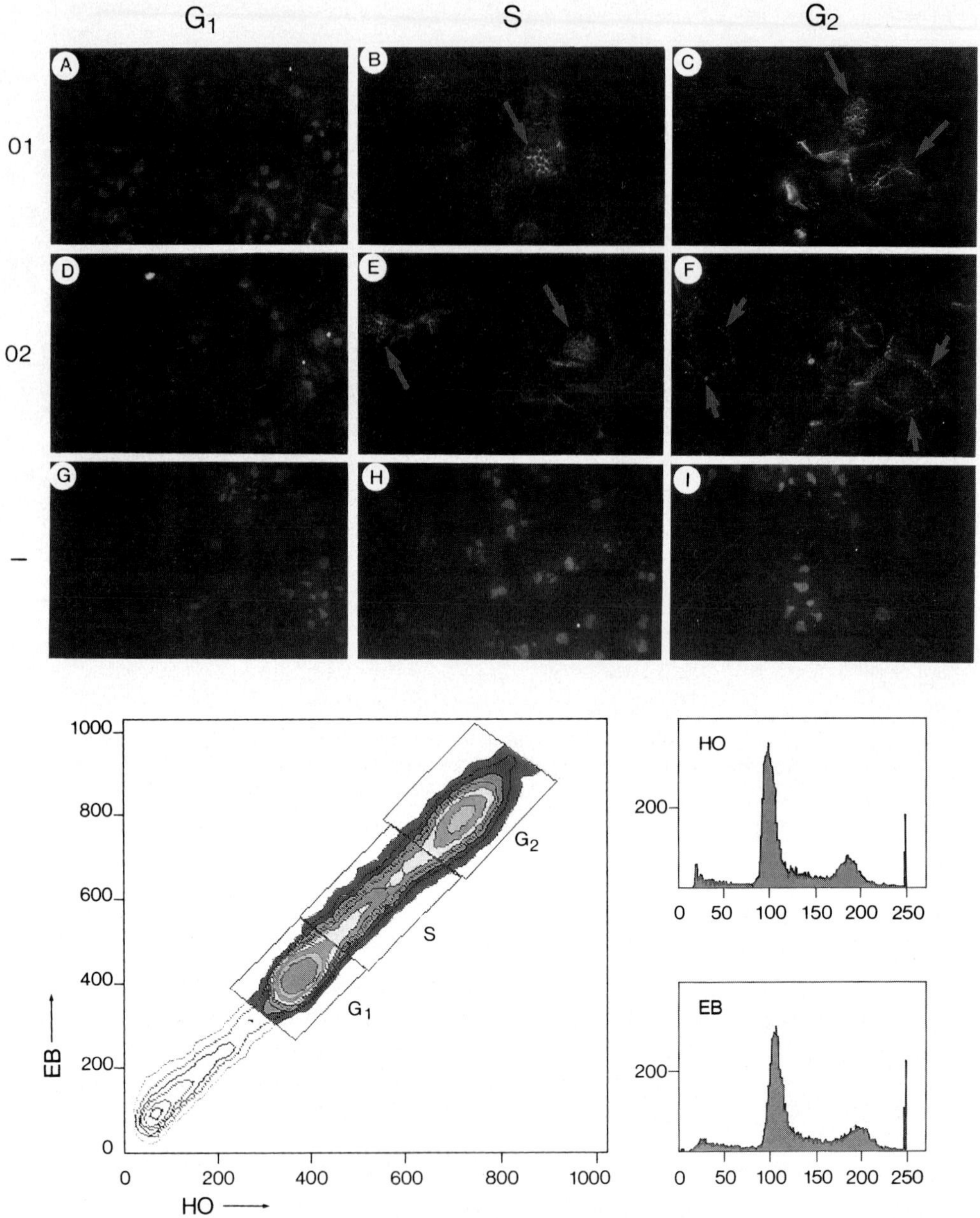

Fig. 6. Cell cycle compartmental specific sorting: HeLa cells were stained with Hoechst (*HO*) and ethidium bromide (*EB*), following the methods described [1]. Stained cells were subjected to flow cytometric analysis and sorting in a Becton-Dickinson FACstar plus. The wavelengths are 450–500 nm for Hoechst, and above 600 nm for EB. The *lower left panel* shows the fluorescence linear channel of x-axis of Hoechst fluorescence and the y-axis of EB fluorescence. The two *lower right panels* show the linear channel of x-axis of HO or EB vs linear scale of y-axis of number of

phase progression factor, stimulating the majority of resting B cells to enter the cell cycle. In contrast, IL5 has little effect on resting B cells. It acts as a co-competence factor, stimulating predominantly low-density and pre-activated B cells. Although γ-interferon has no effect by itself, when added to B cell cultures 36 h after anti-μ stimulation, it is an S-phase progression factor [1].

Two Restriction Points for Normal B Cells

Based on the above data, we propose that there are two restriction points for B cell activation: one at the transition from G_0 to G_1 phase and one at the transition from G_1 to S phase [3, 4]. We still have no real model of transgenic B cell activation. Most transgenic B cells do not respond to lymphokine stimulation plus either antigen or anti-μ (Chen, submitted).

More Applications of Cell Cycle Assays

There must be many proteins that vary in expression through the cell cycle. We are interested in studying the expression pattern of DNA binding proteins with the cell cycle technique described above. It is possible to assay the expression of DNA binding proteins during the cell cycle. A big advantage of this approach is that we could physically separate specific compartment nuclei. We have used transcriptional factors, octamer transcriptional factors (OTF) [8], and oncogene protein *myc* as examples. The progress of our study is discussed below:

Sorting of Compartment-Specific Nuclei

In order to optimize the conditions, we started with sorting of nuclei from HeLa cells. We treated HeLa cells with NP-40, doubly stained the cells with Hoechst and ethidium bromide, and then visualized them on the screen of flow cytometer. This gives the type of profile shown in the lower left panel of Fig. 6. We then gated and sorted nuclei from G_1, S, and G_2 compart-

←

events. **A–I** show the immunofluorescence staining of the rabbit anti-recombinant POU domain (*O1*), Gt_2 rabbit anti-recombinant OTF1 (*O2*), or rabbit normal serum (−) on sorted cells from compartment G_1, S, and G_2. 1×10^5 to 1×10^6 cells each of G_1, S, and G_2 were collected, and cytocentrifuged onto microscopic slides. The cells were fixed in acetone, stained first with rabbit anti-OTF, and then with FITC-labelled human anti-rabbit antibodies (9). The intensity of immunofluorescence was evaluated under UV illumination on a Zeiss Axiovert 35M using the appropriate excitation filters (100×)

ments, collected the nuclei, cytospinned them onto microscopic slides, fixed, and stained with FITC-labelled antibodies (Fig. 6A–I). The red fluorescence is ethidium bromide or Hoechst; the green fluorescence is FITC-labelled anti-OTF antibodies.

At G_1, there is no green color detected inside the nuclei, only the red DNA. Only very faint greenish staining is visable in the cytoplasm surrounding the nuclei. When S phase nuclei are stained, about half of them are covered with a "nest-like" bright green color. This is especially strong with anti-OTF_1 staining (Fig. 6B and E, arrows). When cells from the G_2/M are stained, most of them show the same nest-like, green staining. In addition, there are chains of bead-like bright green fluorescence at the nuclear membrane (Fig. 6C and F, arrows).

Confocal Microscopic Localization of OTF Protein

Figure 7 was obtained with confocal microscopy. With mitotic nuclei, OTF protein is brightly stained at the nuclear envelope. Thus, nuclear OTF proteins seem to be cell cycle regulated. They are *not* expressed in G_1. They are partially expressed in S, and they accumulate in G_2/M.

These data are only partially consistent with reports of Roeder et al. [9]. Namely, we both described the onset of OTF protein in S, but the finding of OTF accumulation in G_2/M is new. We do not know yet whether our observation has any correlation with the cell cycle regulated subnuclear compartments PIKA [10], or the interphase nuclear matrix [11] or metaphase chromosome scaffold [12]. It remains open whether anti-OTF antibodies recognize an additional epitope that becomes accessible during mitosis.

Since the sorting and staining procedures are feasible, the next sets of experiments that we would like to do are the sorting of primary B cells after anti-μ+factor (especially, IL4) stimulation. We found that there is preferential distribution of cells in G_1 after anit-μ+IL4 stimulation, and would like to characterize them further at the molecular level [2].

Analysis of myc Expression in Normal B Cells by Three-Parameter Cell Cycle Assay

While sorting will be useful for biochemical studies, it would be preferable to use a three-parameter technique for analytical work. The last set of data presented here shows our progress in developing such a three-parameter cell cycle assay. After anti-μ+LPS treatment for 3 days, B cells were stained with three colors: Hoechst, 7AAD, and anti-myc antibodies [8]. We detected both myc-positive B cells (Fig. 8, upper left panel) and myc-negative B cells (Fig. 8, upper right panel).

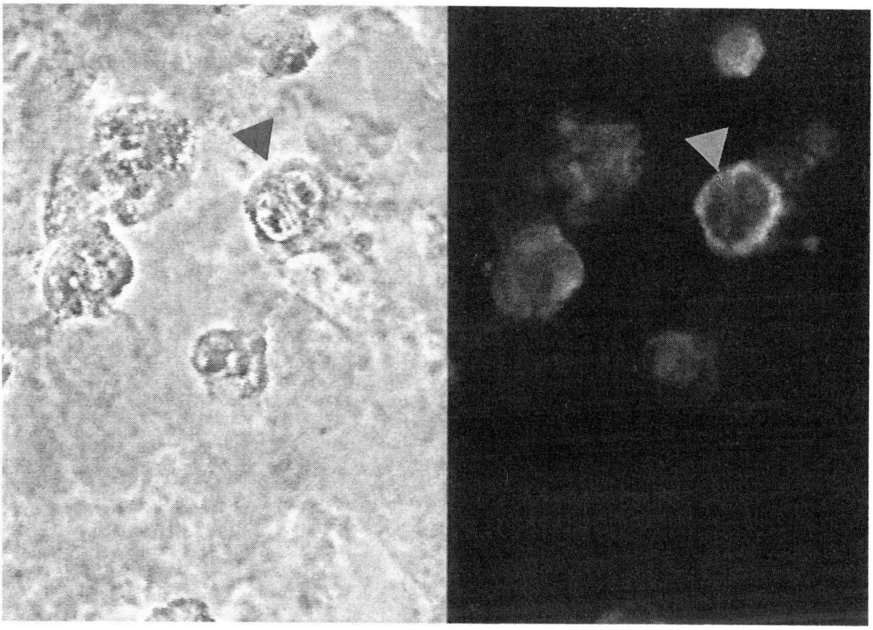

A B

Fig. 7A,B. Confocal microscopic examination of OTF location in the dividing nucleus. HeLa cells were fixed with acetone, and stained first with rabbit anti-OTF antibody and then with FITC-labelled human anti-rabbit antibodies. The intensity of immunofluorescence was examined under UV illumination on a Zeiss Axiovert 35M microscope using the appropriate excitation filters and the Confocal Imaging System MRC-500 (Bio-Rad, Glattburg, Switzerland). **A** shows phase contrast, and **B** shows immunofluorescent micrograph, the *arrow* pointed to a dividing cell (100×). Since cells were not enriched at the G_2/M, the frequency of dividing cells is very low (0.1%)

When B cells are in G_0/G_1 of the first cycle, they are myc negative. When they are stimulated, they enter S and G_2, and are myc positive. After the first division they split into two daughter cells, with approximately equal populations at G_1 of the second cycle: one population is myc positive and the other is myc negative. When the daughter cells enter S and G_2 of the second cycle, they are all myc positive. After the second division into granddaughter cells, they split again into two equal populations at G_1 of the third cycle: one population is myc positive and the other is myc negative. When the granddaughter cells enter S and G_2 of the third cycle, they are all myc positive again. Therefore, myc is expressed in every compartment, *except* in G_0 and G_0/G_1 of the second and third cycles. The reason for saying G_0/G_1 of the second and third cycles is that loss of myc in the daughter cells may be correlated to their return to the resting phase (G_0). With the current BrdU/Hoechst technique, these two phases are indistinguishable.

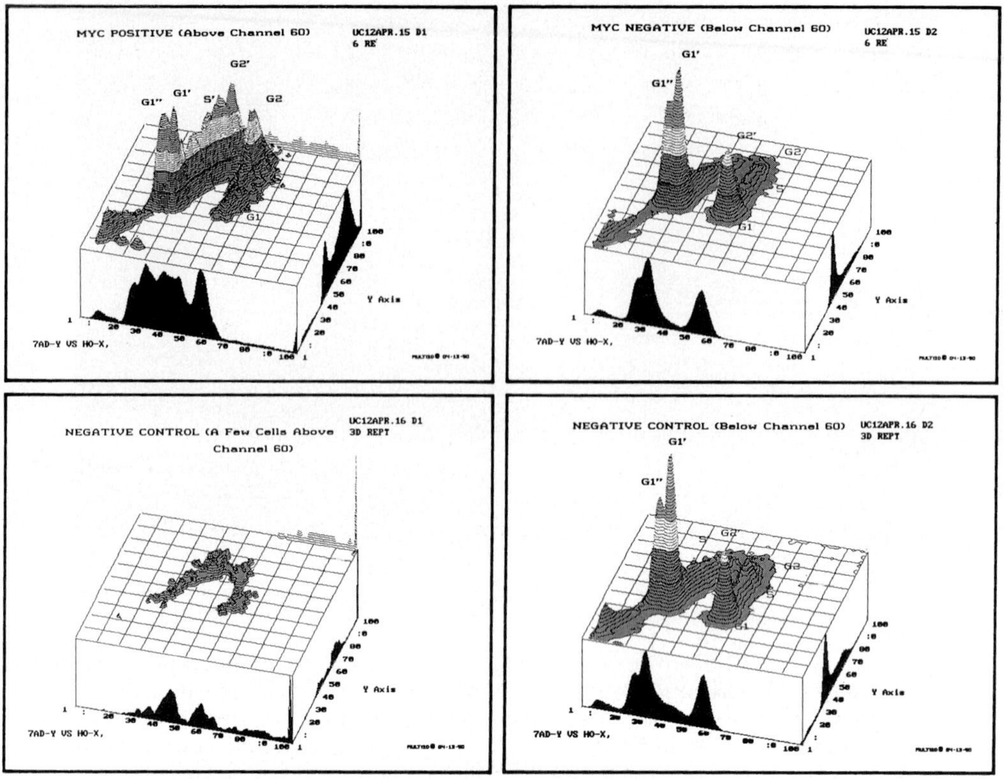

Fig. 8. Three-parameter cell cycle progression pattern of normal B cells stimulated with anti-μ+LPS for 60 h in the presence of BrdU during the culturing. The nuclei were stained with three dyes: x-axis represents Hoechst fluorescence, y-axis represents 7AAD fluorescence. The third parameter represents fluorescence by rabbit anti-mouse myc antibodies, doubling stained with FITC-labelled mouse anti-rabbit antibodies. Cells are divided into myc positive (above channel 60), shown in the *upper left panel*, and myc negative (below channel 60) shown in the *upper right panel*. *Lower panels* are the negative controls, i.e., with normal rabbit serum. There are cells at the background level (blue color), and the mountains represent the percentage of cells in each particular compartment

Lack of Correlation of myc Expression and Apoptosis in Normal B Cells

We do not understand the split pattern of B cell populations whenever they enter G_1/G_0 of cycles. However, both myc-positive and myc-negative cells are *not* in the apoptotic comparment – apoptotic cells are shown in blue color at the lower left corner toward zero scale. The apoptotic B cells are not myc positive. It seems that there is no correlation between myc expression and the apoptosis in normal B cell populations. The observation by Yao and Scott [13] that anti-sense myc oligonucleotides could block the apoptosis induced by anti-μ treatment seems to be a different event: perhaps it occurs only in the cases of lymphomas. On the other hand, apoptosis is a rapid event of approximately 1–3 h. Myc is only needed for the onset of apoptosis, and is then rapidly destroyed in the apoptic cells.

Summary

Using two-parameter flow cytometry assay, we have analyzed the pattern of progression of B cells from IgM-transgenic mice through the cell cycle. We have compared their response to anti-μ or antigen with the response of normal B cells to anti-μ. Treatment of normal mouse B cells with anti-μ stimulates a proportion of them to proliferate into two daughter cells. As expected, treatment with antigen alone can stimulate transgenic B cells to proliferate; indeed, it is a better activator than anti-μ, since four (grand-)-daughter cells are produced. But transgenic B cells respond differently from normal B cells in many respects, such as cell cycle pattern to other stimuli, calcium influx, and PI changes. Some but not all of these effects can be explained if the transgenic B cells are not truly resting normal cells. In other words, they have been previously activated.

Combining cell sorting and immunofluorescent staining methods, we showed that transcriptional factors such as OTF are cell cycle regulated. They do not express at G_1. The expression begins at S, and accumulates at G_2/M. In a three-parameter cell cycle assay, we have detected the expression of myc in normal B cell cycles after anti-μ+LPS activation. We found that myc expressed in B cells of all compartments with the exception of resting B cells and a portion of B cells arrested at G_1 of each cycle. We could *not* detect myct expression in apoptotic B cells.

Acknowledgements. We wish to thank Fiona McConnell for calcium influx measurement; Marcus Dessing, Helga Seyschab, and Martin Poot for two-parameter cell cycle measurement; Holger Hoehn for introducing us to the field of cell cycle analysis; Peter Rabinovitch for three-parameter cell cycle analysis, Ursula Storb, Georges Koehler, and David Baltimore for transgenic mice; James Kenny for sharing of unpublished data; Robert N. Eisenman for anti-myc antibodies; Thomas Gerster for anti-OTF antibodies; and Ulrich Deuschle and Charley Steinberg for helpful discussion and critical reading of this manuscript. The Basel Institute for Immunology was founded and is supported by F. Hoffmann-La Roche, Basel, Switzerland.

References

1. Seyschab H, Friedl R, Schindler D, Hoehn H, Rabinovitch PS, Chen U (1989) Eur J Immunol 19:1605–1612
2. Seyschab H, Hoehn H, Rabinovitch PS, Chen U (1991) Eur J Immunol 21: 2153–2160
3. Chen U (1990) Cytokines 3:1–23
4. Chen U (1992) Immunobiology 185:366–379
5. Storb U, Pinkert C, Arp B, Engler P, Gollahon K, Manz J, Brady W, Brinster R (1986) J Exp Med 164:627–641
6. Carsetti R, Köhler G, Lamers MC (1993) Eur J Immunol 23:168–178
7. Kenny JJ, Sieckmann DG, Freter C, Hodes, R, Hathcock K, Longo DL (1992) Curr Top Microbiol Immunol 182:95–103
8. Chen U, Scheuermann RH, Wirth T, Gerster T, Roeder RG, Harshman K, Berger C (1991) Nucleic Acids Res 19:5981–5989
9. Roberts SB, Seail N, Heintz N (1991) Science 253:1022–1026
10. Saunders WS, Cooke CA, Earnshau WC (1991) J Cell Biol 115:919–931
11. Berezney R, Coffey D (1974) Biochem Biophys Res Commun 30:1410–1419
12. Lewis CD, Laemmli UK (1982) Cell 29:171–181
13. Yao X, Scott W (1993) Immunol Rev 132:163–186

Pit Cells: Some Observations on Their Ultrastructure in Patients with Carcinoma and Viral Hepatitis Compared with Pit Cells in Rats Treated with Biological Response Modifiers

M. Gulubova, M. Ganeva, K. Todorova, and I. Vasilev

Introduction

The pit cells were first described by Wisse et al. [10] in rat liver and peripheral blood, and were so named because the profile of their granules resembled the pits of fruit. For a long time they were observed only in rat and mouse liver and other organs [3, 4, 8, 9]. At first they were supposed to be endocrine cells [10]; however, it is now generally accepted that they are natural killer (NK) cells [3, 6, 8, 9]. Some authors [4, 5], using the rabbit antiserum to asialo GM1 (a surface marker for murine NK cells), have scrutinized immunoelectron microscopically NK activity of rat pit cells. Since pit cells are NK cells it is assumed [9] that they play an important role in antitumor and antiviral defence.

Little is known about human pit cells. They have been obtained mainly by liver lavage and perfusion [2]. Pit cells were first described in human liver in patients with autoimmune hepatitits [7].

The purpose of the present study is to characterize pit cells in human liver and to compare the morphological features of their activity with the same signs of pit cells in rats treated with biological response modifiers (BRMs). We look for them in patients with liver malignancies, where in our opinion pit cells increase in number in liver sinusoids and are activated.

Materials and Methods

Patients

We studied five patients, all of whom had provided informed consent. Wedge liver biopsy specimens were obtained during surgery. Some of them were immersed in 4% glutaraldehyde solution and postfixed in 1% osmium tetroxide (OsO_4). The ultrathin sections were examined under an electron microscope (OPTON EM 109).

Patients suffered from the following diseases: sigmoid carcinoma, endometrial carcinoma, gastric carcinoma, hepatocellular carcinoma, and viral hepatitis. There were no liver metastases in the first three cases.

Animals

Male Wistar rats were used at ages between 7 and 10 weeks. As a BRM we used Polyerga (Hor Fer Vit Pharma, Oldenburg, Germany), which is commercially available. It contains soluble glycopeptides 30 μg per 1 ml (molecular weight 250–1050). The preparation was injected intramuscularly in a dose of 0.20 ml/kg body weight. The animals were sacrificed as follows: group 1, 24 h after injection; group 2, 48 h after injection; group 3, 4 days after injection; group 4, 1 week after injection; group 5, controls – untreated. Each group consisted of two animals.

Preparation of Rat Liver Tissue for Light and Electron Microscopy. Livers were perfused through the portal vein at a rate of 10 ml per min, with 0.1 *M* phosphate buffer supplemented with 2% sucrose (pH = 7.4) for a few seconds. After that the perfusion was continued for 3–4 min with the same buffer containing 1.5% glutaraldehyde. We took tissue blocks from two liver lobes from the fixed blanched zones. Vibratome sections of 70–100 μm thickness were cut. Tissue sections were rinsed in buffer and incubated for endogenous peroxidase demonstration in 0.1% diaminobenzidine +0.02% hydrogen peroxide in 0.1 *M* phosphate buffer, at pH 6.9, and for 1 h at room temperature. Then sections were rinsed in buffer and postfixed in 1% OsO_4 for 2 h, at 4°C. The sections were embedded in Epon to allow semithin and ultrathin sections to be cut.

Cell Counting

The cytochemical staining for endogenous peroxidase in the rough endoplasmic reticulum and nuclear envelope allowed recognition of Kupffer cells [3], and easier determination of pit cells attached to Kupffer cells. The number of lymphocytes was counted light microscopically on semithin sections, at one and the same magnification per five fields of vision in each section. Two semithin sections were cut from each Epon block. Two Epon blocks were made from each liver (ten animals, 20 Epon blocks, 40 semithin sections in total).

Results

We identified pit cells using the descriptions offered by various authors [2, 6, 7, 10].

General Features of Human Pit Cells

We established that in patients with neoplasia of different locations without liver metastases, hepatic sinusoids were filled with an increased number of

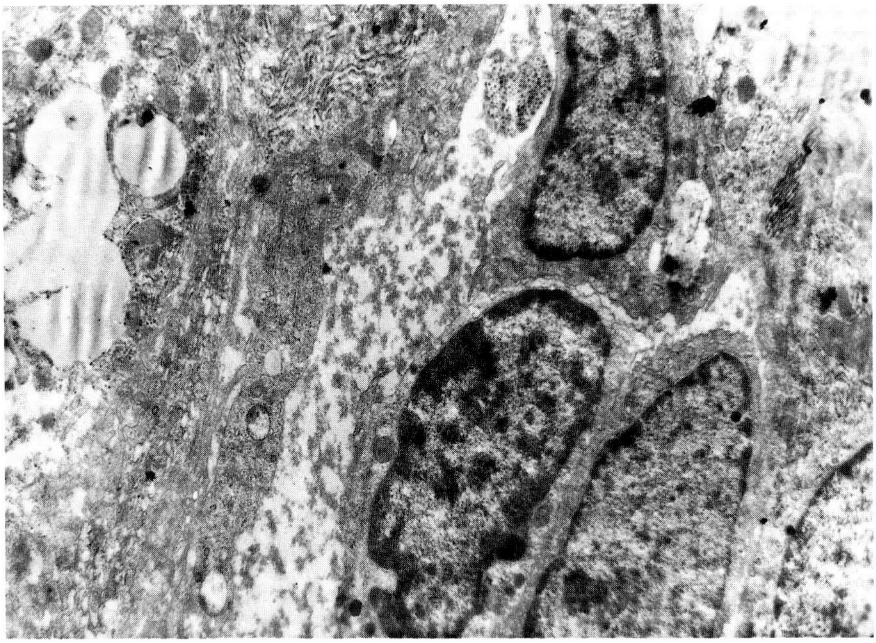

Fig. 1. Pit cell attached to Kupffer cell in sinusoidal lumen. ×4000

lymphocytes. Pit cells were located mainly in sinusoidal lumen, sometimes attached to the endothelial or Kupffer cells. Their nuclei contained highly condensed chromatin and one nucleolus. The form of the nuclei was oval or indented. The cytoplasm was pale with a small number of organelles (Fig. 1). The latter were concentrated at one end of the nucleus. The cytoplasm formed projections without any organelles. These pseudopodia penetrated between cells of the sinusoidal wall. The granules were from 1–2 to 5–6 in number per cell. They were three types: (a) granules with a dense core, a smooth limiting membrane, and a narrow halo beneath it; (b) granules with a dense core and a wide halo; (c) granules containing small vesicles in addition to the dense material. In comparison to rat pit cells, in human ones we have found less rod-cored vesicles and multivesicular bodies. We consider these pit cells to be resting.

In two patients with hepatocellular and gastric carcinoma, pit cells were in close contact with hepatocytes. We consider them to be active (Fig. 2). They contained more organelles than the resting ones. Their granules counted from 6 to 10 in number, situated at one aspect of the nucleus, near the contact area. In the contact zone there was a thinner subplasmalemmal actin coat. Rod-cored vesicles were from 2–3 to 5 in number, and were situated next to microtubules.

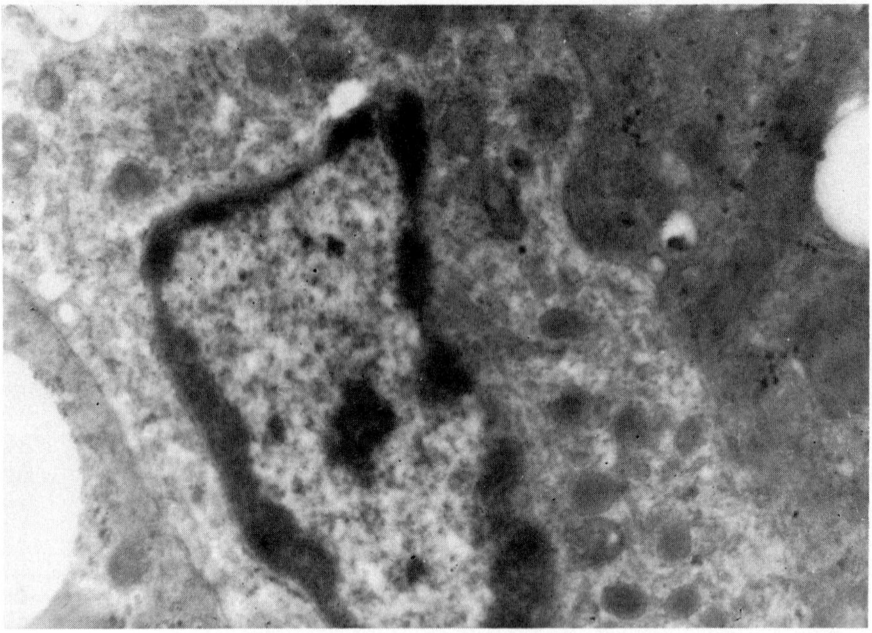

Fig. 2. Pit cell in contact with hepatocyte. Cell organelles are at one pole of the nucleus. Characteristic granules, rod-cored vesicles, microtubules. ×11 000

General Features of Rat Pit Cells

After treatment with a BRM, pit cells increased in number, especially between 4 and 7 days. They were situated mainly in sinusoids, attached to endothelial or Kupffer cells. Pit cells had cytoplasmic projections. Their granules were more numerous than in human pit cells – from 7 to 10 in number. Rod-cored vesicles were found too (Fig. 3). The granules of rat pit cells were almost spherical, being either homogeneous or composed of a very dense core surrounded by a layer of lower electron density. They were negative for endogenous peroxidase.

Discussion

We consider that there are two types of pit cells in human liver: resting and active. Active pit cells were in contact with hepatocytes. They demonstrated pronounced cell polarity, with many organelles situated next to the contact area. The resting pit cells had a few organelles and were located in the middle of the sinusoidal bloodstream. This is a strategic position necessary for them to exert their function.

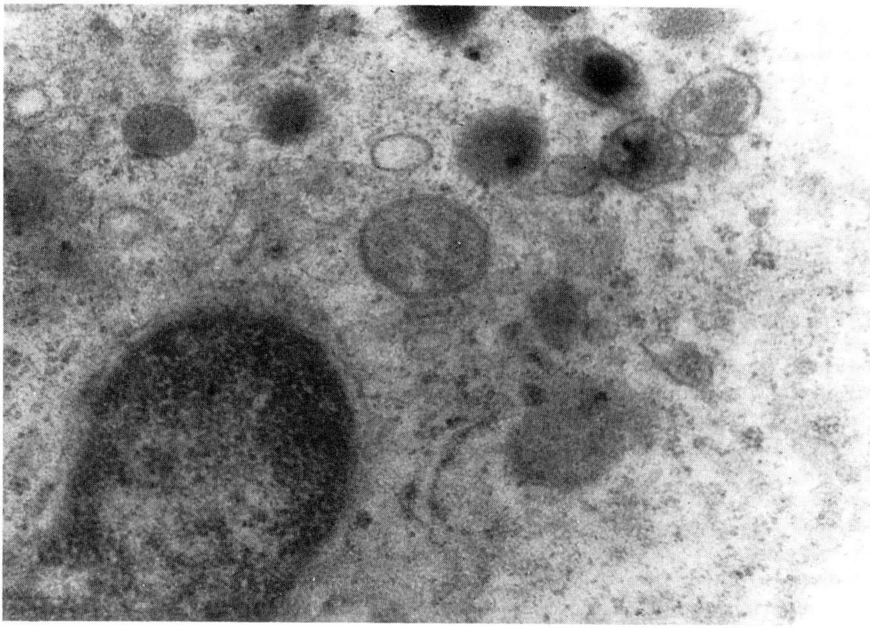

Fig. 3. Three types of pit cell granules in rat liver. ×18 500

We have found an increased number of pit cells and lymphocytes in sinusoids, in neoplasia, and after BRM treatment. This fact supports the hypothesis that pit cells have increased NK and tumoricidal activity [1, 3].

References

1. Borden EC, Sondel PM (1990) Lymphokines and cytokines as cancer treatment. Cancer 65:800–814
2. Bouwens L, Brouwer A, Wisse E (1989) Ultrastructure of human hepatic pit cells. In: Wisse E, Knook DL, Decker K (eds) Cells of the hepatic sinusoid. The Kupffer Cell Foundation, Rijswijk, pp 471–476
3. Bouwens L, Wisse E (1988) Tissue localization and kinetics of pit cells or large granular lymphocytes in the liver of rats treated with biological response modifiers. Hepatology 8:46–52
4. Dan C, Kaneda K, Wake K (1986) Pit cells and liver-associated natural killer activity following administration of OK-432. In: Kirn A, Knook DL, Wisse E (eds) Cells of the hepatic sinusoid, vol 1. The Kupffer Cell Foundation, Rijswijk, pp 427–432
5. Enzan H, Iwamura S, Watanabe S, Saibara T, Ohnishi S, Yamamoto Y, Yamamoto H, Hara H (1989) Immunoelectron microscopic identification of pit cells in the rat and mouse livers. In: Wisse E, Knook DL, Decker K (eds) Cells of the hepatic sinusoid. The Kupffer Cell Foundation, Rijswijk, The Netherlands, pp 479–480

6. Kaneda K, Dan C, Wake K (1983) Pit cells as natural killer cells. Biomed Res 4:567–576
7. Kaneda K, Kurioka N, Seki S, Wake K, Yamamoto S (1984) Pit cell-hepatocyte contact in autoimmune hepatitis. Hepatology 4:955–958
8. Kaneda K, Kataoka M, Kishiye T, Yamamoto H, Wake K (1991) The intracellular distribution of cell organelles in natural killer cells during the cytolysis of bound tumor cells, with special reference to the rod-cored vesicles. Arch Histol Cytol 54:69–79
9. Vanderkerken K, Bouwens L, Wisse E (1989) Heterogeneity and differentiation of pit cells or large granular lymphocytes of the rat. In: Wisse E, Knook DL, Decker K (eds) Cells of the hepatic sinusoid. The Kupffer Cell Foundation, Rijswijk, pp 456–461
10. Wisse E, van 't Noordende JM, van der Meulen J, Daems WT (1976) The pit cell: description of a new type of cell occurring in rat liver sinusoids and peripheral blood. Cell Tissue Res 173:423–435

Mediators

The Polymorphonuclear Neutrophil: A Newly Recognized Participant in the Immune Response

M.L. Rodrick

A large body of evidence exists to show that, following major injury or surgery, patients may become immunosuppressed and this may lead to increased susceptibility to life-threatening infections [1–4]. Recent research by numerous investigators has shown that the secretion of the proinflammatory cytokines IL-1, TNF, and IL-6 are markedly elevated in patients following major injury and that this may lead to some of the clinical effects seen in these patients, such as a process of systemic inflammation leading to multiple organ dysfunction (MOD) [5]. Clinical trials of agents which block endotoxin and TNF are currently underway in these patients. Most of this work has focussed on the monocyte/macrophage as the major participant in the proinflammatory cytokine cascade and as a modulator of the immune response of lymphocytes. The goal of this paper is to suggest that the other major phagocytic cell, the polymorphonuclear neutrophil (PMN), has that same potential.

Human PMNs have important functions in host defense against invading microorganisms. They may be activated as a result of interaction between ligands and membrane receptors on the cell surface followed by processes of transmembrane signalling such as an increase in intracellular Ca^{++} concentration, translocation of protein kinase C, and phosphoinositide turnover. The ligands may be bacterial products such as *Escherichia coli* lipopolysaccharide (LPS) or *Staphylococcus aureus* delta toxin [6] or exogenous or endogenous mediators such as cytokines.

PMNs May Modulate the Immune Response In Vitro and In Vivo

In addition to the important role of the PMNs in response to bacterial invasion by chemotaxis, phagocytosis, and killing, the PMNs' interactions with the mononuclear cells involved in the immune response have been of interest to a small number of researchers for at least 15 years. Studies have been carried out in human and murine systems (Table 1).

A number of studies of the effect of PMNs or factors released from these cells on the blastogenic response of lymphocytes suggested that the PMNs could have a suppressive effect [7, 8]. The addition of 24%–51%

Table 1. The PMN as an immune cell

Finding	Author
Present Ag	Fitzgerald et al. 1983 [46]
Bear Ia-like antigen	Ross et al. 1978 [54]
May up- or down-regulate T cell response to IL-2 secretion	Rodrick et al. 1986 [23]
Modulation of in vivo cell-mediated immunity	Lamster et al. 1980 [18]
Make mRNA and new protein and secrete cytokines in response to stimuli, e.g., LPS:	
IL-1	Lindemann et al. 1984 [28]; Tiku et al. 1986 [26]; Lord et al. 1991 [29]
TNF-α	Dubravec et al. 1990 (31); Djeu et al. 1990 [32]
IL-6	Cicco et al. 1990 [36]
GCSF	Ichinose et al. 1990 [35]
IL-8	Strieter et al. 1990 [38]
IFN-α	Shirafuji et al. 1990 [55]

PMNs to cultures containing lymphocytes caused a decreased response to the T cell mitogen phytohemagglutinin (PHA) as well as inhibition of the mixed lymphocyte reaction (MLR). There was a dose-response relationship as the inhibitory effect was increased with an increase in numbers of PMNs added to the cultures. Similar effects could be seen with the soluble products of the autologous PMNs used in these studies. Hsu et al. [9] found that PMNs or sonicates of PMNs inhibited lymphocyte reactivity. The factor was found to be resistant to freeze-thawing, nondialyzable, and noncytotoxic and its effect was reversed by washing cells treated with it. Later it was shown [10–12] that PMNs can down-regulate natural killer (NK) and cytotoxic T cell activity. Zoschke and Staite [13] reported that LPS-activated PMNs suppressed the blastogenic response of human lymphocytes to Con A in a manner that was catalase-reversible. They found that the suppression occurred at ratios of lymphocytes to PMNs found in peripheral blood. They also found that progeny lymphocytes from the suppressed cultures contained an increased T helper to T suppressor ratio compared with the original cultures or control cultures, suggesting an immunoregulatory role for the PMNs in chronic inflammation.

In contrast, other investigators have reported an enhancement of lymphocyte blastogenesis following addition of PMNs or factors released by PMNs to cultures. Wilson [14] found that purified lymphocyte preparations (>95% pure) displayed only 50%–33% of the response of cultures which contained 30%–60% PMNs. Similarly, the response could be gradually enhanced by the addition of increasing numbers of purified PMNs. Jones [15] found that the addition of increasing percentages of PMNs led to increased blastogenesis in a two-way MLR. Tchorzewski et al. [16] suggested that PMN lysosomes caused lymphocytes to undergo blast transformation. Their immunochemical analysis showed that the factor was not an enzyme but a lysosomal protein. They also [17] showed that pretreatment of human lymphocytes with freeze-thaw lysates of autologous peripheral blood PMNs enhanced the blastogenic response of lymphocytes to PHA.

Work reported as early as 1980 by our laboratory showed that mouse peritoneal exudate PMNs (>95% pure) recruited 3–4 h after IP injection of stimulants could modulate both in vitro and in vivo immune responses in syngeneic systems [18–20] including cell- and complement-dependent cytotoxicity and rejection of skin grafts. PMNs recruited by thioglycollate (TPMNs) were more metabolically active than those recruited by glycogen (GPMNs) and also the two different cell populations had different effects on the immune responses of syngeneic splenocytes. Furthermore the soluble products of PMNs elicited by glycogen (GPMN-S) (after in vitro culture for as little as 1 h) were found to enhance lymphocyte responses to PHA as well as LPS, indicating a potential effect on both T and B cell responses. On the other hand, TPMNs did not produce an enhancing factor for the PHA response until the cells had been in culture for 24 h and this factor (TPMN-S) had no effect on the response of lymphocytes to LPS. Thymocyte responses to PHA were facilitated by all supernatants, indicating an IL-1-like nature for the secreted products of PMNs. When the supernatants were diluted, a loss of enhancing activity occurred as expected but, unexpectedly, a suppressive effect was observed in both TPMN-S and GPMN-S. The two activities were able to be separated by gel chromatography [21]. Similarly, Yoshinaga et al. [22] found a PMN derived T cell potentiation factor which eluted from Sephadex G-75 at a molecular weight (MW) range of 12–24 kDa. The material potentiated PHA-stimulated thymocytes but did not support an IL-2 dependent cell line, indicating again that it was like IL-1, not IL-2. We have shown that normal human PMNs added to cultures of autologous peripheral blood mononuclear cells could enhance the response to PHA and secretion of IL-2 in these cultures [23].

PMNs Make and Secrete Cytokines

PMNs are present in greater numbers than any other leukocyte in the circulating blood of humans, are the first cells to respond, and the first circulating cell to be increased in numbers in response to an inflammatory or infectious challenge. Yet the possible importance of PMNs as cytokine producers has been largely ignored until recently [24]. One reason for this may be that the PMN has been thought to be an "end" cell, not capable of new protein synthesis after its release from the hematopoietic organs into the circulation. Careful investigation of the literature indicates that this is not the case.

In 1984 Goto et al. [25] demonstrated that an IL-1-like lymphocyte stimulating factor was produced at inflammatory sites and the level of this substance at the site was correlated with the infiltration of PMNs. In 1986 it was shown by Tiku et al. [26] that normal human PMNs can make and secrete IL-1 as measured by the thymocyte costimulator assay. The PMN cell population was shown to be >99% pure PMN with <1% contaminating mononuclear cells. Jack and Fearon [27] showed that circulating PMNs can make mRNA and secrete new proteins. In 1988 Lindemann et al. [28] showed that human PMNs produce IL-1 and mRNA for IL-1 in response to recombinant human granulocyte/macrophage colony stimulating factor (GMCSF). It was shown by Lord et al. [29] that PMNs make both IL-1α and IL-1β.

In 1989, Yamazaki et al. [30] showed that PMNs made a cytotoxic product similar to TNF. In 1990 our laboratory published the first report that PMNs make and secrete TNF-α [31]. In this work we showed that the PMN population was >99% pure granulocytes, and that a number of monocytes corresponding to 20% contamination did not, under our culture conditions, secrete as much TNF as the PMNs did, showing that the TNF was not produced by a contaminating population of monocytes/macrophages. We also showed that the TNF was biologically (cytotoxic for the L-M cell line) as well as antigenically active (by ELISA for TNF-α). It was also demonstrated that mRNA for TNF was not made for at least 1 h in culture in response to LPS stimulation, suggesting that the TNF was not stored, but newly made protein. These results were corroborated by independent work of Djeu et al. [32], who showed that TNF was produced by PMNs and inhibited by protein synthesis and RNA inhibitors, again suggesting that new protein was being made by the PMNs in culture. Earlier it had been shown that TNF can stimulate PMNs, suggesting that these cells make autoregulatory molecules [33]. More recently, Bazzoni et al. [34] demonstrated TNF mRNA accumulation and secretion by human PMNs following phagocytosis of opsonized yeast.

Other investigators have shown that several other cytokines may be secreted by PMNs but have not shown evidence for new mRNA for these cytokines. Ichinose et al. in 1990 [35] demonstrated that PMNs make and release GCSF in response to LPS after at least 24 h of culture. Supernatants of unstimulated cells did not have detectable levels of GCSF. No significant cell death occurred in 24-h cultures as measured by trypan blue exclusion or the more sensitive assay of LDH content of cell culture medium, indicating that the cells were not dying and releasing previously made cytokine.

Cicco et al. [36] reported that human PMNs can make and secrete IL-6 in response to stimulation by GMCSF. This activity was neutralized by antibody to IL-6. They also showed that PMNs could be induced to synthesize transcripts for IL-6 indistinguishable in size from IL-6 mRNA produced by activated human macrophages. We have confirmed the production of IL-6 by PMNs in response to LPS (Horgan et al., unpublished). Furthermore,

Henschler et al. [37] have shown that PMNs express functional receptors for IL-6. They found that IL-6 receptor expression was down-regulated by pretreatment of the PMNs with GMCSF.

PMNs have also been shown to make and secrete IL-8 a cytokine that attracts PMNs to an inflammatory focus, suggesting yet another autoregulatory process [38].

These investigations have shown that the PMN is not an "end" cell, but one capable of making and secreting proteins which have been shown to have effects on the immune response and to participate in the body's response to infection.

Until now it was thought that the monocytes were responsible for the majority of the production of these cytokines by circulating blood cells but it must now be considered that the PMN, a much more numerous cell (60%–90% of peripheral leukocytes in humans), may be a major contributor. Furthermore, following infection, PMNs increase markedly in the peripheral blood to as much as 10 times their usual number and they migrate early after infection to sites of inflammation. In fact it has been shown by Meszaros et al. that PMNs are found in large numbers in the liver following an endotoxin challenge in rats and may contribute as much cytokine synthesis as the Kupffer cells there [39].

PMNs May Be Divided into Subsets

Subsets of PMNs have been described by others. PMNs may express receptors for complement (CR) CR1 and CR3 [40] and for the Fc region of immunoglobulin G (FcR-I, -II, and -III). The CD18 integrin family of leukocyte receptors (CD11a/CD18, CD11b/CD18, and CD11c/CD18) are found on PMNs and mediate their adhesion to endothelial cells [41]. Another adhesion molecule in the selectin family, LAM-1, has been found on PMNs [42]. PMNs also express receptors for products of arachidonic acid as evidenced by the finding by Goldman and Goetzl [43] of receptors for leukotriene B_4 (LTB_4).

Variations in subsets of lymphocytes and monocytes have been shown to have effects on the immune response. Variation in subsets of PMNs have been identified in the autoimmune disease systemic lupus erythematosus [44] and more recently in patients following thermal injury [45]. PMNs share many cell surface molecules with monocytes, including FcRI, -II, and III (CD64, CD32, and CD16 respectively) and CR1 and CR3. Buckle et al. [40] have found that cell surface receptors on both PMNs and monocytes can be induced by interferon-γ and the CSFs. PMNs can be induced to express FcRI by IFN-γ. FcRII is constitutively expressed by PMNs but was not significantly altered by treatment with IFN-γ or any of the CSFs tested (human GCSF, GMCSF, and MCSF). However, FcRIII was enhanced on PMNs by IFN-γ, GMCSF, and GCSF but not for all individuals, indicating that there is individual variation in receptor induction. Using a panel of monoclonal antibodies to CD14 these investigators were not able to find evidence of MHC class II expression on any PMNs before or after induction with IFN-γ or any of the CSFs, suggesting a marker for monocytes which is finally different from PMNs. However, there is some controversy about this lack of MHC class II expression as Ia has been identified on murine peritoneal PMNs [47] and on human PMNs by others [48]. It was also observed that constitutive expression of FcRIII by PMNs decreased after 14 h in culture but did not do so in IFN-γ or CSF treated PMNs, suggesting that cytokines might alter the turnover of this receptor on PMNs rather than causing induction of new molecules. Further evidence to support this theory was given by Ichinose et al. [35], who showed that treatment of PMNs with either LPS or GCSF maintained the phenotype of PMNs in culture for 24 h compared to control cells. In unstimulated PMNs, expression of CD16 (FcRIII) was markedly reduced by 24 h of culture, whereas either GCSF or LPS stimulated PMNs maintained or had an enhanced expression of this antigen.

The leukocyte integrins consist of molecules originally referred to as LFA-1, Mac-1 or CR3 and p150/95 [48]. Each is a heterodimer consisting of a unique α-chain of 180, 165, 150 kDa and designated by reactivity with monoclonal antibodies as CD11a, CD11b, and CD11c noncovalently bound to a common CD18 95-kDa chain. The surface marker LAK-1 (Leu 8), also found on PMNs, belongs to another family of cellular adhesion molecules, the selectins. Griffin et al. [42] have shown that activation of PMNs in vitro with GMCSF, PMA LPS, or TNF, but not GCSF, caused loss of LAM-1 from the surface while at the same time up-regulating the expression of CD11b on those cells, again showing that expression of surface markers on PMNs is differentially regulated.

Clinical relevance of the PMN subsets CR3 (CD11b) and FcR (CD16) was shown by Babcock et al. [45] in thermally injured patients. They found that PMNs from patients who developed sepsis had decreased levels of $CD16{+}CD11^{+}$ PMNs compared to preinfection values and this decrease correlated with susceptibility to infection. They did not find any correlation in these patients between $CD35^{+}$ PMNs and sepsis. Work from our laboratory [49, 50] has previously shown that patients following major thermal injury have increased levels of $CR1^{+}$ and $CR3^{+}$ PMNs in their circulation compared with normal controls. It was also found that the PMNs from these patients had decreased functional capacity in their ability to respond to chemotactic stimuli. Inherited deficiency of the adhesion molecules described above has been found and these patients are subject to recurrent infections [51]. A report by Fischer et al. [52] demonstrated that a girl with deficiency in the integrin complex had abnormal phagocytic cell function, but also had decreased cytolytic T cell function, defective antibody production and deficient cytokine production.

How Is PMN Cytokine Secretion Regulated?

Our investigations have shown (Rodrick and Dubravec, unpublished) that the PMN secretion of IL-1 may be down-regulated by addition of exogenous PGE_2, suggesting a role for the arachidonic acid pathway in regulation of cytokine secretion by this cell. Furthermore, IL-1 secretion by the PMNs in response to LPS was up-regulated by the cyclooxygenase inhibitor indomethacin, showing that the endogenous activation of this pathway has a role in this regulation. Numerous investigators have shown that PMN secretion of cytokines may be regulated by another cytokine which may be a PMN product itself, leading to an autoregulatory pathway [33, 36, 53]. Investigation of this regulation is currently being carried out with the intent of defining the role of PMN cytokine secretion and immune regulation.

In summary, our results and those of others have shown that the PMN is capable of making and secreting cytokines involved in the immune response and have suggested that PMNs may have immunomodulatory effects, depending on the stimulus used to activate them. Furthermore, variations in subsets of PMNs as well as in cytokine secretion have been found in several disease states. Hopefully, in the future the importance of this "forgotten" cell will be more appreciated in clinical settings, especially in the immune abnormalities following injury.

References

1. Baker CC (1986) Immune mechanisms and host resistance in the trauma patient. Yale J Biol Med 59:387–393
2. McRitchie DI, Girott M, Rotstein OD, Teodorczyk-Injeyan JA (1990) Impaired antibody production in blunt trauma: Possible role for T-cell dysfunction. Arch Surg 125:91–96
3. Wolfe JHN, Saporoschetz I, Young AE, O'Connor NE, Mannick JA (1981) Suppressive serum, suppressor lymphocytes and death from burns. Ann Surg 193:513–520
4. Moss NM, Gough DB, Jordan AL, Grbic JT, Wood JJ, Rodrick ML, Mannick JA (1988) Temporal correlation of impaired immune response after thermal injury with susceptibility to infection in a murine model. Surgery 104:882–887
5. Demling R, LaLonde C, Saldinger P, Knox J (1993) Multiple organ dysfunction in the surgical patient: pathophysiology, prevention and treatment. Curr Probl Surg 3:347–412
6. Kasimir S, Schonfeld W, Alouf JE, Konig W (1990) Effect of *Staphylococcus aureus* delta-toxin on human granulocyte functions and plateletactivating-factor metabolism. Infect Immun 58:1653–1659
7. Walker RI, Fowler I (1965) Granulocyte inhibition of human peripheral blood lymphocyte growth in vitro. Exp Cell Res 38:379–385
8. Bach ML, Bach FH, Widmer M, Oranen H, Wolbers WH (1971) Lymphocyte reactivity in vitro. VII. The effect of polymorphonuclear leukocytes on lymphocyte response. Transplantation 12:283–286

9. Hsu CCS, Wu MYB, Rivera-Arcilla J (1979) Inhibition of lymphocyte reactivity in vitro by autologous polymorphonuclear cells (PMN). Cell Immunol 48:288–295
10. El-Hag A, Clark RA (1984) Down-regulation of human natural killer activity against tumors by the neutrophil myeloperoxidase system and hydrogen peroxide. J Immunol 133:3291–3297
11. Kay HD, Smith DL (1983) Regulation of human lymphocyte-mediated natural killer (NK) cell activity. I. Inhibition in vitro by peripheral blood granulocytes. J Immunol 130:475–483
12. Petrie HT, Klassen LW, Kay HD (1984) Inhibition of human cytotoxic T lymphocyte activity in vitro by autologous peripheral blood granulocytes. J Immunol 134:230–234
13. Zoschke DC, Staite ND (1987) Suppression of human lymphocyte proliferation by activated neutrophils or H_2O_2: surviving cells have an altered T helper/T suppressor ratio and increased resistance to secondary oxidant exposure. Clin Immunol Immunopathol 42:160–170
14. Wilson DB (1966) Analysis of some of the variables associated with proliferative response of human lymphoid cells in culture. J Exp Zool 162:161–170
15. Jones AL (1966) The effect of polymorphonuclear leukocytes on the blastoid transformation of lymphocytes in mixed leukocyte cultures. Transplantation 4: 337–343
16. Tchorzewski H, Sulowska Z, Denys A (1973) A new lymphocyte transforming factor derived from the lysosomes of polymorphonuclear leukocytes. Experientia 29:481–483
17. Tchorzewski H, Sulowska Z (1980) The mitogenic and enzymatic activities of polymorphonuclear leukocyte (PMNL) lysosomal proteins examined in vitro. Arch Immunol Ther Exp 28:1–8
18. Lamster IB, Sonis ST, Mirando DM, Kolodkin AB, Rodrick ML, Wilson RE (1980) Modification of in vitro and in vivo immune function by acute inflammatory cells. Transplantation 30:244–250
19. Rodrick ML, Lamster I, Sonis S, Wilson RE (1980) Effect of neutrophils on antibody synthesis in mice. J Dent Res 59:460
20. Rodrick ML, Lamster IB, Sonis ST, Pender SG, Kolodkin AB, Fitzgerald JE, Wilson RE (1982) Effects of supernatants of polymorphonuclear neutrophils recruited by different inflammatory substances on mitogen responses of lymphocytes. Inflammation 6:1–11
21. Rodrick M, Sonis S, Lamster I, Fitzgerald J, Wilson RE (1981) Immune regulation by soluble factors from PMN. Fed Proc 40:770
22. Yoshinaga M, Ohkawara S, Nakayama S, Goto F (1983) Characteristics of PMN-derived helper T cell potentiation factor in an inflammatory site. In: Oppenheim J, Cohen S (eds) Interleukins, lymphokines and cytokines. Academic, New York
23. Rodrick ML, Wood JJ, O'Mahony JB, Davis CF, Grbic JT, Demling RH, Moss NM, Saporoschetz I, Jordan A, D'Eon P, Mannick JA (1986) Mechanisms of immunosuppression associated with severe nonthermal traumatic injuries in man: production of interleukin 1 and 2. J Clin Immunol 6:310–318
24. Lloyd AR, Oppenheim JJ (1992) The Poly's lament: the neglected role of the polymorphonuclear neutrophil in the afferent limb of the immune response. Immunol Today 13:169–172
25. Goto K, Nakamura S, Goto F, Yoshinaga M (1984) Generation of an interleukin-1 like lymphocyte stimulating factor at inflammatory sites: correlation with the infiltration of polymorphonuclear leukocytes. Br J Exp Pathol 65:521–532
26. Tiku K, Tiku ML, Skoskey JL (1986) Interleukin-1 production by human polymorphonuclear neutrophils. J Immunol 136:3677–3685

27. Jack RM, Fearon DT (1988) Selective synthesis of mRNA and proteins by human peripheral blood neutrophils. J Immunol 140:4286–4293
28. Lindemann A, Reidel D, Oster W, Meuer SC, Dietmar B, Mertelsmann RH, Herrmann F (1984) Granulocyte/macrophage colony stimulating factor induces interleukin 1 production by human polymorphonuclear neutrophils. J Immunol 140:837–839
29. Lord PCW, Wilmoth LMG, Mizel SB, McCall CE (1991) Expression of interleukin-1α and β genes by human blood polymorphonuclear neutrophils. Am J Pathol 141:397–407
30. Yamazaki M, Ikenami M, Sugiyama T (1989) Cytotoxin from polymorphonuclear leukocytes and inflammatory ascitic fluids. Br J Cancer 59:353–355
31. Dubravec DB, Spriggs DR, Mannick JA, Rodrick ML (1990) Circulating human peripheral granulocytes synthesize and secrete tumor necrosis factor alpha. Proc Natl Acad Sci USA 87:6758–6761
32. Djeu JY, Serbousek D, Blanchard DK (1990) Release of tumor necrosis factor by human polymorphonuclear leukocytes. Blood 76:1405–1409
33. Klebanoff SJ, Vadas MA, Harlan JM, Sparks LH, Gamble JR, Agosti JM, Waltersdorph AM (1986) Stimulation of neutrophils by tumor necrosis factor. J Immunol 136:4220–4225
34. Bazzoni F, Cassatella MA, Laudanna C, Rossi F (1991) Phagocytosis of opsonized yeast induces tumor necrosis factor-alpha mRNA accumulation and protein release of its mature protein. J Leukoc Biol 5:223–228
35. Ichinose Y, Hara N, Ohta M, Aso H, Chikama H, Kawasaki M, Kubota I, Shimizu T, Yagawa K, (1990) Recombinant granulocyte colony-stimulating factor and lipopolysaccharide maintain the phenotype of and superoxide anion generation by neutrophils. Infect Immun 58:1647–1652
36. Cicco NA, Lindemann A, Content J, Vandenbussche P, Lubbery M, Gauss J, Mertelsmann R, Herrmann F (1990) Inducible production of interleukin-6 by human polymorphonuclear neutrophils: role of granulocyte-macrophage colony-stimulating factor and tumor necrosis factor-alpha. Blood 75:2049–2052
37. Henschler R, Lindemann A, Brach MA, Mackensen A, Mertelsmann RH, Hermann F (1991) Expression of functional receptors for interleukin-6 by human polymorphonuclear leukocytes. Downregulation by granulocyte-macrophage colony stimulating factor. FEBS Lett 283:47–51
38. Strieter RM, Kasahara K, Allen R, Showell HJ, Standiford TJ, Kunkel SL (1990) Human neutrophils exhibit disparate chemotactic factor gene expression. Biochem Biophys Res Commun 173:725–730
39. Meszaros K, Bojta J, Bautista AP, Lang CH, Spitzer JJ (1991) Glucose utilization by Kupffer cells, endothelial cells and granulocytes in endotoxemic rat liver. Am J Physiol 260:G7–G12
40. Buckle AM, Jayaram Y, Hogg N (1990) Colony-stimulating factors and interferon-gamma differentially affect cell surface molecules shared by monocytes and neutrophils. Clin Exp Immunol 81:339–345
41. Cobbold S, Hale G, Waldmann H (1987) Non-lineage, LFA-1 family and common leucocyte antigens: new and previously defined clusters. In: McMichael AJ, Beverley PCL, Cobbold S, Crumpton MJ, Gilks W, Gotch FM, Hogg N, Horton M, Ling N, MacLenan ICM, Mason DY, Milstein C, Spiegelhalter D, Waldmann H (eds) Leucocyte typing III. White cell differentiation antigens. Oxford University Press, Oxford, p 788
42. Griffin JD, Spertini O, Ernst TJ, Belvin MP, Levine HB, Kanakura K, Tedder TF (1990) Granulocyte-macrophage colony-stimulating factor and other cytokines regulate surface expression of the leucocyte adhesion molecule-1 on human neutrophils, monocytes and their precursors. J Immunol 145:576–584

43. Goldman DW, Goetzel EJ (1984) Heterogeneity of human polymorphonuclear leukocyte receptors for leukotriene B4: identification of a subset of high affinity receptors that transduce the chemotactic response. J Exp Med 159:1027–1041
44. Buyon JP, Shadick N, Berkman R, Hopkins P, Dalton J, Weissmann G, Winchester R, Abramson SB (1988) Surface expression of Gp 165/95, the complement receptor CR3, as a marker of disease activity in systemic Lupus erythematosus. Clin Immunol Immunopathol 46:141–149
45. Babcock GF, Alexander JW, Warden GD (1990) Flow cytometric analysis of neutrophil subsets in thermally injured patients developing infections. Clin Immunol Immunopathol 54:117–125
46. Fitzgerald JE, Sonis ST, Rodrick ML, Wilson RE (1983) Interaction of Ia antigen-bearing polymorphonuclear leukocytes and murine splenocytes. Inflammation 7:25–33
47. Lukacs K, Cohen DA, Kaplan AM (1986) HLA-Dr-unrestricted accessory cell function in human neutrophils. Clin Immunol Immunopathol 38:344–349
48. Sanchez-Madrid F, Nagy J, Robbins E, Simon P, Springer TA (1983) A human leucocyte differentiation antigen family with different alpha subunits and a common beta subunit: the lymphocyte function associated antigen (LFA-1) the C3bi complement receptor (OKM1, Mac-1) and the p150.95 molecule. J Exp Med 158:1785–1803
49. Moore FD Jr, Davis C, Rodrick ML, Fearon DT, Mannick JA (1987) Neutrophil activation after thermal injury as assessed by complement receptor upregulation. N Engl J Med 314:948–952
50. Davis CF, Moore FD Jr, Rodrick ML, Fearon DT, Mannick JA (1987) Neutrophil activation after burn injury: contributions of the classic complement pathway and of endotoxin. Surgery 102:477–484
51. Anderson DC, Springer TA (1987) Leucocyte adhesion deficiency: an inherited defect in the Mac-1, LFA-1 and p150,95 glycoproteins. Annu Rev Med 38:175–194
52. Fischer A, Seger R, Durandy A, Grospierre B, Virelizier JL, Le Deist F, Griscelli C, Fischer E, Kazatchkine M, Bohler MC et al. (1985) Deficiency of the adhesive protein complex lymphocyte function antigen 1, complement receptor type 3, glycoprotein p150.95 in a girl with recurrent bacterial infections. Effects on phagocytic cells and lymphocyte functions. J Clin Invest 76:2385–2892
53. Strieter RM, Kasahara K, Allen RM, Standiford TJ, Rolfe MW, Becker FS, Chensue SW, Kunkel SL (1992) Cytokine-induced neutrophil-derived interleukin-8. Am J Pathol 2:397–407

IL-6 Changes After Surgical Stress

M.L. Vuotto, A. Barbarisi, E. Bresciano, M. Fratta, M.T. Ielpo, M. Mosti, and D. Mancino

Some events, such as trauma, alter the physiological state of an organism, thus causing stress. Many studies show that there are early neuroendocrine immune changes involving the adrenal gland that cause increased glucocorticoid plasma levels and catecholamine release. This mechanism is unrelated to the nature or amount of stressful signals [1]. Glucocorticoids are immunosuppressive agents. They can modulate the immune response by acting directly on cells and/or indirectly on production and activity of various cytokines [1, 2].

The relationship between the immune system and the hypothalamic-pituitary-adrenal axis (HPA axis) is still unclear. Recently it has been suggested that some cytokines can play an important role as messengers between the immune and neuroendocrine systems. Cytokines may modulate secretion and activity of many hormones produced under stress. They probably act by stimulating the HPA axis through the release of corticotropin-releasing factor (CRF) [3, 4]. It is becoming increasingly clear that leukocytes, in response to an immune stimulus, can themselves produce neurohormones and neuropeptides such as enkephalins and endorphins.

Surgical stress modifies the immune response by suppressing specific and nonspecific components of host defense. Postoperative conditions have been compared to "acquired immunodeficiency." The magnitude of this phenomenon can be related to surgery complexity and duration. It has also been shown that serious trauma is followed by alterations in prostanoid synthesis and in cytokine secretion as well as by "stress hormone" plasma level increases. It seems that the changes in cytokine secretion could play a key role in the immunologic and metabolic state after surgical trauma. It is believed that many unfavorable post-traumatic conditions, such as extensive tissue damage, could depend on excessive or untimely cytokine release.

Many authors have observed increased secretion of TNF, IL-1, and IL-6 by macrophages in response to various injuries. In addition, it has been shown that plasma levels of these cytokines increase after major surgery, especially during sepsis, and there is a correlation between elevated cytokine levels and severity of infection [5–7].

In previous investigations we demonstrated that moderate surgical stress induces increased levels of human IL-1α and IL-1β in vitro in the early postoperative period [8, 9]. The aim of the present study was to evaluate the effects of mild surgery on IL-6 serum levels and its secretion by human monocytes in vitro.

Materials and Methods

Population

Thirty patients (15 men and 15 women; mean age 35 years) were included in the study. Informed consent was obtained and no remuneration was offered. All those with immune disease or recent blood transfusions and those who had regularly taken immune-modulating drugs or narcotics in the 6 months preceding the study were excluded, as were subjects with jaundice, excised spleen, recurrent or local infection, nutritional deficiency, metabolic disease, neoplasia, and liver or renal disease. The sera of all subjects were screened for anti-HIV antibodies and HBsAg.

After evaluating operative risk following ASA classification (with no one exceeding class I), patients had clean or clean-contaminated elective surgery with the same team [10]. Operations lasted no more than 120 min. Standardized general anesthesia was always used. No blood transfusions were given.

Second-generation cephalosporins were given. Blood was drawn prior to surgery (PreO) and on the 2nd and 7th postoperative (PO) days. Sera was stored at −20°C until used.

Monocyte Cultures

Mononuclear cells were taken from samples of peripheral blood by Ficoll-Paque fractioning (Pharmacia, Uppsala, Sweden). The isolated cells were washed three times with phosphate-buffered saline and then resuspended, at a final concentration of 2×10^6 cells/ml in RPMI 1640 complete medium (Flow Laboratories, Irvine, Scotland), containing 2.5% heat-inactivated fetal calf serum, 2 m*M* L-glutamine, and antibiotics. Aliquots of 1 ml cell suspensions were distributed into 24 sterile well dishes (Falcon, Oxnard, USA) and incubated at 37°C in 5% CO_2 in air. After 2 h the nonadherent cells were removed by washing with warm RPMI 1640 incomplete medium (without serum, glutamine, and antibiotics). Approximately 90% of the adherent cells (ACs) were esterase-positive and had the typical monocyte morphology after Giemsa staining. Their viability was evaluated by the trypan blue exclusion test.

IL-6 Production

The AC from each well were incubated for 24 h at 37°C in 5% CO_2 in air with 1 ml of RPMI 1640 complete medium with or without 20 μg/ml LPS

(*E. coli* O55:B55; Difco Laboratories, Detroit, Mich., USA). After incubation the supernatants were collected, centrifuged at 250 g for 10 min, and stored at −20°C until used.

Il-6 Assay

IL-6 levels in sera and in supernates of cells cultures were determined by RIA method. Results was expressed as pg/0.1 ml of IL-6.

Statistical Analysis

Results were evaluated by the Student's *t* test.

Results

Supernatants of human peripheral blood monocyte cultures, incubated without LPS, showed no significant increase in IL-6 levels.

LPS-stimulated monocytes markedly increased IL-6 secretion on PO2. IL-6 levels in the same cell culture conditions declined on PO7, but did not return to baseline (Table 1).

IL-6 serum levels remained almost unchanged on both the 2nd and 7th postoperative days (Table 2).

Conclusion

Surgical stress induces an early immune depression that seems to play a central role in producing various postoperative complications, such as slow wound healing, severe drug-resistant infections, and septic shock. There is also evidence that many unfavorable post-traumatic conditions are not due

Table 1. IL-6 supernatant levels of monocyte cultures from surgical patients

Days after surgery	IL-6 (pg/0.1 ml ± SD)	
	RPMI 1640	RPMI 1640 + LPS
0	32 ± 19	1495 ± 858
2	30 ± 15	2111 ± 778*
7	95 ± 79	1796 ± 384**

* $P < 0.05$ vs PreO
** $P < 0.05$ vs PO2

Table 2. IL-6 serum levels in surgical patients

Days after surgery	0	2	7
IL-6 (pg/0.1 ml ± SD)	14 ± 7	14 ± 5	17 ± 8

to an impaired host response. These could depend on an overwhelming response of combined biological systems and their mediators ("stress hormones" and cytokines) [11]. In consequence, an abnormal "neuroimmune hormone" secretion after surgical stress can mediate a large number of postoperative immunologic and metabolic disorders.

The increased IL-6 secretion in vitro by human LPS-activated monocytes appears to be a surgery-linked phenomenon.

The unchanged IL-6 plasma levels in the postoperative period may be due to increased or activated serum inhibiting factors, such as glucocorticoids and catecholamines. In addition, there may be a feedback loop between IL-6, CRF production, and glucocorticoid secretion in vivo, as shwon for IL-1. Finally, the constant postoperative IL-6 plasma levels may have been due to the positive clinical evolution of our patients.

References

1. Khansari DN, Murgo AJ, Faith RE (1990) Effects of stress on the immune system. Immunol Today 11:170–175
2. Bateman A, Singh A, Kral T, Solomon S (1989) The immune hypothalamic-pituitary-adrenal axis. Endocr Rev 10:92–112
3. Perlstein RS, Mougey EH, Jackson WE, Neta R (1991) Interleukin-1 and interleukin-6 act synergistically to stimulate the release of adrenocorticotropic hormone in vivo. Lymphokine Cytokine Res 10:141–146
4. Hooghe-Peters E, Velkeniers B, Vanhaelst L, Hooghe R (1991) Interleukin-1, interleukin-6: messengers in the neuroendocrine immune system? Pathol Res Pract 187:622–625
5. Marano MA, Fong Y, Moldawer LL, Wei H, Calvano SE, Tracey KJ, Barie PS, Manogue K, Cerami A, Shires GT, Lowery SF (1990) Serum cachetin/tumor necrosis factor in critically ill patients with burns correlates with infection and mortality. Surg Gynecol Obstet 170:32–38
6. Grzelak I, Olszewski WL, Rowinski W (1989) Blood mononuclear cell production of IL-1 and IL-2 following moderate surgical trauma. Eur Surg Res 21: 114–122
7. Guo Y, Dickerson C, Chrest FJ, Adler WH, Munster AM, Winchurch RA (1990) Increased levels of circulating interleukin-6 in burn patients. Clin Immunol Immunopathol 54:361–371
8. Vuotto ML, Bresciano E, Mancino D, Ielpo MT, Mosti M, De Martino G, Barbarisi A (1991) In vitro production and secretion of IL-1 by human monocytes after surgical trauma. In: Faist E, Meakins J, Schildberg FW (eds) Host defense dysfunction in trauma, shock and sepsis. Springer, Berlin Heidelberg New York, pp 651–654

9. Bresciano E, Barbarisi A, Gazzerro P, Ielpo MT, Mosti M, Vuotto ML (1992) Influenza dello stress chirurgico sulla secrezione in vitro di IL-1α e IL-1β da monociti umani. Surg Immunity 5:54
10. National Academy of Sciences-National Research Council, Division of Medical Sciences (1984) Ad hoc committee on trauma postoperative wound infections: the influence of ultraviolet irradiation of the operating room and various other factors. Ann Surg 160 Suppl [2]:1
11. Baue AE (1993) Progress in trauma care through understanding the cell biology of injury. In: Faist E, Meakins J, Schildberg FW (eds) Host defense dysfunction in trauma, shock and sepsis. Springer, Berlin Heidelberg New York, pp 3–13

Does Epidural Analgesia During Labor Alter Postpartum Maternal IL-6 Serum Levels?

R.F. De Jongh, M.J. Puylaert, W. Ombelet, H. Vandeput, R. Heylen, E. Bosmans, R. Berghmans, and H. Suzuki

Recent studies suggest that cytokines can participate in the pathophysiology of normal and abnormal pregnancy and parturition. Interleukin 6 (IL-6), an early and integral responder in the cascade of host mediators after injury, exerts multiple biological activities which comprise the induction of fever, the modulation of the synthesis of acute-phase proteins by the liver, activation of B and T lymphocytes, and the stimulation of hemopoietic progenitor and stem cells.

In our study, 20 patients received epidural analgesia with top-ups of 10 ml bupivacaine 0.125% with epinephrine 1/800 000 and 1 μg/ml sufentanyl (group epi). The epidural catheter was placed on the patients' demand. Patients without pain relief or pentazocine 30 mg IM formed the control group (group cont, $n = 31$).

Venous blood was obtained (1) after hospital admission, (2) just after parturition, (3) ±12 h postpartum, and (4) 24 h postpartum. Serum was stored at −20°C until IL-6 determination (ELISA). EDTA blood was used for leukocyte, platelet, and hematocrit investigations (Coulter counter).

The results of the study are shown in Figs. 1 and 2.

White cell count increased after parturition with a significant difference between the groups 12 h postpartum. Leukocyte demargination or release out of the bone marrow seems to be altered by the epidural analgesic technique.

IL-6 levels were increased postpartum and returned to normal after 24 h. Compared to the group cont, in the group epi IL-6 levels were 300% ($P < 0.001$) and 50% ($P < 0.05$) higher after parturition and 12 h postpartum respectively. IL-6 levels 24 h postpartum were correlated with IL-6 levels at admission, indicating that the modulating immunological processes were terminated. Maternal IL-6 levels just after delivery were correlated with the duration of labor, duration of oxytocin administration, anesthetic group, and number of previous abortions.

To explain these findings one must look for the *sources of IL-6* in maternal blood:

- Monocytes, macrophages, endometrial stroma cells, and fibroblasts
- IL-6 in amniotic fluid (amniotic-maternal blood barrier, 200 pg/ml before labor to 800 pg/ml during labor)

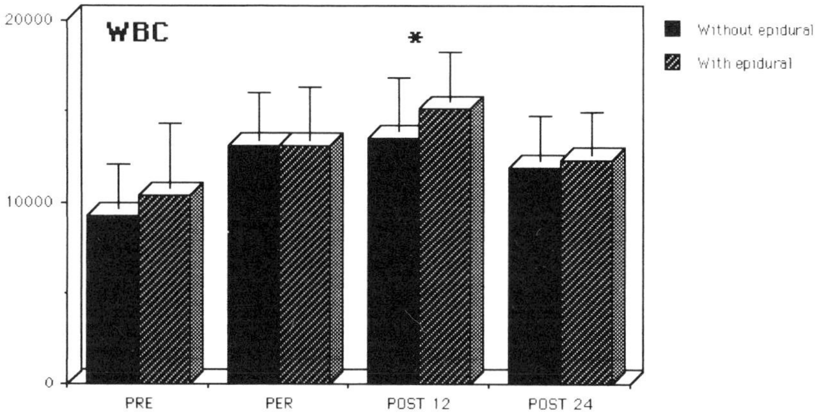

Fig. 1. Maternal white blood cell count (*WBC*) at time of admission (*pre*), just after delivery (*per*), 12 h postpartum (*post 12*), and 24 h postpartum (*post 24*). *Asterisk* denotes significant difference at $P \leqslant 0.05$

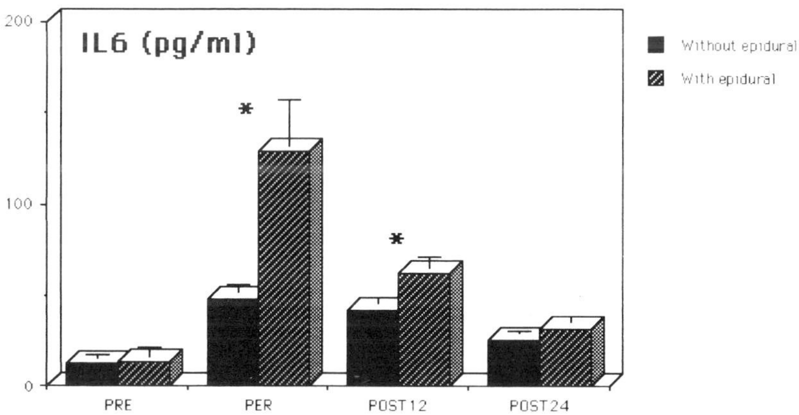

Fig. 2. Maternal IL-6 at time of admission (*pre*), just after delivery (*per*), 12 h postpartum (*post 12*), and 24 h postpartum (*post 24*). *Asterisks* denote significant differences at $P \leqslant 0.05$

- Activated smooth muscles (uterine contractility?)
- Cervical ripening with polymorphonuclear cell activation and destruction of connective tissue
- Endotoxin production following microbial invasion into the uterus
- Hormonal changes that influence the production of several cytokines (neuroendocrine-immunological interaction, central or peripheral level)

Immunological stress measured by serum IL-6 levels seemed to be altered by *epidural analgesia*. Explanations for this finding include biases in the study design, and direct and indirect effects of the epidural analgesic technique on the maternal immunological and hormone system.

1. *Bias*: The study was not randomized or blinded. Epidural analgesia was given on patient demand. The duration of labor and the duration of oxytocin administration were longer in this group. Moreover it is possible that oxytocin stimulation was augmented after pain relief. Patients who required epidural analgesia probably had lower stress and pain thresholds or different serum hormone levels.

2. *Direct effects*: Bupivacaine stimulates uterine contractility; however, blood levels of this drug were extremely low using 0.125% of this local anesthetic in the epidural space. All patients with epidural analgesia received at least 1 l Ringer's lactate to maintain stable hemodynamics, inducing moderate hemodilution. Sympathetic output and, to a lesser degree, parasympathetic output are decreased by epidural techniques. This can influence the contractions of the uterus. Moreover changes in uterine vascular resistance can influence the "wash out" of IL-6.

3. *Indirect effects*: Epinephrine and cortisol can suppress IL-6 production. Blood levels of both hormones were found to be lower in patients with epidural pain relief. In contrast, estrogens, known to be potent inhibitors of IL-6 production, were significantly higher in the epidural-treated women.

It is concluded that labor induces immunological activation, or the immune system plays a key role in inducing labor. Epidural analgesia, prolonged labor, and prolonged oxytocin stimulation seem to stimulate IL-6 production. Maternal IL-6 blood levels tend to normalize after 24 h.

References

Cruickshank AM, Fraser WD, Burns HJ et al. (1990) Response of serum interleukin-6 in patients undergoing elective surgery of varying severity. Clin Sci 79:161

Heinrich PC, Castell JV, Andus T (1990) Interleukin-6 and the acute phase response. Biochem J 265:621–636

Vinatier D, Tiffet O, Dufour P et al. (1992) Cytokines et grossesse: physiologie. J Gynecol Obstet Biol Reprod (Paris) 21:535-543

The Effect of Epidural Analgesia During Labor on the Immune System. Part 2. Neonatal Blood IL-6 Levels

M.J. Puylaert, R.F. De Jongh, W. Ombelet, H. Vandeput, R. Heylen, E. Bosmans, R. Bergmans, and H. Suzuki

Birth is a stressful event for the child. A lot of physiological changes happen during the early extrauterine period to make an independent existence possible. He must breathe air, change his circulatory pattern, maintain his body temperature, limit the invasion of microorganisms, ingest, digest, and assimilate food for activity and growth, provide new routes for excretion of metabolic end products, restrict the hemorrhage of trauma, and expand his hematopoietic system. In these processes, cytokines might play an important role.

IL-6 is a pleiotropic cytokine which plays an important role in host defense against stress and infection. Together with IL-3, granulocyte-macrophage colony-stimulating factor, and erythropoietin, IL-6 belongs to the factors that control granulopoiesis, monocytopoiesis, and erythropoiesis [3–5, 7, 8, 10, 11].

In fetal life, IL-6 induces the active cycling and expansion of hematopoietic progenitor cells, granulocytes, and monocytes. Here GM-CSF seems to play a minor role [4, 7]. After birth, abnormalities of plasma cytokines including IL-6 may contribute to increased susceptibility to infection in neonates [10]. Measurement of cytokine levels may be useful to predict the neonatal course and outcome and to reflect the perinatal stress.

We investigated whether the type of analgesia given to the mother in the peripartal period influenced the plasma IL-6 level of the child. Cord blood samples were obtained from 51 neonates with a gestational age between 37 and 41 weeks at the time of delivery. None of the children or the mothers showed infectious complications. All mothers had a vaginal delivery. Epidural analgesia (intermittent bupivacaïne 0.125% with epinephrine and $1\,\mu$g/ml sufentanil) was administered on request to 20 patients. The second group of mother ($n = 31$) received no pain relief or an intramuscular injection with 30 mg pentazocine. The protocol was approved by the local ethics cmmittee.

Table 1 shows the characteristics of the neonates. Cord blood samples were placed in pyrogen-free dry test tubes. Serum and blood cells were separated at 4°C (5 min, 1000 *g*) and kept frozen at −20°C. IL-6 was determined with the ELISA method.

Table 1. Characteristics of neonates

Weight (mean)	No		3339 g
	Epi		3346 g
Sex/weight	No	F	3387 g
		M	3298 g
	Epi	F	3358 g
		M	3338 g
Placental weight	No	F	620 g
		M	625 g
	Epi	F	745 g
		M	681 g
Induction	19/51, among whom 11 mothers received an epidural catheter		

No, No pain relief or i.m. pentazocine; Epi, epidural analgesia

Results

No significant difference could be found between the neonates in terms of body weight, sex vs body weight ratio, or placental weight.

Serum Cytokines and Type of Delivery. No significant difference was found between IL-6 levels in the blood of neonates of mothers who received epidural analgesia during delivery and IL-6 levels in the blood of neonates of mothers who did not receive such analgesia. However, a 300% increase in IL-6 levels was seen in maternal blood postdelivery. The levels were markedly higher in mothers who had received epidural analgesia than in those who had not: 45.55 + 26.89 pg/ml (mean + SEM) vs 18.25 + 3.83 ($P = 0.11$, unpaired t test).

Serum Cytokines of the Neonate/Mother. Stepwise regression analysis showed that 43% of the difference in neonatal IL-6 levels was accounted for by the maternal IL-6 level upon admission to the hospital and after delivery (relationship between predelivery maternal level and neonatal level: $P = 0.001$; relationship between perdelivery maternal level and neonatal level: $P = 0.013$).

Serum Cytokines of the Neonate and Amniotic Fluid IL-6 Level. The level of IL-6 in the amniotic fluid was found, on the basis of stepwise regression analysis, to have no predictive value for the IL-6 level of the neonate.

Discussion

Although the difference was not significant, IL-6 levels were higher in neonates of mothers who received epidural analgesia. However, the difference was much more marked within the maternal group. Our findings indicate that there is a partial barrier to IL-6 delivery through the placenta. Since all of our pregnancies were at term, we may conclude that the children all had a normal ability to produce IL-6 of their own [4, 5, 10].

In amniotic fluid, maternal and fetal macrophages are found during infection, both of which can be responsible for the increase in IL-6 during infection. No statistical correlation could be found between the amniotic and neonatal IL-6 [9, 11]. Since we had 51 normal noninfectious pregnancies, we assume that the IL-6 found in the amniotic fluid is mainly maternally produced due to the labor, although further investigation is necessary.

The epidural anesthesia as we provided it to the mothers dose not alter the umbilical blood flow. Thus the difference in IL-6 between maternal and neonatal blood was not induced by an impaired blood flow [1, 6, 12].

From this study we may conclude that the type of anesthesia given to the mother does not change the outcome for the child. Possibly the IL-6 level of the mother on admission to the hospital could be of predictive value for the child's IL-6 level and thereby his outcome. A lot of questions still remain, such as the effects of premature labor and infection, and a lot of work still needs to be done.

References

1. Albright GA, Jouppila R, Hollmén A et al. (1981) Epinephrine does not alter human intervillous blood flow during epidural anesthesia. Anesthesiology 54(2): 131–135
2. Dudley DJ, Trautman MS, Araneo BA et al. (1992) Decidual cell biosynthesis of interleukin-6 regulation by inflammatory cytokines. J Clin Endocrivol Metab 74(4):884–889
3. Gardner JD, Liechty KW, Christenses RD (1990) Effect of interleukin-6 on fetal hematopoietic progenitors. Blood 75(11):2150–2155
4. Liechty KW, Christensen RD (1990) In vivo effect of interleukin-6 on cycling status of haematopoietic progenitors from adults and neonates. Pediatr Res 28(4):323–326
5. Liechty KW, Koenig JM, Mitchell MD et al. (1991) Production of interleukin-6 by fetal and maternal cells in vivo during intraamniotic infection and in vitro after stimulation with interleukin 1. Pediatr Res 29(1):1–4
6. Marx FG, Patel S, Berman JA et al. (1986) Umbilical blood flow velocity waveforms in different maternal positions and with epidural analgesia. Obstet Gynecol 68(1):61–64
7. Meister B, Herold M, Mayr A et al. (1993) Interleukin-3, interleukin-6, granulocyte-macrophage colony-stimulating factor and erythropoietin cord blood levels of preterm and term neonates. Eur J Pediatr 152:569–573
8. Miller LC, Isa S, LoPreste G et al. (1990) Neonatal interleukin-1B, interleukin-6, and tumor necrosis factor: cord blood levels and cellular production. J Pediatr 117(6):961–965
9. Romero R, Avila C, Santhanam U, Sehgai PB (1990) Amniotic fluid interleukin 6 in preterm labor. J Clin Invest 85:1392–1400
10. Schibler KR, Liechty KW, Whithe WL et al. (1992) Defective production of interleukin-6 by monocytes: a possible mechanism underlying several host defense deficiencies of neonates. Pediatr Res 31(1):18–21

11. Santhanam U, Avila C, Romero R et al. (1991) Cytokines in normal and abnormal parturition elevated amniotic fluid interleukin-6 levels in women with premature rupture of membranes associated with intrauterine infection. Cytokine 3(2):155–163
12. Smedstad KG (1989) Controversies in obstetric anaesthesia. Can J Anaesth 36(3):S20–S25

Risk Factors

Risk Factors for the Development of Surgical Infection

E.W. TAYLOR

Every operation in surgery is an experiment in bacteriology.
Lord Moynihan

Infection is the most common post-operative complication and over half the patients who die on surgical wards die of infective complications. Many of the invasive procedures we use to assist in the management of patients are associated with infection and the recent EPIC study of the risk of nosocomial infections in intensive care units has shown that intravenous, central venous and arterial pressure lines, urinary catheters, endotracheal intubation and mechanically assisted ventilation are all associated with a high incidence of infection [1].

The probability of a patient developing infection is proportional to the bacterial contamination which occurs at operation and to the competence of the immune system of that patient to resist the contamination. Risk factors for infection can be divided into those related to the contamination, which could be considered exogenous factors, and those associated with the host resistance, i.e., endogenous risk factors.

Bacterial contamination itself may be exogenous or endogenous when the contamination occurs from an external source or from the bacteria already colonizing the patient. Many of the factors associated with protecting the patient from exogenous contamination such as the use of theatre overshoes [2], gloves [3], masks [4], head gear [5], wound dressings [6], etc. are of little proven value yet have entered the mythology of the operating theatre. Increasingly such measures are seen as protective of the health care staff against blood-borne diseases rather than protective of the patient [7].

Many factors in the preparation of the patient before surgery influence the risk of post-operative infection. The operation should be through an area of skin free from infective lesions and the skin should be adequately prepared. Shaving offers little other than aesthetic benefit but if done is best done in the immediate pre-operative period [8]. Where the colon is to be opened at operation controversy continues to exist as to whether pre-operative oral antibiotics in addition to parenteral perioperative prophylaxis are of value or not. In a recent study in the author's unit ciprofloxacin was given orally on the pre-operative day to remove the gram-negative aerobic bacilli from the gut – a form of selective decontamination, with considerable reduction in the incidence of wound infection, intra-abdominal abscess and septicaemia [9].

The use of wound and intra-peritoneal drains continues to be controversial but there is increasing evidence that their use is associated with a higher incidence of post-operative infection [10, 11]. The drain may provide a portal of entry for bacteria and the material of the drain may act as a foreign body in the tissues, reducing immunocompetance.

An early return to enteral nutrition in the immediate post-operative period may be associated with a lower incidence of wound infection, intra-abdominal abscess formation and other infective complications [12]. In addition early nutrition may prevent villous atrophy of the intestinal mucosa, reduce the incidence of bacterial translocation and lead to a more rapid return of gastro-intestinal function.

There is substantial evidence that, as the level of bacterial contamination of the wound increases, be that contamination of exogenous or endogenous origin, so the incidence of post-operative infection also increases [13]. This has led to the standard classification of wounds into clean, clean contaminated, contaminated and dirty [8].

Host resistance is the other main determinant of the incidence of post-operative infection and evidence has accumulated in the last few years that blood transfusion, particularly whole blood, is a suppressor of immune competence [14, 15]. Similarly, a prolonged pre-operative in-patient stay and the presence of remote infection at the time of operation are associated with an increased incidence of post-operative infection [16]. The patient's overall fitness for anaesthesia is a reflection of their ability to resist bacterial contamination and the American Society of Anesthesiology grading is a good indicator of the risk posed by the patient's underlying condition.

Hayley [17] assessed 75 potential risk factors for predicting post-operative infection and found that, by a process of co-linearity, these could be reduced to four: an abdominal operation, an operation lasting more than 2 h, operations classified as contaminated or dirty, and patients who had

Table 1. Percentage incidence of infection comparing traditional wound classification with a multivariate risk index in 59 352 randomly selected hospitalized patients. [Source: Haley RW (1991) Nosocomial infections in surgical patients: developing valid measures of intrinsic patient risk. Am J Med 91 (Suppl 3B): 1455–1515]

Wound classification	Simplified risk index (no. of risk factors)				
	Low	Medium	High		
	0	1	2	3	4
Clean	1.1	3.9	8.4	15.8	–
Clean contaminated	0.6	2.8	8.4	17.7	–
Contaminated	–	4.5	8.3	11.0	23.9
Dirty		6.7	10.9	18.8	27.4

three or more concomitant diagnoses. Cross-tabulating the incidence of these risk factors with the standard classification of clean, clean contaminated, contaminated and dirty in a cohort of 58 498 patients showed that the risk index may be a more important assessment of risk than the standard contamination classification (Table 1).

Culver et al. [18] confirmed these findings in a further 84 961 patients and have refined the risk factors to three: an ASA grade of 3, 4 or 5; an operation classified as contaminated or dirty; and duration of the operation greater than *T* hours, where *T* is specific to each operation.

An assessment of the risk posed by the procedure performed and by the individual patient is essential whenever audit or trials are undertaken in which post-operative infection is the end point in the assessment of any aspect of patient care, or of the efficacy of antibiotic prophylaxis or therapy.

References

1. Rennie MJ (1993) EPIC: infection in intensive care in Europe. Br J Intensive Care 3:27–36
2. Humphreys H, Marshall RJ, Ricketts VE, Russell, Reeves DS (1991) Theatre over-shoes do not reduce operating theatre floor bacterial counts. J Hosp Infect 17:117–23.
3. Dodds RDA, Guy PJ, Peacock AM, Duffy SR, Barker SGE, Thomas MH (1988) Surgical glove perforation. Br J Surg 75:966–968
4. Gunevall TG (1991) Post-operative wound infections and surgical face masks: a controlled study. World J Surg 15:383–388
5. Humphreys H, Russell AJ, Marshall RJ, Ricketts VE, Reeves DS (1991) The effect of surgical theatre head-gear on air bacterial counts. J Hosp Infect 19: 175–181
6. Chrintz H, Vibits H, Corditz TO, Harreby JS, Waaddegaard P, Larsen SO (1989) Need for surgical wound dressing. Br J Surg 76:204–205
7. Shanson DC, Taylor EW, Gill ON, Hughes SPF, Speller DCE, Chisholm GD, Emmerson AE (1992) Risk to surgeons and patients from HIV and hepatitis: guidelines on precautions and management of exposure to blood or body fluids. Br Med J 305:1337–1343
8. Cruse PJE (1992) Classification of operations and audit of infection. In: Taylor EW (ed) Infection in surgical practice, Oxford University Press, Oxford
9. Taylor EW, Lindsay G, the West of Scotland Surgical Infection Study Group (1994) Selective decontamination of the colon before elective colorectal operations. World J Surg (in press)
10. Simchen E, Rozin R, Way Y (1990) The Israeli study of surgical infection of drains and the risk of wound infection in operations for hernia. Surg Gynecol Obstet 170:331–337
11. Rao GN (1988) Predictive factors in local sepsis after splenectomy for trauma in adults. J R Coll Surg Edinb 33:68–70
12. Kudsk KA, Croce MA, Fabian TC, Minard G, Tolley EA, Poret HA et al. (1992) Enteral versus parenteral feeding. Effects on septic morbidity after blunt and penetrating abdominal trauma. Ann Surg 215:502–511
13. Raahave D, Friis-Moller A, Bjerre-Jepsen K, Thiis-Knudsen J, Rasmussen LB (1986) The infective dose of aerobic and anaerobic bacteria in post-operative wound sepsis. Arch Surg 121:924–929

14. Tartter PI (1989) Blood transfusion and post-operative infections. Transfusion 29:456–459
15. Jensen LS, Anderson A, Fristrup SC, Holme JB, Hrid HM, Kraglund K et al. (1990) Comparison of one dose versus three doses of prophylactic antibiotics, and the influence of blood transfusion, on infectious complications in acute and elective colorectal surgery. Br J Surg 77:513–518
16. Garibaldi RA, Cushing D, Lerer T (1991) Risk factors for post-operative infection. Ann J Surg 91 [Suppl 3B]:158–163
17. Haley RW (1991) Nosocomial infections in surgical patients: developing valid measures of intrinsic patient risk. Am J Med 91 [Suppl 3B]:145–151
18. Culver DH, Horan TC, Gaynes RP, Martone WJ, Jarvis WR, Emori TG et al. (1991) Surgical wound infection rates by wound class, operative procedure and patient risk index. Am J Med 91 [Suppl 3B]:152–157

Anergy and Postoperative Septic Complications

M. CAINZOS, J.A. ALCALDE, M. BUSTAMANTE, J. POTEL, and J.L. PUENTE

Introduction

In the last 15 years a number of studies have demonstrated that patients exhibiting preoperative disturbances of delayed hypersensitivity response are at increased risk for developing major septic complications during the postoperative period [1–11].

The strength of the correlation between anergy and major postoperative sepsis has been increasingly recognized since the mid-seventies, and is now accepted by most surgeons. This is due in part to the standardization of the skin test methodology.

The aim of this study was to evaluate the relationship between anergy and the development of postoperative septic complications in patients undergoing surgery for intra- and extra-abdominal pathology.

Patients and Methods

A prospective study was carried out over a 5-year period (1984–89) on 1201 subjects: 929 patients and 272 controls.

The control group comprised 272 individuals (136 men, 136 women), in good general health and with no history of weight loss or drug treatment. The age of the subjects ranged from 21 to 92 years (mean + SD: 51.9 + 19.8 years).

The surgical group consisted of 929 patients (526 men, 403 women) ranging in age from 14 to 91 years (mean + SD: 59.1 + 22.4 years). These patients were admitted for elective general and gastrointestinal surgery. Patients were included in the study only if they had been free of preoperative septic complications, except for patients with Crohn's disease or ulcerative colitis . With the exception of those patients with ulcerative colitis or Crohn's disease the study participants had not received previous treatment with corticosteroids, radiotherapy, or chemotherapy and had undergone no other surgery in the 3 months prior to the operation.

Multitest IMC was used to assess delayed hypersensitivity. This instant multipuncture kit consists of an acrylic device bearing eight heads, seven of which contain 0.03 ml of each of the following antigens: tetanus, 550 000

Merieux units (MU)/ml; diphtheria, 1100000 MU/ml; *Streptococcus* (group C), 2000 MU/ml; tuberculin, 300000 IU/ml; *Candida*, 2000 MU/ml; *Tricophyton*, 150 MU/ml; and *Proteus mirabilis*, 150 MU/ml. The eighth head, which contains a 70% weight/volume glycerol solution, is a control.

Antigens were injected into the volar aspect of the forearm and results read at 48 h. A positive response was defined as a cutaneous papule with a mean diameter of 2 mm or more. On the basis of the results of the skin test and age, patients were segregated into three groups (immunocompetent, relatively anergic, and anergic). Patients less than 70 years of age were considered immunocompetent (IC) or normergic with a mean papule diameter of more than 10 mm in males and more than 5 mm in females, relatively anergic (RA) or hypoergic with a mean papule diameter of 2–5 mm in females and 2–10 mm in males, or anergic when there was no response or when papule diameter was less than 2 mm for all antigens. Patients more than 70 years of age (whether male of female) were considered immunocompetent (IC) with a mean papule diameter of 5 mm or more, relatively anergic (RA) with a mean papule diameter between 2 and 4 mm, or anergic (A) when there was no response or when the papule diameter was less than 2 mm for all antigens. All patients were admitted to hospital at least 2 days prior to the operation.

The surgical procedures were classified in to four groups in order of increasing seriousness and risk [12]: group I, herniorrhaphy, exploratory laparotomy, etc; group II, cholecystectomy, mastectomy, etc: group III, partial gastrectomy, hemicolectomy, etc: and group IV, esophagectomy, hepatectomy, Puestow's procedure, etc.

Prophylactic antibiotics were administered to patients with gastric cancer and to those undergoing colorectal and biliary surgery with a high risk of developing infection (more than 60 years of age, jaundice, and obstruction of the biliary tract).

The patients were monitored daily for clinical signs of septic complications during the postoperative period and, on an ambulatory basis, for 4 weeks after discharge. Major sepsis was defined as intra-abdominal abscess, bacteremia, lung infection, anastomotic fistula, septic shock, and death from sepsis. Wound infections were viewed as minor septic events. Intra-abdominal abscess was detected during surgery, on autopsy, or after percutaneous drainage and was confirmed by culture. Bacteremia was defined as fever with repeatedly positive blood cultures. Lung infection was defined as fever with pulmonary infiltrate visible in roentgenograms and requiring antibiotic therapy. Anastomotic fistula was detected radiologically. Wound infection was defined as pus in the surgical wound requiring drainage.

Statistical analysis was carried out with the chi-squared test with Yate's correction. P values equal to or less than 0.05 were considered significant.

Table 1. Delayed hypersensitivity test: results

	Control group (n = 272)	Patient group (n = 929)	χ^2	P
Immunocompetent (IC)	194 (71.3%)	483 (51.9%)	32.45	<0.001
Relative anergy (RA)	52 (19.1%)	257 (27.7%)	8.03	<0.01
Anergy (A)	26 (9.6%)	189 (20.3%)	17.03	<0.001
RA + A	78 (28.7%)	446 (48.0%)	32.45	<0.001

Table 2. Patients not undergoing surgery: diagnoses

Carcinoma of the thyroid	1
Benign thyroid pathology	2
Breast cancer	1
Hernias	2
Cancer of the esophagus	12
Benign pathology of the esophagus	2
Cancer of the stomach	3
Gastroduodenal ulcer	2
Benign pathology of the stomach	2
Cancer of the gastrointestinal tract	3
Benign pathology of the small intestine	1
Cancer of the colon and rectum	5
Benign pathology of the colon/rectum	16
Extrahepatic biliary lithiasis	30
Cancer of the liver and biliary tree	2
Benign pathology of the liver	3
Portal hypertension	3
Cancer of the pancreas	7
Benign pathology of the pancreas	5
Retroperitoneal tumors	1
Other	8
	112

Results

There were significant differences between controls and patients in the proportion of subjects assigned to each group (IC, RA, and A) (Table 1)

Of the 929 patients studied, 112 did not undergo surgery. Forty were classified as immunocompetent, 36 as relatively anergic, and 36 as anergic. Table 2 shows the clinical diagnoses of these patients. The 40 patients classed as immunocompetent were discharged without septic complications, but five (13.9%) of the anergic and one of the relatively anergic patients developed major sepsis and shock, and five of these six patients died (Table 3).

Eight hundred and seventeen patients underwent surgery. Table 4 shows the clinical diagnoses for this group. Skin testing indicated immuno-

Table 3. Patients not undergoing surgery: clinical outcome

Immunocompetent (IC) $n = 40$	40 (100%)	Discharged without septic complications
Relative anergy (RA) $n = 36$	35 (97.2%)	Discharged without septic complications
	1 (2.8%)	Septic shock and death
Anergy (A) $n = 36$	31 (86.1%)	Discharged without septic complications
	4 (11.1%)	Septic shock and death
	1 (2.8%)	Septic shock

IC vs A, $\chi^2 = 8.00$ $P < 0.01$

Table 4. Patients undergoing surgery: diagnoses

Patients with extra-abdominal pathology (n = *108*)	
Carcinoma of the thyroid	4
Benign thyroid pathology	28
Cancer of the parotid gland	5
Benign parotid gland pathology	1
Breast cancer	45
Benign breast pathology	2
Hernias	19
Other	4
Patients with intra-abdominal pathology (n = *709*)	
Cancer of the esophagus	33
Benign pathology of the esophagus	7
Cancer of the stomach	140
Gastroduodenal ulcer	34
Benign and malignant pathology of	6
gastrointestinal tract	109
Cancer of colon and rectum	
Benign pathology of colon/rectum	17
Extrahepatic biliary lithiasis	264
Cancer of liver and biliary tree	17
Benign pathology of the liver	9
Portal hypertension	7
Cancer of the pancreas	33
Benign pathology of the pancreas	23
Other malignant tumors	2
Other benign conditions	8

competence in 446 patients, relative anergy in 218, and anergy in 153. Table 5 shows the incidence of major septic complications during the postoperative period: with respect to both major septic complications alone and major septic complications plus wound infection, there were statistically significant differences between the IC and A groups. There were also statistically significant differences between the IC, RA, and A groups in bacteremia, septic shock, and death from sepsis (Table 6).

Table 5. Postoperative septic complications in patients undergoing surgery for intra- or extra-abdominal pathology ($n = 817$)

	Immunocompetent (IC)	Relatively anergic (RA)	Anergic (A)
Major septic Complications*	446/22 (4.9%)	218/22 (10.1%)	153/26 (16.9%)
Major septic complications plus wound infection**	446/62 (13.9%)	218/34 (15.6%)	153/33 (21.6%)

* IC vs RA, $\chi^2 = 7.16$ $P < 0.01$
IC vs A, $\chi^2 = 21.55$ $P < 0.0001$
** IC vs A, $\chi^2 = 5.34$ $P < 0.05$

Table 6. Types of postoperative septic complications recorded following surgery for intra- or extra-abdominal pathology

	Immunocompetent (IC)	Relatively anergic (RA)	Anergic (A)
Wound infection	31 (6.9%)	14 (6.4%)	7 (4.6%)
Intra-abdominal abscess	5 (1.1%)	3 (1.8%)	3 (1.3%)
Anastomotic fistula	2 (0.4%)	4 (1.8%)	2 (1.3%)
Lung infection	6 (1.3%)	2 (0.9%)	5 (3.3%)
Bacteremia*	2 (0.4%)	8 (3.7%)	4 (2.6%)
Septic shock**	2 (0.4%)	8 (3.7%)	9 (5.6%)
Death***	4 (0.9%)	9 (4.1%)	10 (6.5%)

* IC vs RA, $\chi^2 = 7.67$ $P < 0.01$
IC vs RA + A, $\chi^2 = 10.67$ $P < 0.01$
** IC vs RA, $\chi^2 = 12.06$ $P < 0.001$
IC vs A, $\chi^2 = 17.79$ $P < 0.0001$
*** IC vs RA, $\chi^2 = 5.70$ $P < 0.02$
IC vs A, $\chi^2 = 12.92$ $P < 0.001$

Among the 817 patients who were operated on, 108 presented extra-abdominal pathology, and in this group there was no significant difference between IC, RA, and A patients in the rate of major septic complications in the postoperative period (Table 7). Similarly, no significant differences were observed in the rate of wound infection.

Among the 709 patients presenting with intra-abdominal pathology there were significant differences in the rate of major postoperative septic complications between the IC and RA groups ($P < 0.05$), and between IC and A groups ($P < 0.0001$) (Table 8). There was also a significant difference between IC and A patients when major septic complications and wound

Table 7. Incidence of major septic complications in patients undergoing surgery for extra-abdominal pathology (n = 108)

	Number	Complications
Immunocompetent (IC)	71	0 (0.0%)
Relative anergy (RA)	22	0 (0.0%)
Anergy (A)	15	1 (6.7%)

P = NS

Table 8. Incidence of major septic complications in patients undergoing surgery for intra-abdominal pathology (n = 709)

	Number	Complications
Immunocompetent (IC)	375	22 (5.9%)
Relatively anergic (RA)	196	22 (11.2%)
Anergic (A)	138	25 (18.1%)

IC vs RA, χ^2 = 5.35 P<0.05
IC vs A, χ^2 = 16.87 P<0.0001

infection were considered together. The rate of major postoperative septic complications was 14.9% in the IC group and 22.5% in the A group (P < 0.05).

Of the 817 patients who underwent surgery, 101 were classified as group I for surgical risk, 393 as group II, 271 as group III, and 52 as group IV. In group I major septic complications were observed only in 1.9%, although major septic complications plus wound infection were observed in 8.9%. On the other hand, in group IV the rate of major septic complications was 34.6% and that of major septic complications plus wound infections, 46% (Table 9).

Table 10 shows the incidence of major septic complications in IC, RA, and A surgical patients in each of the surgical risk groups. Statistically significant differences were found between IC and A patients in both group II (P < 0.001) and group (P < 0.001).

Discussion

In recent years the increased use of multiple broad-spectrum antibiotics combined with the correct application of antibiotic prophylaxis has led to a significant reduction in rates of postoperative infection. Nevertheless, some patients still develop postoperative septic complications, and these complications often cause death. This suggests that exquisite surgical technique and

Table 9. Grade of surgical procedure and major postoperative septic complications (n = 817)

Grade of surgical procedure	Major septic complications	Major septic complications plus wound infections
I (n = 101)	2 (1.9%)*	9 (8.9%)**
II (n = 393)	18 (4.6%)*	41 (10.4%)**
III (n = 271)	32 (11.8%)*	55 (20.3%)**
IV (n = 52)	18 (34.6%)*	24 (46.2%)**

*I vs III, χ^2 = 8.88 $P < 0.01$
I vs IV, χ^2 = 63.75 $P < 0.0001$
II vs III, χ^2 = 12.96 $P < 0.001$
II vs IV, χ^2 = 59.74 $P < 0.0001$
III vs IV, χ^2 = 17.58 $P < 0.0001$
**I vs III, χ^2 = 6.16 $P < 0.02$
I vs IV, χ^2 = 29.29 $P < 0.0001$
II vs III, χ^2 = 12.91 $P < 0.001$
II vs IV, χ^2 = 43.06 $P < 0.0001$
III vs IV, χ^2 = 14.82 $P < 0.001$

Table 10. Grade of surgical procedure, delayed hypersensitivity response, and major postoperative septic complications

Grade	Immunocompetent	Relative anergy	Anergy
I (n = 101)	56/0 (0.0%)	29/1 (3.4%)	16/1 (6.2%)
II (n = 393)	228/5 (2.2%)	96/5 (5.2%)	69/8 (11.6%)
III (n = 271)	135/9 (6.7%)	74/9 (12.2%)	62/14 (22.6%)
IV (n = 52)	27/8 (29.6%)	19/7 (36.8%)	6/3 (50.0%)

II: IC vs A, χ^2 = 11.51, $P < 0.001$
IC vs RA + A, χ^2 = 5.98, $P < 0.02$
III: IC vs A, χ^2 = 11.36, $P < 0.001$
IC vs RA + A, χ^2 = 6.93, $P < 0.01$

antibiotic prophylaxis are not sufficient to prevent postoperative septic complications in some patients. Further studies are clearly needed to identify the risk factors associated with postsurgical complications.

The pioneering studies by the McGill group over the last 15 years have introduced the word "anergy" into the surgical lexicon and have shown the importance of preoperative disturbances of cell-mediated immunity in increasing the risk of developing major septic complications during the postoperative period. The early findings of this group were not initially accepted by other investigators in the field, due in part to their small sample size [13, 14]. The recent introduction of a homogeneous system to evaluate delayed hypersensitivity response (Multitest IMC) has allowed various authors to confirm the relationship between preoperative anergy and major postoperative sepsis.

We studied 929 patients who had undergone intra- and extra-abdominal general surgery. Our results confirm the correlation between anergy (or relative anergy) and postoperative sepsis. We also found that anergic patients who did not undergo surgery had a 14% risk of septic complications (septicemia via intravenous catheters or as a result of lung infection), in most cases (11%) leading to death.

Detailed analysis of our results suggests that anergy or relative anergy in patients who undergo extra-abdominal surgery does not significantly affect the risk of postoperative major sepsis. However, because most of these patients underwent group I surgery (the lowest in surgical risk), the importance of disturbances in cell-mediated immunity was also investigated in patients undergoing intra-abdominal (i.e., higher risk) surgery.

This analysis shows that anergic or relatively anergic patients undergoing high-risk intra-abdominal surgery (risk groups III and IV) are significantly more likely to develop postoperative major sepsis. This is in agreement with the results obtained by Scharckert et al. [10] and underlines the importance of environmental factors.

The importance of preoperative anergy appears to be clear to most surgeons who have studied large groups of patients. What remains to be resolved, is how best to help this subgroup of patients, which may represent up to 80% of jaundiced patients [15–17] and 56% of patients with gastric cancer [18]. Moesgaard and Lykkegaard-Nielsen [19] demonstrated that increasing the period of prophylactic antibiotic administration to anergic patients does not reduce the incidence of either major septic complications or death due to sepsis.

It is possible that the problem is in part associated with an increased polymorphonuclear leukocyte (PMN) adherence and decreased PMN chemotaxis [20–22]. But more recent studies (by the same authors [23, 24] do not confirm this view. Until the precise cause of anergy in these patients is better understood, it will be difficult to find a clinically effective treatment for anergy or to prevent the development of postoperative sepsis in anergic patients.

While we await new studies which may provide a key to the restoration of an adequate immunomodulatory system, it is clearly necessary to pay very careful attention to surgical antisepsis procedures for anergic patients.

In conclusion, the Multitest IMC is an appropriate method for assessing delayed hypersensitivity response in the surgical patient. Our results confirm those of Christou et al., who compared the conventional method of skin testing with the Multitest IMC [25].

References

1. MacLean LD, Meakins JL, Taguchi K et al. (1975) Host resistance in sepsis and trauma. Ann Surg 182:207–217
2. Meakins JL (1977) Host defense mechanisms: evaluation and roles of acquired defects and immunotherapy. Can J Surg 18:259–268
3. Pietsch JB, Meakins JL, MacLean LD (1977) The delayed hypersensitivity response: application and clinical surgery. Surgery 82:349–355
4. Christou NV, Meakins JL (1979) Delayed hypersensitivity in surgical patients: a mechanism for anergy. Surgery 86:78–85
5. Johnson WC, Ulrich F, Meguid MM et al. (1979) Role of delayed hypersensitivity in predicting preoperative morbidity and mortality. Am J Surg 137:536–542
6. Daly JM, Dudrick SJ, Copeland EM III (1980) Intravenous hyperalimentation. Effect of delayed cutaneous hypersensitivity in cancer patients. Ann Surg 192: 587–592
7. Heimann TM, Aufses AH Jr (1984) Surgical complications and skin test reactivity in patients with inflammatory bowel disease. Arch Surg 119:885–887
8. Revhaug A, Giercksky KE (1984) Preoperative cutaneous hypersensitivity reaction related to postoperative complications following elective surgery. Acta Chir Scand 150:279–283
9. Christou NV (1985) Host defense mechanisms in surgical patients: a correlative study of the delayed hypersensitivity skin test response, granulocyte function and sepsis in 2202 patients. Can J Surg 28:39–49
10. Scharckert HK, Betzler M, Zimmermann GE et al. (1986) The predictive role of delayed cutaneous hypersensitivity testing in postoperative complications. Surg Gynecol Obstet 162:563–568
11. Cainzos M, Potel J, Puente JL (1989) Correlation between anergy and postoperative sepsis in surgical patients. Value of multitest. Surg Res Commun 4:299–305
12. Christou NV, Rode H, Larsen D et al. (1984) The walk-in anergic patients. How best to assess the risk of sepsis following elective surgery. Ann Surg 119: 438–444
13. Brown R, Hamid J, Patel N et al. (1980) The delayed hypersensitivity response as a prediction of the outcome of surgical operation-dogma disputed. Br J Surg 67:368
14. Ausobsky JR, Bean P, Proctor J, Pollock AV (1982) Delayed hypersensitivity testing for the prediction of postoperative complications. Br J Surg 63:346–348
15. Cainzos M, Potel J, Puente JL (1988) Anergy in jaundiced patients. Br J Surg 75:147–149
16. Cainzos M, Potel J, Puente JL (1989) Anergy in patients with biliary lithiasis. Br J Surg 76:169–172
17. Cainzos M, Alcalde JA, Potel J, Puente JL (1990) Variations in the cellular immune response as a function of total bilirubin. Surg Res Commun 7:285–299
18. Cainzos M, Alcalde JA, Potel J, Puente JL (1989) Anergy in patients with gastric cancer. Hepatogastroenterology 36:36–39
19. Moesgaard F, Lykkegaard-Nielsen M (1989) Preoperative cell-mediated immunuty and duration of antibiotic prophylaxis in relation to postoperative infectious complications. A controlled trial in biliary, gastroduodenal and colorectal surgery. Acta Chir Scand 155:281–286
20. Christou NV, Meakins JL (1979) Neutrophil function in surgical patients: two inhibitors of granulocyte chemotaxis associated with sepsis. J Surg Res 26: 355–364

21. Christou NV, Meakins JL (1979) Neutrophil sunction in surgical patients: in vitro correction of abnormal neutrophil chemotaxis by levamisole. Surgery 85: 543–548
22. Meakins JL, Christou NV, Shizgal HM, MacLean LD (1979) Therapeutic approaches to anergy in surgical patients. Ann Surg 190:286–296
23. Christou NV, Tellado JM (1989) In vitro polymorphonuclear neutrophil function in surgical patients does not correlate with anergy but with "activating" processes such as sepsis or trauma. Surgery 106:718–724
24. Tellado JM, Giannias B, Kapadia B et al. (1990) Anergic patients before elective surgery have enhanced nonspecific hostdefense capacity. Arch Surg 125:49–53
25. Christou NV, Boisvert G, Broadhead M, Meakins JL (1985) Two techniques of measurement of the delayed hypersensitivity skin test response for the assessment of bacterial host resistance. World J Surg 9:798–806

The Relationship Between Platelet, Lymphocyte and Monocyte Counts, Sepsis and Survival in Polytrauma Patients

T. Mózes, T. Mészáros, J. Wille, and G. Berentey

Introduction

Trauma is frequently followed by septic complications, including adult respiratory distress syndrome (ARDS) and multiple organ failure, which remain major causes of morbidity and mortality [1, 2]. This clinical observation may lead to the conclusion that trauma induces decreased resistance to infection [3]. It seems that many of the immunological and inflammatory abnormalities noted after trauma may be due to the disturbance of monocyte-macrophage/lymphocyte interaction [3]. The resulting impairment of the host defence mechanism has its clinical correlate because there is enhanced susceptibility of trauma patients to infections. In our department 69% of the deaths after polytrauma were due to septic multiple organ failure in 1992. The aim of this study was to assess the importance of variations in levels of platelets, monocytes and lymphocytes in patients at risk of developing post-traumatic septic complications.

Materials and Methods

Thirty-eight patients sustaining severe trauma during a 1-year period between January and December 1992 were evaluated retrospectively in the Department of Traumatology, Semmelweis University of Medical Sciences, Budapest, Hungary. Patients were assigned an Injury Severity Score (ISS) using the method of Baker et al. [4].

Platelet, monocyte and lymphocyte counts were measured by a haematology analyser on the day of trauma and on days 1, 5, 10, 15 and 20 after trauma.

Statistical analysis. All values are expressed as means ± SEM. The data were evaluated by a non-parametric two-way analysis of variance (Friedman test) followed by the Wilcoxon-Wilcox test to identify differences between measurements performed on the day of trauma and at different times after trauma. The Mann-Whitney U test was performed to evaluate the differences between the groups. A P value of 0.05 or less was considered statistically significant for all tests.

Results

The characteristics of the survivors and non-survivors are presented in Table 1 and Fig. 1. There were no significant differences between groups with regard to age, sex and ISS. Mean ISS was 33 ± 2. Four of the severely injured patients died within 24 h of arrival in the department due to the combination of head, thoracic and abdominal injuries (ISS 62 ± 8). The remaining nine patients died due to sepsis, ARDS and multiple organ failure. Sepsis was defined using clinical evidebces of infection [5]. Of the 25 survivors of severe trauma, 12 had septic complications. Septic complications were defined as any form of localized inflammation and/or infection without generalized signs of infection like superficial and/or deep wound infection, bone infection (osteitis, osteomyelitis) etc.

All patients requiring surgical interventions received standard surgical care and postoperative intensive care unit treatment (early stabilization and mechanical ventilation).

Platelet count declined in 5 days after trauma in all three groups. In non-survivors it remained at sustained low levels. However, in survivors, independently of the quality of outcome, platelet count returned to a supranormal level in 10 days following severe trauma (Fig. 2).

Table 1. Characteristics of survivors and non-survivors

	Non-survivors	Survivors: septic	Survivors: non-septic
Age (yr)	48 ± 5	35 ± 5	39 ± 5
Sex	9 m; 4 f	8 m; 4 f	6 m; 7 f
Antibiotic	100%	100%	50%
Onset of sepsis (day)	2.9 ± 0.6	6.4 ± 1.2	–

m, Males; f, females

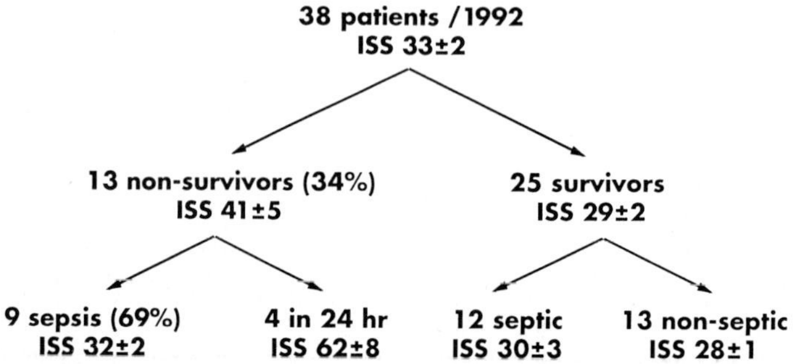

Fig. 1. Outcome in the 38 patients

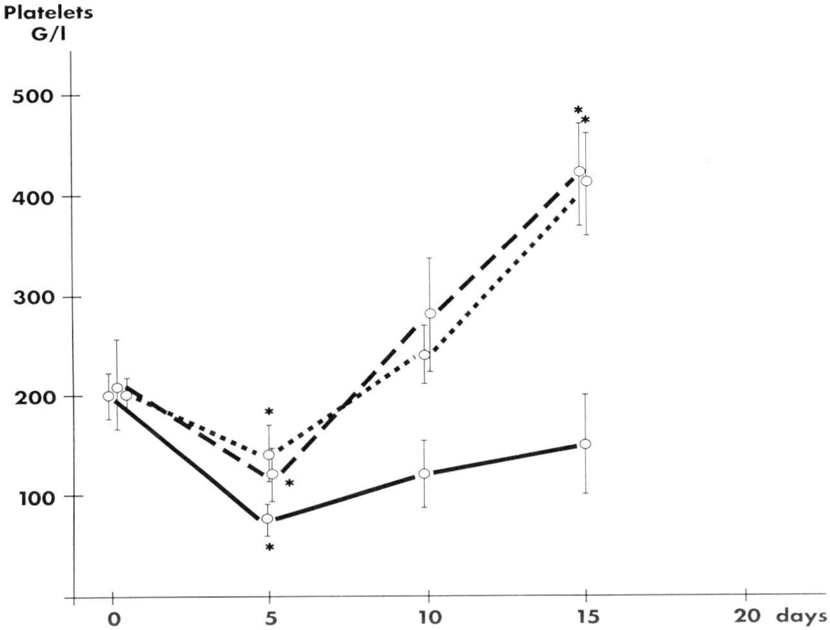

Fig. 2. Effect of severe trauma on the platelet count. *Solid line* indicates non-survivors; *interrupted line* indicates septic survivors; *dotted line* indicates non-septic survivors. *Asterisk* denotes significantly different from baseline values ($P < 0.05$)

Severe and sustained lymphopenia was found in non-survivors from the day of trauma until death. In survivors with septic complications a similarly severe lymphopenia also occurred; however, the lymphocyte count returned to baseline levels in 15 days following trauma. In survivors without any septic complications this improvement in lymphopenia occurred within 5 days after trauma (Fig. 3).

The monocyte count remained unchanged on the day of trauma in all three groups. In non-survivors there was a decrease in monocyte count, while a marked increase was observed at 5 days after trauma in non-septic survivors. In septic survivors this elevation in monocyte count occurred at 15 days following trauma (Fig. 4).

Discussion

Three different outcomes were observed in polytrauma patients treated in our department; non-survivors and survivors with and without septic complications. The occurrence of septic complications, including death due to sepsis, seems to be independent of the severity of trauma. No differences were observed in Injury Severity Score in regard of outcome. Platelet count

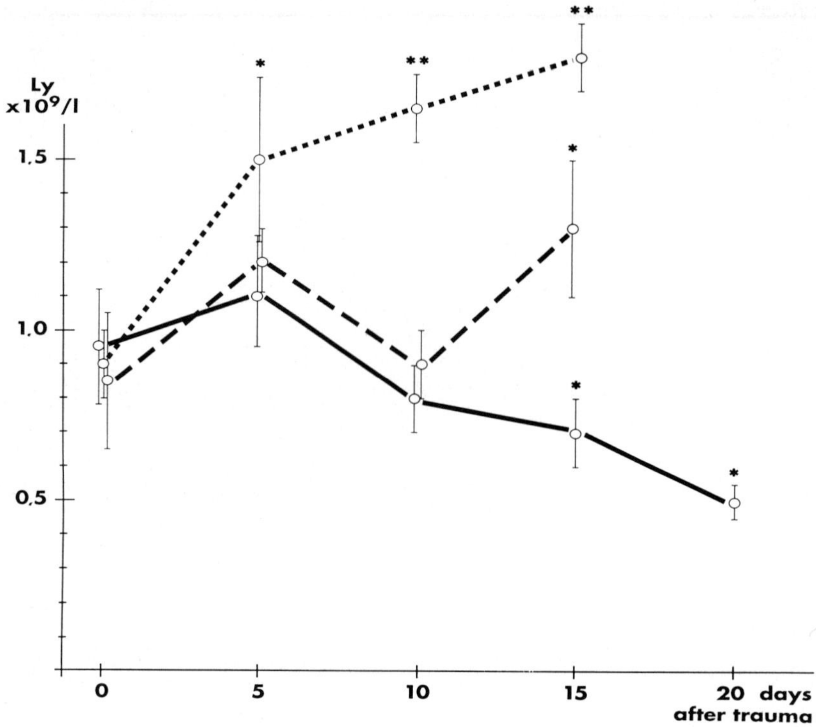

Fig. 3. Effect of severe trauma on lymphocyte (*Ly*) counts. Other details as for Fig. 2

may serve as a predictor of survival following severe trauma; however, it is not discriminative between septic and non-septic survivors. In this respect, lymphocyte and monocyte counts seem to be more relevant prognostic indicators of sepsis and death following severe injury.

The mechanisms behind thrombocytopenia and lymphocytopenia remained uncovered. Increased destruction or a decrease in production of these cells or both may be possible. Furthermore, it is also unclear whether the fall in the count of these cells is the cause or consequence of post-traumatic septic complications. Nevertheless, it has been demonstrated that the alteration of cell-mediated immunity following trauma is mainly due to the disruption of monocyte/lymphocyte interaction [3]. The trigger for the disturbance of monocyte function is not completely understood. Bacterial endotoxins, either leaking directly from the gut into the portal circulation or produced by intestinal bacteria translocated from the gut in response to injury and/or ischaemia, are well-known stimuli of monocytes [6]. However, tissue hypoxia on systemic or local levels, cellular destruction from ischaemia and trauma are also able to influence monocytes [6]. Taken together, it seems that independently of triggering mechanisms, septic complications,

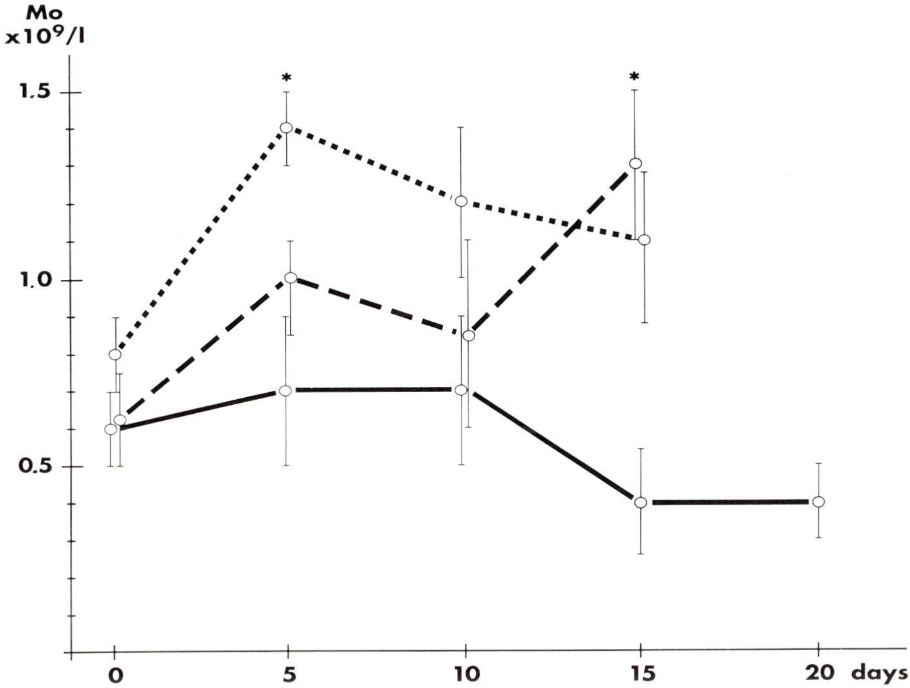

Fig. 4. Effect of severe trauma on monocyte (*Mo*) counts. Other details as for Fig. 2

including multiple organ failure, most probably result from interactions between monocytes and lymphocytes.

In summary, severe and sustained lymphopenia was found in non-survivors due to sepsis following severe trauma. In septic survivors lymphopenia recovered in 15 days after trauma, while in non-septic survivors this improvement occurred within 5 days following trauma.

References[1]

1. Faist E (1993)
2. Hoch RC (1993)
3. Ninnemann JL (1989)
4. Baker SP (1974)
5. Bone RC (1991)
6. Deitch EA (1992)

[1] References available from the author.

CD4+ Lymphocytes as a Prognostic Indicator of Surgical Infection in the Immunodepressed Patient

C. Emparan, V. Portugal, J.E. Bilbao, A. Apecechea,
J.A. Carnicero, I. Iturburu, and J. Mendez

Introduction

Surgical procedures on patients with severe immune deficiencies are increasing. The fact that an immunocompromised state is a major factor in the pathogenesis of infection makes it imperative that the clinician has an adequate working knowledge of the host's antibacterial defense systems and how they are affected by surgery.

Today, one of the most important groups undergoing surgical procedures are the HIV-infected patients. The number of seropositives is growing, and diagnostic and therapeutic procedures involving the surgeon are increasing. These patients have severe immune depression characterized by a progressive fall in the CD4+ lymphocyte population, which produces a well-known disease pattern characterized by the progressive onset of opportunistic infections and AIDS-related neoplasms, such as Kaposi's sarcoma and non-Hodgkin's lymphoma.

In order to elucidate the effects that such an immune status has on the environment of surgical infection, and the kind of wound infections that a decreased number of CD4+ lymphocytes would produce in patients undergoing surgical procedures, lymphocyte populations have been studied and correlations performed with the incidence of infection.

Patients and Methods

Seventy patients with HIV infection (91.4% of whom were intravenous drug abusers, 4.2% heterosexual contacts, and the other 4.2% homosexuals) underwent surgical biopsies for enlarged lymph nodes. Counts of the lymphocyte population (CD11+, CD4+, CD8+) and white blood cells (with neutrophils) were done prior to the lymph node biopsy. Surgery was performed in 90% with local anesthesia in the cervical (70%) or axillary zone (21%). The nodes were studied histologically and tissue cultures were done. Whenever wound infection was suspected, surgical drainage was performed and microbiological cultures done.

Based on previous studies the patients were classified into three different risk groups, depending on the number of CD4+ cells found in blood:

1. *Group A* ($n = 26$) was composed of patients with more than 500 cells per milliliter of blood. This group had a low incidence of AIDS-related diseases. The histological results of the lymph node examinations revealed follicular hyperplasia a stage in the progression of HIV infection known as progressive generalized lymphadenopathy. The neutrophil count averaged ca. 5100 cells/ml of blood ($\bar{x} = 5124$).

2. *Group B* ($n = 24$) was composed of those patients who had a CD4+ count of 200–500 cells. In southern Europe, this group presents AIDS-related infections. The results of lymph node biopsies revealed tuberculous adenitis, staged in the CDC classification as CDC-IV-C2. The neutrophil count in group B averaged ca. 3800 cells ($\bar{x} = 3.785$).

3. *Group C* ($n = 20$) comprised those patients who had a count of less than 200 CD4+ cells per milliliter of blood. This group of patients with severe immune deficiency usually show severe infections caused by opportunistic microbiological agents, and lymph node biopsies reveal AIDS-related neoplasms. In our experience the most common neoplasm found is Hodgkin's lymphoma. The prognosis of these patients is survival for less than 1 year. The neutrophil count was 2500 cells/ml, close to the normal values.

Results

The infection rate in the 70 patients was 5.71%, and in all the cases there was a positive correlation between the cultures obtained from the lymph node and the organism infecting the wound. In such cases the kind of surgery would not be classified as "clean surgery."

In group A there were two wound infections caused by *Staphylococcus aureus*. The microbiological culture of the lymph nodes biopsied also identified the same bacteria. This group of patients presented what we consider a "typical" wound infection, and the infection rate in the group was 7.69%. This percentage could be considered as close to the normal rate of wound infection in similar surgical procedures performed by our surgical team.

In group B there were no wound infections.

Group C presented two wound infections caused by *Mycobacterium tuberculosis*. The infection rate in this group was 10%. Both patients presented cold abscesses, released during the surgical procedure, and surgery was considered "dirty." The wound cultures also showed mycobacteria.

Statistical analysis revealed no significant differences between the three groups.

Discussion

CD4+ lymphocytes play a major role in the evolution of immune depression and clinical evolution in HIV-infected patient. In fact, the Walter-Reed staging classification attributes to the number of CD4+ cells a causal significance in the evolution to AIDS. In their experience there could be two different groups of patients: those who have more than 400 cells/ml of blood, and those who have less than 400.

As CD4+ cells play a major role in the extent of the cytotoxic response and in the suppression of the immune response to wound infection, we have selected a group of patients undergoing a homogeneous surgical procedure under local anesthesia which would not interfere with the immune response. The group comprised patients with a similar age (26 years), sex (80% males), and risk group (91.4% IVDUs); there were differences only in the CD4+ cell count and in the neutrophil count caused by the suppression of the activity of the lymphocyte population.

Even though immune defects do not occur in isolation, in our model it is easy to determine whether a particular abnormality is a primary event of clinical importance, and the decreased neutrophil count a secondary immune abnormality depending on the decreased rate of CD4+ lymphocytes and the subsequently increased suppressive response.

As wound infection is generally caused by extracellular bacteria, the immune response depends more on neutrophils than on lymphocytes. The most important effector cell recruited by the inflammatory response is the neutrophil, whose primary function is the detection, ingestion, and destruction of bacteria and fungi that have penetrated the local defenses and invaded viable tissue.

The response to intracellular bacteria such as *Mycobacterium tuberculosis* depends directly on lymphocytes, especially the CD4+ population. We have found "typical" wound infections in our group A, which is characterized by a reasonable immune level of CD4+ lymphocytes. This group presented what we can call a reasonable level of CD4+ cells and a neutrophil count close to 5100 cells/ml of blood. An infection rate of 5% with lymph node cultures positive for *Staphylococcus* and wound infections caused by the same bacteria can be considered a reasonable result for this kind of surgical procedure.

In group C, with a severe deficiency of CD4+ cells, we found a high incidence of "atypical" wound infections caused by *Mycobacterium tuberculosis*. As they presented a decreased rate of CD4+ cells, they had a neutrophil count lower than that found in group A. The incidence of wound infection was higher, but there was no statistically significant difference from the other groups, and this can be considered a good result if we take note that the lymph node biopsies were defined by the surgeon as drainage of a cold abscess.

Conclusions

The number of CD4+ lymphocytes in blood cannot be used as a prognostic indicator of wound infection by itself, but it does correlate with the incidence of opportunistic infections in patients undergoing lymph node biopsies. In patients with a low CD4+ count, decreased neutrophil counts are usual, and a high incidence of surgical infection can be anticipated. Nevertheless, in our experience, minor surgical procedures in patients with HIV infections do not have a high incidence of wound infection. Further study is required in patients undergoing major surgical procedures, because it is generally accepted that the extent of the injury is directly related to the magnitude of the immunosuppression.

Immunologic Monitoring in Patients with Glioma Treated Neurosurgically

A.G. Kaprelyan, N.M. Mincheva, K.T. Metodiev, D.M. Minchev, and D.S. Cholakov

About 50% of intracranial tumors derive from the brain parenchyma; most of these arise from the glia, preferentially from the astroglia (astrocytomas) and to a lesser extent from the oligodendrocytes (oligodendrogliomas). Gliomas are classified into four grades, each grade of tumor exerting a certain influence on overall immune reactivity. Grade I (pilocytic astrocytomas) and grade II (fibrillary, protoplasmatic, gemistocytic astrocytomas) are slow-growing tumors, whereas grade III (anaplastic astrocytomas) and grade IV (glioblastomas) are fast growing. This is obviously of essential importance for surgical treatment, diagnosis, and prognosis (including prediction of complications). Within this context, immunologic monitoring has a major role to play.

Materials and Methods

A total of 12 patients with gliomas were studied. The gliomas were diagnostically verified in the clinics of neurology and neurosurgery, followed by application of a modified model of immunologic monitoring which included dynamic control of the immune status. The following were monitored: macrophage activity (NBT test), T-helper and T-suppressor activity, the mitochondrial enzymes succinate dehydrogenase (SDH) and α-glucose-6-phosphate dehydrogenase (α-GPDH), complement C3 component, and lysozyme in serum; morphologic analysis of intraoperative biopsy materials was also performed. The immunologic monitoring was performed several times: when the patient was admitted to the clinic, before operation, intraoperatively, after operation, and during the follow-up period.

Analysis and Discussion

Malignant gliomas cause suppression of the systemic immune system; furthermore the brain is considered an immunologically privileged site. There are several mechanisms by which a tumor can escape immune surveillance, including (a) coating of cells with glucosaminoglycans; (b) secretion of T-cell suppressor factor/transforming growth factor β-2, which suppresses T-lymphocyte activation systematically and, after infiltration into the tumor, locally; and (c) attainment of tumor necrosis factor-α resistance by amplified expression of the *her2/erb*-B2 oncogene.

In the present study the authors established suppression of the immune response in all cases at the time of admission to the clinic. Table 1 shows the background results of the monitoring at the time of hospitalization.

In healthy subjects the levels of the parameters investigated are as follows: 180–240 IU for NBT test, >1.0 for T-h/T-s, 18–20 FG for SDH, 9–11 FG for α-GPDH, 1080–1100 μg/ml for C3, and 15–18 μg/ml for lysozyme in serum. It is thus obvious that all of the patients with gliomas were immunologically suppressed upon admission.

However, we considered that it might be interesting to examine the immune status of patients with different grades of glioma. Of the 12 patients, seven had slow-growing tumors (grades I + II) while five had fast-growing ones (grades III + IV). Analysis of the results obtained preoperatively revealed that some of the parameters (T-helper and T-suppressor cell activity, SDH, and α-GPDH) showed significantly lower levels in patients with grade III or IV tumors than in those with grade I or II tumors (Table 2).

Table 1. Results of immunologic monitoring of patients at the time of their admission to the clinic (results are presented as averages for the 12 patients)

Test	Result
NBT test[a]	104.0 IU
T-h/T-s[b]	0.82
SDH[c]	11.34
α-GPDH	6.28
C3	736.0 μg/ml
Lysozyme/serum	10.6 μg/ml

[a] Measured spectrophotometrically
[b] Ratio between the absolute number of T-helper (T-h) and T-suppressor (T-s) cells
[c] Measured in FG (formazan granules)

Table 2. Differences in immunoreactivity of patients with slow-growing (SGT) and fast-growing (FGT) tumors[a]

Group	T-h/T-s	SDH	α-GPDH
FGT	0.74	9.86	4.98
SGT	0.89	12.88	7.56

[a] The remaining tests (NBT test, C3 and serum lysozyme) did not show noteworthy differences between patients from the two groups

Table 3. Immunoreactivity of patients with fast-growing (FGT) or slow-growing (SGT) tumors 10 days postoperatively

Group	NBT	T-h/T-s	SDH	GPDH	C3	Lysozyme
FGT	148.0	0.92	14.52	8.66	894.0	13.7
SGT	162.0	0.98	16.32	9.40	974.0	15.1

Intraoperatively and 24h after tumor excision all patients showed a similar level of immunoreactivity to that before operation, but whereas the values in respect of immunoregulatory cells (helper and suppressor T-lymphocytes), both enzymes (SDH and α-GPDH), and C3 were essentially unchanged, the level of NBT macrophage activity and lysozyme content were considerably higher: NBT at 136IU and lysozyme at 18 μg/ml. These tests are nonspecific and the aforementioned results were probably due to the operative trauma, which may exert an influence over natural resistance factors.

In later periods after operation the patients with slow-growing gliomas showed significantly quicker normalization of their parameters than those with fast-growing gliomas. Table 3 shows the results of immunologic monitoring 10 days postoperatively.

As is known from the available literature and from our previous studies, it is quite important to analyze the degree of immunoreactivity (high, average, low) of each patient, thus providing a possibility of predicting clinical complications and identifying stages of the disease (cancer, infections, etc.). In terms of immunoreactivity our patients could be divided into two types: low responders ($n = 7$) and high responders ($n = 4$). One of the patients (with grade IV glioma) was unclassified due to fluctuation in his basic immune data. It is well established that patients with lower immunoreactivity more frequently experience infectious complications. We aim to study the influence of the immune status on postoperative convalescence. It appears that patients with higher immunoreactivity recover better after operation and that their immunologic monitoring parameters show values nearer to normal. However, this is speculation and, of course, such a conclusion requires future detailed studies. In any case, there is undoubtedly a very close link between the immunoreactivity and the clinical status of patients with glioma.

References

1. Bhondeley MK et al. (1988) Imbalances in T-cell subpopulations in human gliomas. J Neurosurg 68:589–593
2. Lissyanii NI et al. (1991) Changes of the immune status in patients with brain tumors before and after operation. J Collect Authors Russia 19–21

3. Drannik GN, Metodiev KT, Nenov DS, Baran EY (1989) Renal transplantation efficiency is dependent on pretransplantation immunologic monitoring. Transplant Proc 21(1):17
4. Roszman T et al. (1991) Modulation of T-cell function by gliomas. Immunol Today 12:10
5. Hossfeld DK, Sherman CD, Love RR, Bosch FX (1990) Manual of clinical oncology, 5th edn. Springer, Berlin Heidelberg New York, p 392

Therapy Modalities (1)

High-Dose Immunoglobulins for Prophylaxis of Severe Sepsis

L. Dominioni, A. Imperatori, R. Gennari, and R. Dionigi

Septic complications continue to rank among the main causes of morbidity and mortality in surgical and trauma patients, in spite of recent improvements in the modalities of intensive case treatment. Several studies have shown that the tendency to develop postoperative infections, and especially the risk of developing septic episodes with fatal outcome, is influenced not only by bacterial contamination occurring during the operation or as a result of trauma, but also by a condition of immunologic deficit and impaired acute-phase response [1–3].

Severe infectious complications are characterized by a septic acute-phase response; this may end with the resolution of infection or may progress to the condition of septic shock or multiple organ failure (MOF), determining fatal outcome [4]. It is relevant that the mortality of patients with septic shock has not changed in the past 20 years; it ranges between 30% and 80%, depending upon the causative organisms, the overall condition of the patient, and the adequacy of treatment [5, 6].

Numerous new therapeutic modalities which have been proposed to improve the results of treatment of severely septic patients, including immunotherapy with polyvalent intravenous immunoglobulins (IVIG). The strategies of passive immunotherapy with IG can be subdivided into three main groups, according to the nature of the substance used: (1) polyvalent IG, isolated from pooled donor blood; (2) hyperimmune globulin, derived either from selected screened donors or from plasmapheresis of immunized volunteers; (3) monoclonal antibodies [7]. We will review the information available on immunoprophylaxis and immunotherapy of sepsis with polyvalent IVIG.

The rationale for the use of IVIG to treat severe infections stems from in vitro and animal studies documenting that high-dose IG enhance opsonization and phagocytosis of pathogenic bacteria [8, 9]. Moreover, recent clinical studies have shown that in septic patients the phagocytic function of circulating polymorphonuclear neutrophils (PMN) is defective; the degree of such impairment correlates to the severity of the septic state [10].

The beneficial effect of administering high-dose IG in the septic patients can be twofold: (1) the polyvalent IG provides large quantities of antibodies against invading pathogens; the IG bound to the pathogens can "opsonize" (facilitate) their phagocytosis; (2) the opsonization of phagocytosis by exogenously administered polyvalent IG would be of special importance in those patients who present a significant defect of their phagocytic function, when they are challenged by a large bacterial invasion.

Theoretically, before proceeding to passive immunotherapy with high-dose IG, due to the relevant cost of this drug it would be necessary to demonstrate that a deficit of antibodies against the pathogens responsible for the infection exists, or a deficit of phagocytosis which responds to IG therapy should be shown. However, the clinical use of polyvalent IG has been very empirical so far. In fact, for more than 10 years, since IVIG became available, high-dose IG have been given to septic patients or to patients at high risk of developing severe infections only on the basis of an estimated potential advantage of providing an "extra quantity" of antibodies to combat infection, whithout actually assessing the status of the patient's humoral immunity and phagocytic function. Several clinical studies have reported the use of high-dose IVIG in trauma and surgical patients, both for prophylaxis of infections in patients at risk and for treatment of established infection. The interpretation of some of these studies is difficult because they were not blind, or appropriate control groups were lacking. We will report here only the results of clinical trials carried out prospectively, with control groups.

The first placebo-controlled, randomized study of prophylaxis of bacterial infections with polyvalent IVIG in patients at risk following multiple trauma was reported by Glinz et al. in 1985 [11]. One hundred and fifty severely traumatized patients requiring ICU treatment were prospectively randomized to receive either polyvalent IVIG (Sandoglobulin-Sandoz, IgG) or albumin (as placebo control). Among the 76 patients receiving IVIG (36 g in divided doses over 12 days) the incidence of infections was significantly lower ($P = 0.0217$) than in the 74 controls, mainly due to a significantly decreased incidence of pneumonia ($P = 0.0111$). A marked reduction (32%) of the therapeutic use of antibiotics was observed in the IVIG group; however, the mortality was not significantly different in the two groups (Table 1). This study is important because for the first time it documented: (1) a beneficial effect of IVIG for prophylaxis of infections; (2) no side-effects of the administration of IVIG in large doses in patients who already has normal IG plasma levels. As a further comment on the results of this study, it must be noted that the overall dose of IVIG given was not very high (approx. 0.5 g/kg b.w.); thus a more pronounced favorable effect in terms of reduction of mortality might have been missed because the IVIG dose was suboptimal. It is currently accepted that an adequate high dose of IVIG for prophylaxis or treatment of severe infections is approx. 1 g/kg b.w. given in single doses or a small number of dose fractions [12].

In 1988 Mao et al. [13] also observed a beneficial effect of the early administration of polyvalent IVIG (Endobulin-Immuno, IgG) in the prevention of surgical and post-traumatic sepsis. Thirty-two patients were randomized to receive either polyvalent IVIG (40 g in divided doses, over 10 days)

Table 1. Prophylaxis of sepsis with IVIG

Author	No. pts.	Blind study	Mortality (%)		Significance
			IVIG	Placebo	
Glinz et al. [11]	150	Yes	30	20	NS
Mao et al. [13]	32	Yes	13	24	NS
Lehmkuhl et al. [14]	97	Yes	6	10	NS
Collaborative Study Group [6]	220	Yes	15	22	NS

or placebo. Fewer septic episodes and less positive blood cultures were found in the IVIG group; however, mortality was not significantly different (Table 1). Once more it should be noted that the IVIG dosage given in this study is suboptimal by currently accepted criteria; moreover, the small number of patients enrolled actually prevents a sound statistical evaluation of the trial's results.

Lehmkuhl et al. in 1991 [14] reported on the prophylaxis of infections following major intraabdominal surgery, using 5-S immunoglobulins (IgG). They randomized 97 patients in a placebo-controlled, double-blind study, also stratifying patients according to the severity of disease. No difference in mortality was observed (Table 1). The authors reported that the IG-treated patients had a more favorable postoperative course, a decreased need for mechanical ventilation, and a shorter time of recovery from ICU; however, the differences with the control group did not attain statistical significance.

Finally, a multicentric, prospective, placebo-controlled, randomized and double-blind study was carried out to assess the prophylactic value of polyvalent IVIG (Gammagard-Baxter, IgG) given to patients at high risk of postsurgical infections [6]. This large collaborative study was carried out in seven intensive care units in Switzerland, Belgium, and the United States and enrolled 329 patients who could be evaluated. They were randomized into three groups, receiving respectively: (1) IVIG 0.4 g/kg b.w.; (2) hyperimmune globulin (anti core-lipopolysaccharide) 0.4 g/kg b.w.; (3) 25% albumin, 8 ml/kg b.w., as placebo. These doses were repeated weekly, until discharge. Also in this study no significant advantage in terms of reduction of mortality was observed in the IVIG-treated group (Table 1). However, in patients receiving the standard IVIG a significantly lower incidence of acquired infections of all types was observed ($P = 0.03$); especially important was the decrease in incidence of acquired pneumoniae ($P = 0.02$), particularly the decrease of gram-negative pneumoniae ($P = 0.02$). Moreover, in the IVIG group the number of days spent in ICU and the total days of hospitalization were significantly lower (Table 2). The conclusion of this important study is that in selected high-risk ICU patients the prophylactic administration of high-dose IVIG can reduce the incidence of infections.

Table 2. Prophylactic standard polyvalent IVIG (St-IVIG) vs core-LPS IVIG (Co-IVIG) vs placebo in patients at high risk of postsurgical infection [7]

	Placebo	Co-IVIG	St-IVIG	*P*
No. of assessable pts.	112	108	109	
With acquired infection	53	50	36	0.03
With acquired pneumoniae	29	23	14	0.02
With GN pneumoniae	15	17	5	0.02
With systemic episodes	12	13	13	NS
Overall mortality (%)	22	20	15	NS
Stay in hospital (days)	29	24	21.50	0.06
Stay in ICU (days)	6	5	4	0.02

Table 3. Significant beneficial effects of prophylactic polyvalent IVIG

1. Decreased acquired infection rate ($P = 0.03$ [6]; $P < 0.004$ [15]).
2. Decreased pneumonia rate ($P < 0.02$ [11]; $P = 0.02$ [6]).
3. Reduced ICU stay and hospital stay ($P = 0.06$ [6]).

Another clinical trial of prophylaxis of infections with IVIG deserves mention, although it was not blind and placebo controlled. It is the study of Cafiero et al. [15], which was carried out in patients at risk of sepsis undergoing surgery for colorectal cancer; the results document a significant ($P < 0.004$) reduction in the incidence of postoperative infections in the IVIG-treated group (Sandoglobulin-Sandoz, IgG, approx. 0.3 g/kg b.w.).

In conclusion, high doses of polyvalent IgG, given prophylactically to high-risk patients, have been shown to yield beneficial effects, including a decrease in the occurrence of acquired infections (Table 3).

References

1. Dionigi R, Dominioni L (1992) Sepsis and the immune response. In: Eremin O, Sewell H (eds) The immunological basis of surgical science and practice. Oxford, Oxford, pp 117–132
2. Marshall JC, Christou NV, Horn R et al. (1988) The microbiology of multiple organ failure. Arch Surg 123:309–315
3. Dominioni L, Dionigi R, Zanello L et al. (1987) Sepsis score and acute phase protein response as predictors of outcome in septic surgical patients. Arch Surg 122:141–146
4. Fry DE, Pearlstein L, Fulton RL et al. (1980) Multiple system organ failure. Arch Surg 115:136–140
5. Dominioni L, Dionigi R, Zanello M, Chiaranda M et al. (1991) Effects of high-dose IgG on survival of surgical patients with sepsis scores of 20 or greater. Arch Surg 126:236–240

6. The Intravenous Immunoglobulin Collaborative Study Group (1992) Prophylactic intravenous administration of standard immune globuline as compared with core-lipopolysaccaride immune globulin in patients at high risk of post-surgical infection. N Engl J Med 327:234–240
7. Cometta A (1993) Clinical effects of high doses of polyvalent immunoglobulin in sepsis. 6th Annual Meeting of the Surgical Infection Society Europe, 3–5 June, Varese
8. Fisher G (1983) Functional antibacterial activity of a human intravenous immunoglobulin preparation: in vitro and in vivo studies. Vox Sang 44:262–299
9. Van Furth R, Leijh PCJ
10. Dominioni L, Gennari R, Interdonato PF et al. (1993) Effects of high-dose polyvalent IgG on defective bacterial phagocytosis in severe surgical sepsis. Surg Res Commun
11. Glinz W, Grob PJ, Nydegger UE et al. (1985) Polyvalent immunoglobulins for prophylaxis of bacterial infections in patients following multiple trauma – a randomized, placebo-controlled study. Intensive Care Med 11:288–294
12. Nydegger UE (1992) Clinical relevance of optimal vs maximum doses of prophylactic and therapeutic immunoglobulins. In: Dominioni L, Nydegger UE (eds) Intravenous immunoglobulins today and tomorrow. Royal Society of Medicine Services, London, pp 11–25 (International congress and symposium series, no 189)
13. Mao P, Enrichens F, Olivero G et al. (1989) Early administration of intravenous immunoglobulins in the prevention of surgical and post-traumatic sepsis: a double blind randomized clinical trial. Surg Res Commun 5:93–98
14. Lehmkuhl P, Jeck-Thole S, Dellbrugge J, Pichlmayr I (1990) Effects of immune globulins given following major intraabdominal surgery. Fortschr Anasthesiol Notfall Intensivmed 4:48–52
15. Cafiero F, Gipponi M, Bonalumi U et al. (1992) Prophylaxis of infection with intravenous immunoglobulins plus antibiotic for patients at risk for sepsis undergoing surgery for colorectal cancer: results of a randomized, multicenter clinical trial. Surgery 112:24–31

Perioperative Immunity, Inflammatory Response, and Postoperative Infection in Cardiopulmonary Bypass Patients

H.G. KRESS, R. SILBER, and D. BERGER

Open-heart surgery is a unique form of surgical trauma, as it superimposes the additional effects of cardiopulmonary bypass and hypothermia on conventional operative injury. Since the first open-heart operations, cardiopulmonary bypass (CPB) has been known to contribute to the mortality and morbidity of cardiac surgery. Although modern cardiopulmonary bypass seems to be well tolerated, it can never be truly physiological. During cardiopulmonary bypass, poor tissue perfusion and ischemic damage to the bowel mucosa may result in the translocation of endotoxin and enteric gram-negative bacteria from the gut [1, 2]. Thus, cardiopulmonary bypass patients are at risk for the development of postoperative infections and a "whole-body inflammatory response" resembling septic shock, the so-called post-perfusion syndrome [3].

This article summarizes the results from several prospective clinical studies that focused on some of the very complex and multifaceted pathophysiological mechanisms contributing to such complications.

Infection and Immunity in CPB Patients

Cardiopulmonary bypass has been shown to be associated with a decreased in vitro capacity of cell-mediated and humoral immunity during and shortly after the operation [4]. Functional depression of T and B lymphocytes, impaired natural killer cell activity, and – although not consistently found – decreased capacity of polymorphonuclear leukocytes and the reticuloendothelial system have been described. Severe reductions in complement and immunoglobulin plasma levels are consistent findings after cardiopulmonary bypass.

Although many investigators assume that the occurrence of postoperative infection is related to a preexisting or perioperatively acquired impairment of the immune system, as yet all these in vitro tests of immune functions have failed to reveal a clear preoperative definition of the patient prone to infection after elective open-heart surgery. For example, this could be illustrated by investigating the migratory function of isolated polymorphonuclear neutrophils (PMN) preoperatively and at defined postoperative time intervals after cardiac surgery (Fig. 1). Preoperatively, mean

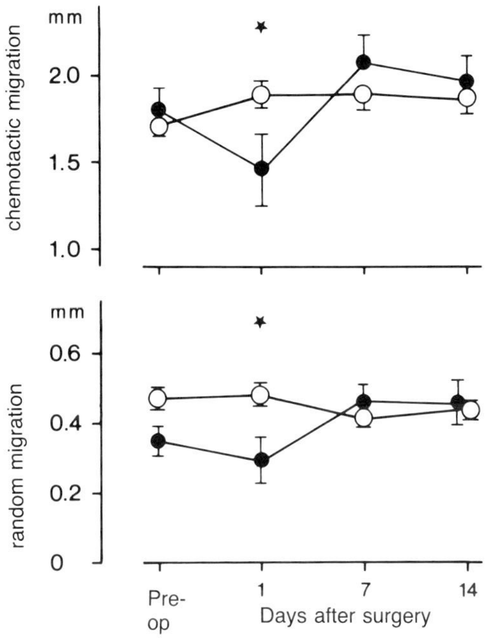

Fig. 1. Mean random and chemotactic neutrophil migration in patients with (*closed circles*) and without postoperative infection (*open circles*). $^*P < 0.05$ by Mann-Whitney U-test. [From 4]

chemotaxis values and random migration were statistically indistinguishable between patients with postoperative infections and those without such complications. On the first postoperative day, however, chemotactic response and random migration significantly decreased in those patients who later developed infections, but remained unchanged or even slightly increased in patients without infection (Fig. 1). Interestingly, this impairment of PMN function occurred not only hours, but even days before the clinical manifestation of typical infectious signs [4].

Mean plasma levels of C-reactive protein (CRP) also differed significantly already at day 1 after surgery, whereas no difference could be found prior to the operation. Thus, no predictive role of the preoperative CRP level could be derived from our data. Postoperative CRP levels, however, continuously decreased in patients without infection, but further increased in those with infectious complications [4].

In the same study we could demonstrate that the preoperative lack of cutaneous delayed-type hypersensitivity (DTH) response to seven standardized recall antigens identifies cardiac patients at increased risk of postoperative infection [4]. Two-thirds of the anergic patients but less than 10% of the relatively anergic or the reactive patients developed infectious complications. This difference in infectious rate was statistically significant at the 0.001 level, and the predictive value of preoperative cutaneous anergy could be confirmed by further studies [5]. Thus, preoperative cutaneous anergy identifies "at-risk" patients who would otherwise have been considered in optimal clinical condition for elective cardiac surgery.

Prophylactic Administration of Intravenous Immunoglobulins (IVIG)

Once the patients at risk have been identified, the question arises of how to protect them from postoperative infection? As already mentioned, a severe and long-lasting reduction in immunoglobulin levels (IgG, IgM) is a consistent finding after cardiopulmonary bypass, and this reduction lasts up to 14 days after the operation.

Therefore, we investigated in a prospective, randomized, and placebo-controlled trial whether or not the prophylactic intravenous application of a commercial human immunoglobulin preparation enriched in IgA and IgM (Pentaglobin, Biotest Pharma GmbH, Frankfurt, FRG) was able to reduce the rate of postoperative infections in this anergic "at-risk" group. Out of 515 patients skin tested before elective cardiac surgery, the 40 anergic patients were allocated randomly to two groups receiving either immunoglobulins or normal saline after their operations. Moreover, 20 patients randomly selected from the 471 DTH reactive individuals formed a third group, expected to represent those at normal infectious risk. For 2 weeks after operation, localized and generalized infections were documented according to CDC criteria by a blindfolded investigator [5].

Not surprisingly, the postoperative reduction in IgG plasma levels was rapidly and effectively reversed by the application of 20 g of the commercially available intravenous immunoglobulin preparation. However, there was also a significant difference in the overall incidence of postoperative infections between the placebo and the immunoglobulin group, as well as between the placebo group and randomly selected reactive patients. Nine out of 21 patients in the placebo group, but only one patient in the immunoglobulin group developed infectious complications ($P < 0.01$). The immunoglobulin group and the reactive patients did not differ in this respect. Interestingly, the immunoglobulin administration also had an effect on the maximal body temperature of patients without infection. The immediate postoperative increase in body temperature often found even in nonseptic cardiac patients was significantly reduced by IVIG administration (Fig. 2). The underlying mechanisms, however, still had to be elucidated.

Endotoxemia and Systemic Inflammatory Response After CPB

Many components of the inflammatory response are stimulated during extracorporeal circulation: platelets and leukocytes, the humoral cascades of

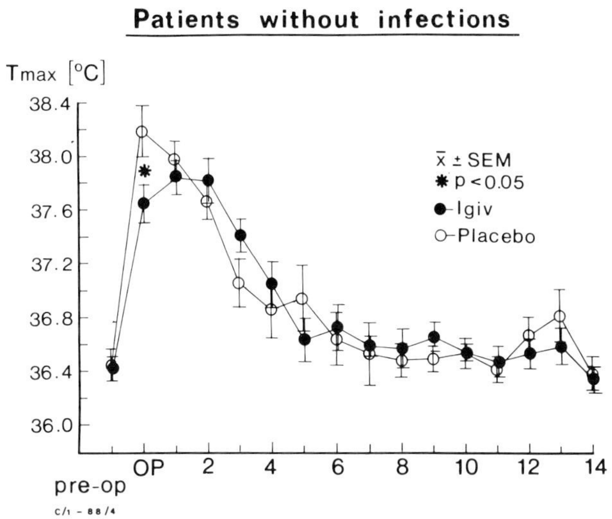

Fig. 2. Postoperative body temperature (daily maximum increase) in patients without infection. Comparison between the placebo and the immunoglobulin (*Igiv*; 20 g) group

coagulation, fibrinolysis, kallikrein, and complement [3]. Activated PMN are trapped in the pulmonary capillaries, followed by the release of proteolytic enzymes and damaging oxygen free radicals. As the pattern of activation during CPB shows striking similarities with the physiological response to endotoxin from gram-negative bacteria [6], it seemed obvious to search for circulating endotoxin in our patients, and to investigate the effects of immunoglobulin administration.

Immediately after the start of CPB the plasma concentration of endotoxin significantly increased, showing a further rise after release of the aortic cross-clamp (Fig. 3). The endotoxin levels remained elevated at least during the first 2 postoperative days, with a second rise 4–6 h after termination of bypass. Surprisingly, however, the administration of IVIG had no effect. Neither the prolonged endotoxemia nor the inflammatory response (IL-6, CRP) was attenuated by the perioperative immunoglobulin prophylaxis. As shown in Fig. 4, the concentration of IL-6 gradually increased after release of the aortic cross-clamp, reaching its peak 2–4 h after termination of bypass.

Nevertheless, the inflammatory response did not remain totally unaffected by the immunoglobulin administration. At the first postoperative day, leukocytosis, especially granulocytosis, was significantly mitigated in the immunoglobulin group, showing a significantly delayed increase in these patients. Furthermore, the daily maximum body temperature of the IVIG group remained consistently below that of the placebo group.

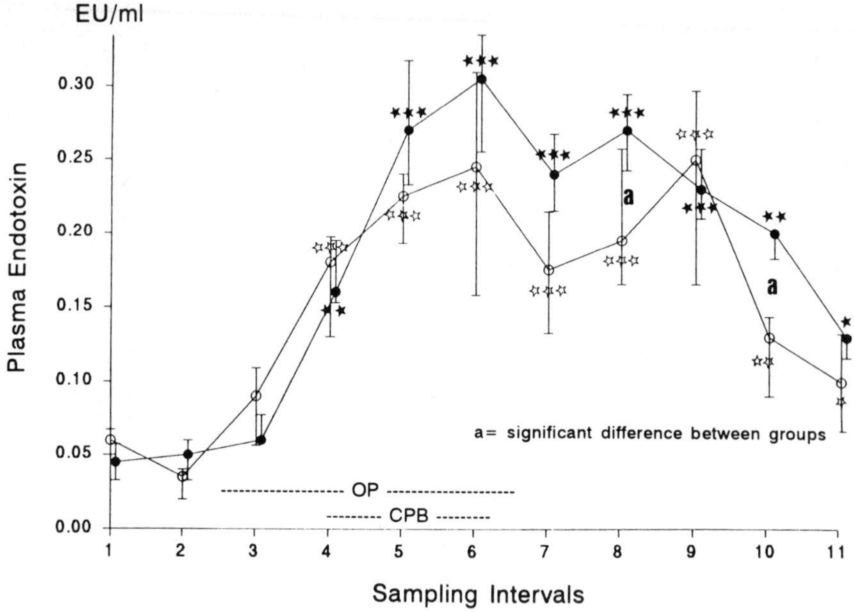

Fig. 3. Median plasma endotoxin levels in patients treated with i.v. immunoglobulin (-●-; $n = 20$) or placebo (-○-; $n = 20$). Circulating plasma endotoxin was measured by one of the authors (D.B.) using a chromogenic modification of the limulus amebocyte lysate (LAL) test [7]. *OP*, operation; *CPB*, cardiopulmonary bypass; sampling intervals: 1 = preoperative day; 5 and 6 = release of aortic cross-clamp and 15 min thereafter; 7–11 = 2, 4, 6, 24, and 48 h after CPB. $^{***}P < 0.001$; $^{**}P < 0.01$; $^{*}P < 0.05$

What Does All This Mean for Our Patients?

Modern CPB, too, continues to be associated with an increased risk of postoperative infection, mainly due to the more or less severe impairment of important cellular and humoral immune functions. As this is especially true for preoperatively anergic patients, these individuals have to be considered an at-risk group for open-heart surgery. However, anergic cardiac patients can be effectively protected by commercial IgM-enriched IVIG.

Poor tissue perfusion and ischemic damage of the bowel mucosa during and after CPB cause a long-lasting, severe endotoxemia that is closely related to a "whole-body inflammatory response" in these patients. Whereas the inflammatory response may be at least marginally affected by IVIG administration, endotoxemia remains unaffected at all. Thus, the protective effect of IgM- and IgA-enriched IVIG in anergic patients does not seem to be mediated by antiendotoxin antibodies occurring at relatively high titers, especially in the IgM fraction of these preparations. On the other hand, it can be concluded from our data that endotoxemia per se does not play a

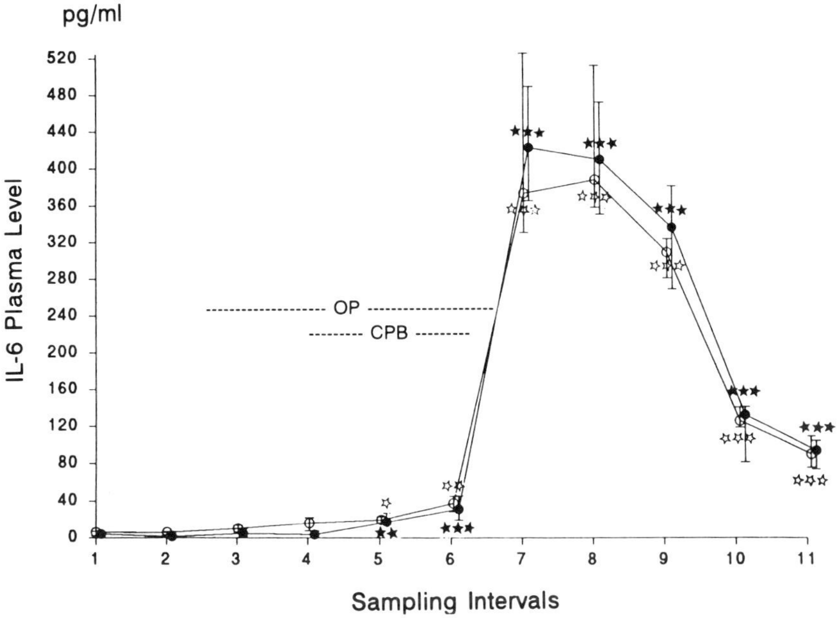

Fig. 4. Median plasma levels of IL-6 in patients treated with i.v. immunoglobulin (-○-; n = 20) or placebo (-○-; n = 20). Circulating IL-6 was determined by ELISA (Dianova, Hamburg, FRG). *OP*, operation; *CPB*, cardiopulmonary bypass; for sampling intervals see Fig. 3

crucial role for the development of postoperative infections in CPB patients. In this respect, immune functions of the host could be of major importance.

References

1. Freeman R, Gould FK (1985) Rises in antibody to enteric gram negative bacilli after open heart surgery: a possible mechanism for postoperative pyrexia. Thorax 40:538–541
2. Freeman R, Gould FK (1985) Prevention of fever and gram negative infection after open heart surgery by antiendotoxin. Thorax 40:846–848
3. Westaby S (1987) Organ dysfunction after cardiopulmonary bypass. A systemic inflammatory reaction initiated by the extracorporeal circuit. Intensive Care Med 13:89–95
4. Kress HG, Gehrsitz P, Elert O (1987) Predictive value of skin testing, neutrophil migration and C-reactive protein for postoperative infections in cardiopulmonary bypass patients. Acta Anaesthesiol Scand 31:397–404
5. Kress HG, Scheidewig C, Elert O (1990) Postoperative passive immunoprophylaxis prevents infections in "at-risk" patients after open-heart surgery. J Cardiothorac Anesth 4 [Suppl 3]:67
6. Berger D, Marzinzig E, Marzinzig M, Beger HG (1988) Quantitative endotoxin determination in blood-chromogenic modification of the limulus amebocyte lysate test. Eur Surg Res 20:128–136

Therapy Modalities (2)

Immunological Consequences of Antibiotic Therapy

D.H. WITTMANN

Antibiotics may interfere with host defense in many ways. They may impact bacterial toxin release and thus alter the response of the host to bacterial challenge including endo- and exotoxinemia. They may also alter the release of various proinflammatory mediators and influence the complex system of immune defense. Antibiotics may alter the action of complement and immunoglobulins. They may interfere with phagocytosis and intracellular killing of bacteria by neutrophils and macrophages, alter monocyte and lymphocyte function, and influence delayed-type hypersensitivity and antibody production. There are reports which also show that antibiotics interfere with allograft rejection in transplant surgery.

There are various theoretical possibilities for antibiotics interfering with host response. Antibiotics may inhibit or suppress, enhance or stimulate, the response of the host to infection. Antibiotics may have no effect at all and variable effects may be seen depending on the method used. Here I will first describe suppression then stimulation and discuss variable effects if observed by the same or different authors and I will state whether no effects have been seen when examined and mention that the specific immune function has been tested when I think it is important.

Antibiotic Effects on Bacterial Toxin Release

There are no reports about inhibition or suppression of toxin release from bacteria by various antibiotics. Endotoxin, the lipopolysaccharide of the outer membrane of bacterial cell wall, is known to induce a burst of reactions into which various cytokines and proinflammatory chemical compounds are involved. Endotoxin is released when bacteria die, and it has been observed clinically that bacteriocidal antibiotics may potentiate bacterial killing and thus be responsible for increased endotoxin release. In fact, increased endotoxin levels have been found by various authors [1–3]. The changes in LPS level parallelled bacteriocidal effects of antibiotics. Dofferhoff et al. [3], for example, saw an increase by 1.8–4.8 times in circulating LPS after exposure of various antibiotics. As an indirect measure, TNF release can be assayed. TNF is produced by macrophages in response to endotoxin challenge via expression of CD-4 and CD-8 receptors and subsequent generation of TNF messenger RNA release [4]. Simon et al. [5] found increased TNF generation following 1-hour exposure of gram-negative bacteria to imipenem, following 2- to 4-h exposure to cefotaxime, ceftazidime, and aztreonam, and following 1.5-h exposure to ciprofloxacin. In a critical analysis of the literature, they also investigate studies that have not been able to demonstrate any clinical effect of endotoxin release following exposure of the bacteria with antibiotics.

In treating infections, this possibility may be complicating the initiation of antibiotic therapy in patients who have high bacterial inoculae at the site of infection such as in diffuse peritonitis. For that reason, authors recommend the use of bacteriocidal antibiotics only when most of the bacteria have been eliminated operatively [6]. Interpretation of the antibiotic stimulated endotoxin release is complicated by the fact, as mentioned before, that not endotoxin but the response to endotoxin creates toxicity. Also, endotoxin release may occur in absence of lysis and even before bacteriolysis takes place [7]. Also, it should be noted at this point that normal serum is bacteriocidal to gram-negative bacteria [8] and consequently serum properties may be blamed for endotoxin release rather than the addition of antibiotics. However, in balancing the information that speaks in favor or against antibiotic induced endotoxin release as a clinical reality, the information available that supports the notion of bacteriocidal antibiotics aggravating septic shock may have the stronger argument.

Meroni et al. [9] and Labro [10] found a down-modulation of TNF and IL-1 following administration of cefodizime. Inhibition of TNF and IL-1 release was true for high concentration of quinolones and macrolides [10]. If cefodizime was given to immune suppressed mice, the interleukin-1 and interferon-γ release was restored to normal, which was interpreted as a positive immune modulation. Further studies are required to assess the immunomodulatory effects of antibiotics and its clinical relevance.

Antibiotic Effects on Immunoglobulins

An inhibition of IgG and IgM synthesis was found by Pulverer [11] for cefotaxime and an enhancement by Roszkowski et al. [12] for ciprofloxacin. Cefotazime, an erythromycin in AIDS patients, did not affect immunoglobulin synthesis [11, 13]. Chloramphenicol and trimetoprime-sulmetoxazole suppress antibody production [14, 15].

Antibiotic Effects on Monocyte Function

Inhibition of monocyte chemotaxis has been observed with gentamycin, tetracyclin, fusidic acid, and TMP, and suppression of the monocyte oxidative burst by cefotaxime by Nielson [16]. Ohnishi et al. [17] saw a stimulation of monocyte activity by release of an activating factor by cefimizole, and Dammacco and Benvestito [18] saw enhancement of monocyte function by cefodizime in patients with multiple myoloma. No effect on monocyte chemotaxis has been observed for penicillin, ampicillin, cefotaxime, ofloxacin, metronidazole, clindamycin, and tobramycin.

Antibiotic Effects on Lymphocyte Function

Inhibition of lymphocyte function has been seen with cefotaxime, clindamycin, tetracyclines, chloramphenicol, TMP, and amphotericin-B [11, 19–23], enhancement for cefotazime in vitro [10] and stimulation of natural killer cells by cefodizime [24]. Other studies showed no effect for cefodizime, ciprofloxacin, or gentamycin [11, 12, 19]. Inhibition of delayed-type hypersensitivity using in vitro models of T-cell function have been reported for piperacillin and cefazoline [25] for cefotaxime [11], and for tetracyclines and erythromycin [25]. Enhancement of delayed-type hypersensitivity seems to occur with amphotericin-B [26] and in immunocompromised patients with cefodizime [25]. No effects were noted with ciprofloxacin by Roszkowski et al. [12] and cefodizime by Pulverer [11], who did not examine immunocompromised patients.

Antibiotic Effects on Neutrophil Function

Most studies indicate that antibiotics may improve bacterial killing of human PMNs (polymorphnuclear leukocytes) when altered by preincubation. Results, however, are conflicting. A very good overview on the subject has been presented by Van den Broek [27]. He categorizes the effects of antibiotics on phagocytosis of microorganisms into the following categories:

1. Antibiotics may interact with microorganism or with phagocytes.
2. Antibiotics may interfere with chemotaxis by changing the production of chemoattractants.
3. Antibiotics may interfere with phagocytosis by interacting with bacterial toxins that inhibit phagocytosis or by altering the ability of phagocytes to produce bacteriocidal moieties.
4. Antibiotics may interact with intracellular killing of phagocytes.
5. Antibiotics may interfere with phagocytic digestion of bacteria.

Stimulation of phagocytosis and killing by neutrophils has been reported for cefaclor, cefotaxime, cefmetazole, cefetamed, and cefodizime [28–32]. Labro et al. [29] observed an increase in the oxidative burst by cefotaxime. In patients with sickle cell anemia, chemotaxis was inhibited [32]. A suppression of phagocytosis and killing by neutrophils was observed for gentamycin, tobramycin, amicacin, clindamycin, and tetracyclines [33–35].

Other antibiotics suppress chemotaxis (aminoglycosides, tetracyclines, fusidic acid, erythromycin, and rifampin and amphotericin-B) [19, 36–40], while random migration has been reported to be suppressed by cefoxitin, cefamandole, cefoperazone [40], and erythromycin [39]. Kaplan and Remington and others report a suppression of chemiluminescence by TMP, chloramphenicol, and amphotericin-B [41–45].

Others have reported inhibitory as well as enhancing effects on neutrophil phagocytosis and killing by tetracyclines, clindamycin, erythromycin, chloramphenicol, and rifampin. The reports are partially contradictory and it becomes very difficult to evaluate the true nature of interaction of antibiotics with neutrophil function. Even reports that show no effect on neutrophil phagocytosis and killing may not disclose the reality because the methods utilized vary greatly and each method examines only a minute aspect of the entire process [35, 46–48]. When looking at phagocytosis and killing by neutrophils, no effect was seen with penicillins, cefotaxime and cefodizime, nalidixic acid, and TMP [11, 19, 47, 49]. Migration was not affected by norfloxacin, pefloxican, or ofloxacin [49], and no effect on neutrophil chemotaxis has been reported for cefotaxime, cefodizime, clindamycin, netilmycin, and some antifungal agents [11, 34, 50–52]. Also, chemiluminescence and the sensitivity of indium-111 scan have been shown not to be affected by antibiotics such as erythromycin, cefotaxime, and cefodizime [51, 52].

Antibiotic Effects on Allograft Rejection

As opposed to infection, in transplant surgery suppression of immune response may be a desirable effect and positively influence survival of transplanted organs. An inhibition of allograft rejection has been reported for trimetoprim [53], for chloramphenicol and fusidic acid [25], and for rifampin. Whether an enhancement of allograft rejection by amphotericin-B as observed by Blanke et al. [26] is a fact that should caution use of antifungal agents in transplanted patients needs further clinical confirmation.

Summary

Overall, the tremendous amount of literature on the subject utilizing a multitude of laboratory and clinical tests gives a conflicting picture. It is impossible to objectively compare the studies and rate them in a scientific manner, and I can only talk about an impression that I have obtained from the study of this literature.

1. Antibiotics do seem to enhance endotoxin release and should not be used before high bacterial numbers can be reduced by surgical elimination.

2. The immune enhancing effect reported by others for newer antibiotics such as cefodizime should undergo the test of prospective controlled clinical trials before a final conclusion is reached.
3. Antibiotics seem to interfere with the delicate interplay of the immune defense system negatively.

The suggestion that antibiotics may negatively influence host defense is supported by numerous studies dealing with prophylaxis of postoperative infections with antibiotics. While antibiotics effectively decrease wound infection rates when given in a timely fashion before the surgical procedure, an increase in infection rate is seen when antibiotics are continued after the wound is closed [54]. A single-shot antibiotic prophylaxis was compared to multiple doses in 1003 patients entered into 27 studies. Twenty-two of 510 cases who received a single dose developed an infection (4.3%), whereas 34 of 493 cases who received multiple injections developed infection (6.9%) [54]. Increased infection rates following multiple dosing may be subtle when looking at individual studies with low numbers, and are then difficult to appreciate; this observation, however, is constant throughout many studies comparing single with multiple doses. Since postoperative antibiotics are not effective (without preoperative dose) [55], increased infections with postoperative administrations of antibiotics must be interpreted as resulting from inhibition of wound healing which involves many of the host defense mechanisms.

References

1. Hurley JC (1992) Antibiotic-induced release of endotoxin: a reappraisal. Clin Infect Dis 15:840–854
2. Shenep JL, Barton RP, Morgan KA (1985) Role of antibiotic class in the rate of liberation of endotoxin during therapy for experimental gram-negative bacterial sepsis. J Infect Dis 151:1012–1018
3. Dofferhoff ASM, Nijland JH, de Vries-Hospers HG et al. (1991) Effects of different types and combinations of antimicrobial agents on endotoxin release from gram-negative bacteria: an in-vitro and in-vivo study. Scand J Infect Dis 23:745–754
4. Dunn DL, Roderich AB (1993) Immunotherapy. Landes, Austin
5. Simon DM, Koenig G, Trenholme GM (1991) Differences in release of tumor necrosis factor from THP-1 cells stimulated by filtrates of antibiotic-killed *Escherichia coli*. J Infect Dis 164:800–802
6. Wittmann DH (1980) Chemotherapeutic principles in difficult-to-treat infections. Infection 8:323–329
7. Tesch VL, Morrison DC (1988) in Surgery. I. Peritonitis. J Immunol 141: 3523–3531
8. Taylor PW (1983) Bactericidal and bacteriolytic activity of serum against gram negative bacteria. Microbiol Rev 47:46–83
9. Meroni PL, Capsoni F, Borghi MO et al. (1992) Immunopharmacological activity of cefodizime in young and elderly subjects in vitro and ex vivo studies. Infection 20:S61–S63

10. Labro M-T (1992) Immunological evaluation of cefodizime: a unique molecule among cephalosporins. Infection 20:S45–S47
11. Pulverer G (1992) Effects of cefodizime and cefotaxime on cellular and humoral immune response. Infection 20:S41–S44
12. Roszkowski W, Ko HL, Roszkowski K et al. (1986) Effects of ciprofloxacin on the humoral and cellular immune responses in balb/c-mice. Zentralbl Bakterial Hyg [A] 262:396–402
13. Ras GJ, Anderson R (1986) An in vitro study of oral therapeutic doses of cotrimoxazole and erythromycin stearate on abnormal polymorphonuclear leucocyte migration. J Antimicrob Chemother 17:185–193
14. Daniel T, Suhrland L, Weisberger A (1965) Suppression of the anamnestic response to tetanus toxoid in man by chlorammphenicol. N Engl J Med 273: 367–369
15. Avrilommi H, Vuori M, Salmi A (1976) Sulphamethoxazole-trimethoprim: effect on antibody response in man. Chemotherapy 22:37–42
16. Nielson H (1989) Antibiotics and human monocyte function. APMIS 97:447–451
17. Ohnishi H, Inaba H, Mochizuki H et al. (1984) Mechanism of action of AC-1370 on phagocyte functions. Antimicrob Agens Chemother 25:88–92
18. Dammacco F, Benvestito S (1992) Effects of cefodizime on non-specific immune functions in patients with multiple myeloma. Infection 20:S64–S66
19. Forsgren A, Banck G, Beckman H et al. (1980) Antibiotic-host defence interactions in vitro and in vivo. Scand J Infect Dis [Suppl 24]:195–203
20. Munster A, Loadholdt C, Leary A et al. (1977) The effect of antibiotics on cell-mediated immunity. Surgery 81:692–695
21. Becker D, Katz J, Metz J (1974) Comparative effects of thiamphenicol and chloramphenicol on haemopoieisis and lymphocyte transformation in vitro in man. Postgrad Med J 50:S88–S94
22. Gaylarde PM, Sarkany I (1978) Suppression of thymidine uptake of human lymphocytes by co-trimoxazole. Br Med J 3:144–146
23. Taernvik A, Ansehn S (1974) Effect of amphotericin B and clotrimazole on lymphocyte stimulation. Antimicrob Agents Chemother 6:529–533
24. Auer IO, Hardoerfer C, Zimmermann I (1992) Cefodizime stimulates subpopulations of cells mediating spontaneous or antibody-dependent cytotoxicity in patients with bacterial infections. Infection 20:S54–S57
25. Labro MT (1993) Immunomodulation by antibacterial agents: is it clinically relevant? Drugs 45:319–328
26. Blanke T, Little J, Shirley S et al. (1977) Augmentation of murine immune responses by amphotericin B1. Cell Immunol 33:180–190
27. Van den Broek PJ (1989) Antimicrobial drugs, microorganisms, and phagocytes. Rev Infect Dis 11:213–241
28. Scheffer J, Knoller J, Cullman W et al. (1992) Effects of cefaclor, cefetamet and Ro 40–6890 on inflammatory responses of human granuloocytes. J Antimicrob Chemother 30:57–66
29. Labro MT, Babin-Chevaye C, Hakim J (1986) Effects of cefotaxime and cefodizime on human granulocyte functions in vitro. J Antimicrob Chemother 18:233–277
30. Rodriguez A, Barriga C, Fuente M (1991) Stimulation of phagocytic processes and antibody-dependent cellular cytotoxicity of human neutrophils by cefmetazole. Microbiol Immunol 35:545–556
31. Feitta A, Bersani C, Bertoletti R et al. (1988) In vitro and ex vivo enhancement of nonspecific phagocytosis by cefodizime. Chemotherapy 34:430–436
32. Kaur P, Walters T, Desposito F et al. (1983) Polymorphonuclear leucocyte chemotactic defects in children with sickle cell anemia. J Allergy Clin Immunol 71:S109

33. Ferrari F, Pagani A, Marconi M et al. (1980) Inhibition of candidacidal activity of human neutrophil leukocytes by aminoglycoside antibiotics. Antimicrob Agents Chemother 17:87–88
34. Sheng F, Freischlag J, Backstrom B et al. (1987) The effects of in vivo antibiotics on neutrophil (PMN) activity in rabbits with peritonitis. J Surg Res 43:239–245
35. Forsgren A, Schmeling D, Quie P (1974) Effect of tetracycline on the phagocytic function of human leukocytes. J Infect Dis 130:412–415
36. Goodhart G (1977) Effect of aminoglycosides on the chemotactic response of human polymorphonuclear leukocytes. Antimicrob Agents Chemother 12:540–542
37. Seklecki M, Quintiliani R, Maderazo E (1978) Aminoglycoside Antibiotics moderately impair granulocyte function. Antimicrob Agents Chemother 13: 552–554
38. Belsheim J, Gnarpe H, Persson S (1979) Tetracyclines and host defense mechanisms: interference with leukocyte chemotaxis. Scand J Infect Dis 11:141–145
39. Nelson S, Summer W, Terry P et al. (1987) Erythromycin-induced suppression of pulmonary antibacterial defenses. Am Rev Respir Dis 136:1207–1212
40. Labro MT, Pochet I, Babin-Chevaye C et al. (1987) Effect of ceftriaxone-induced alterations of bacteria on neutrophil function. J Antimicrob Chemother 20:857–869
41. Kaplan S, Perillie P, Finch S (1969) The effect of chloramphenicol on human leukocyte phagocytosis and Respiration. Proc Soc Exp Biol Med 130:839–843
42. Hauser WE Jr, Remington JS (1982) Effect of antibiotics on the immune response. Am J Med 72:711–716
43. Lehrer R (1973) Effects of colchicine and chloramphenicol on the oxidative metabolism and phagocytic activity of human neutrophils. J Infect Dis 127:40–48
44. Bjorksten B, Ray C, Quie P (1976) Inhibition of human neutrophil chemotaxis and chemiluminescence by amphotericin B. Infect Immun 14:315–317
45. Marmer DJ, Fields BT, France GL et al. (1981) Ketoconazole, amphotericin B, and amphotericin B methyl ester: comparative in vitro and in vivo toxicological effects on neutrophil function. Antimicrob Agents Chemother 20:660–665
46. Forsgren A, Gnarpe H (1973) Tetracycline interference with the bactericidal effect of serum. Nature [New Biol] 244:82–83
47. Korzeniowski OM (1989) Effects of antibiotics on the mammalian immune system. Infect Dis Clin North Am 3:469–478
48. Zeis B (1988) Antimycobacterial drugs and the production of reactive oxidants by polymorphonuclear leucocytes in vitro. Chemotherapy 34:56–60
49. Lombard J, Descotes J, Evreux J (1987) Polymorphonuclear leukocyte chemotaxis little affected by three quinolones in vitro. J Antimicrob Chemother 20:615–617
50. Berger S (1985) The use of antimicrobial agents for noninfectious diseases. Rev Infect Dis 7:357–367
51. Forsgren A (1984) Antimicrobial agents and host defence. Scand J Infect Dis 43:S24–S33
52. Datz F, Thorne D (1986) Effect of antibiotic therapy on the sensitivity of indium-111-labeled leukocyte scans. J Nucl Med 27:1849–1853
53. Ghilchik M, Morris A, Reeves D (1970) Immunosuppressive powers of the antibacterial agent trimethoprim. Nature 227:393–394
54. Wittmann DH, Condon RE (1991) Prophylaxis of postoperative infections. Infection 19:S337–S344
55. National Research Council (1964) Postoperative wound infections: The influence of ultraviolet irradiation of the operating room and of various other factors. Ann Surg 160:S8–S178

Immunomodulation in the Critically Ill Surgical Patient

R.V. Maier

The critically ill surgical patient is at high risk for immune dysfunction. Severe stress states (such as multiple trauma and sepsis) produce a deleterious, potentially lethal, immunologic dichotomy. The uncontrolled disseminated activation of the normally protective immunoinflammatory cascades produces a "malignant systemic inflammation" that leads to diffuse multiple organ bystander injury, progressive organ dysfunction, and ultimate sequential organ failure referred to as multiple organ failure syndrome (MOFS) [1–3]. Concomitantly, this "malignant systemic inflammation" induces a simultaneous prolonged and excessive down-regulatory and ultimately immunosuppressive response. In addition, the diffuse activation of these inflammatory cascades leads to a consumptive depletion of the normal protective mechanisms of the immune system. Thus, the appropriate immunomodulation of the critically ill patient will not only prevent MOFS but also maintain normal host defense mechanisms and prevent nosocomial infections, which further induce the malignant systemic inflammatory response, and ultimate organ failure. A major challenge at present is the inability to identify the most critical abnormal components of the immunologic response present in the critically ill patient. While both our understanding of the underlying pathologic mechanisms and therapeutic options have increased dramatically, we are unable to monitor and specifically identify the immunologic dysfunction occurring to determine the dose, time, and duration for the correct therapy in these complex patients.

While sepsis is the most frequent etiology of "malignant systemic inflammation," other massive inflammatory insults can induce a similar host response, referred to as the "sepsis syndrome" or systemic inflammatory response syndrome [3, 4]. Although major trauma and other isolated severe insults can cause significant physiologic dysfunction it appears that ARDS or MOFS are caused by a recurrent and/or sustained ongoing insult referred to as the double-hit phenomenon. Therapeutic options can focus on prevention of either the initial or the secondary insult of the double-hit phenomenon.

A common initial insult, particularly in the injured patient, is ischemia/reperfusion injury during resuscitation from hypovolemic shock. Activation of the neutrophil during reperfusion with subsequent disseminated adherence and nondiscriminate cytotoxicity is a major effector of ischemia/reperfusion injury [4–6]. The sequence of events involved in this activation process is still incompletely known. However, in vivo studies showing that inhibition of neutrophil adherence provides subsequent protection against diffuse cytotoxicity are encouraging. Approaches to inhibition of neutrophil adherence involve blockage of adherence proteins through use of monoclonal antibodies to either neutrophil membrane CD11/CD18 adhesion complex or to one of multiple adhesion proteins up-regulated in endothelial cells, such as P-selectin or E-selectin [5].

The major focus for immunomodulation in prevention of diffuse malignant inflammatory process has been to modulate the response of the immunoinflammation to potent stimuli, the second hit of the double-hit phenomena in the critically ill surgical patient. The most potent and common stimulus of the immunoinflammatory system is endotoxin. Multiple approaches have been tried to detoxify endotoxin. The use of high-dose polyvalent immunoglobulin therapy has been encouraging in European trials of sepsis. Clinical trials utilizing monoclonal IgM antibody to endotoxin have shown a subpopulation effect in the critically ill hypotensive endotoxemic patient from gramnegative infection [7, 8]. Recent data, however, have demonstrated a potential increase in complications from gram-positive organisms. In addition to endotoxin, increasing understanding of the underlying pathophysiology of multiple organ failure has led to identification of and means of specifically blocking the crucial central components of this inflammatory process. Inhibitors of selected deleterious inflammatory cytokines improve outcome in animal models of sepsis and endotoxemia and are now moving into clinical trials. However, the recently completed trial in septic patients utilizing the interleukin-1 receptor antagonist (IL-1ra), a recombinant product of a normally occurring protein that blocks IL-1 and its receptor interaction [9, 10], did not demonstrate significant improvement in the clinical course. Whether the patient population, dose, or use of only a single mediator inhibitor may explain the failure is unknown. Inhibition of tumor necrosis factor (TNF), another crucial effector molecule, has shown some benefit in animal trials [11]. Use of anti-TNF antibody or the soluble TNF receptor which has been produced by recombinant techniques is currently undergoing clinical evaluation in an attempt to down-regulate the overly aggressive inflammatory response. Similarly, specific inhibitors of platelet activating factor (PAF) have shown a protection against endotoxemia in animals [12, 13]. Overall, however, it is unknown whether any of these directed modalities have a demonstrable benefit in the face of the extremely complex interactive system that has evolved. The potential for a multiple pronged approach to the problem utilizing inhibitors of several mediators to produce ultimate benefit is unproven at present. The use of anti-TNF and IL-1ra, plus/minus inhibition of PAF, may be ultimately needed to shut down the inflammatory destructive process.

The second aspect of the immunologic dysfunction dichotomy, the excessive consumption and depletion of normal host inflammatory responses and excessive feedback down-regulation subsequent to severe injury, is also under study. Reversal of the immunosuppression and up-regulation of the host response to prevent secondary nosocomial infections and other complications is an area of intense investigation. Use of colony stimulating factors, GCSF and GMCSF, which reverse the bone marrow suppression and increase production of neutrophils and other immune cells, has been encouraging in burn models. These studies are now being tested clinically in the human burn. Similarly, interferon-γ (IFN-γ) is being used to reverse the depressed immune response following chemotherapy and severe trauma [14]. While macrophage immune function has been improved, a recent clinical trial in severely injured patients did not significantly reduce infectious complications. In addition, IFN-γ therapy in normal animals led to an excessive response to endotoxin challenge and increased toxicity. Another approach has been inhibition of immunosuppressive agents. Since PGE-2 has been identified as a major effector of the postinjury immunosuppression [15], including bone marrow responses, nonsteroidal anti-inflammatory drugs and other agents to block this effect have been used to reverse both the immunosuppression and the suppression of the bone marrow. Current clinical trials are investigating their effectiveness.

A new exciting field in the care of the critically ill is the use of nutrition as an immunomodulator [16–18]. The stress response involves protein redistribution and a concomitant catabolism of the skeletal muscle and other structural proteins. Recent studies have shown that the catabolism, while good as an acute response, becomes detrimental and destructive when prolonged in the critically ill [19]. The ability of growth hormone to reverse this catabolism and protein and nitrogen wasting has been documented in the burn model, particularly in children. In those cases where growth hormone fails, it appears due to insufficient release of insulin-like growth factor-1 (IGF-1) as a major effector molecule of growth hormone. Recent trials are using recombinant IGF-1 to reverse the detrimental catabolic process and enhance the host immune state [20].

Glutamine, normally a nonessential amino acid, is insufficiently produced during episodes of severe stress and becomes an essential amino acid. Glutamine is tissue trophic to the small intestine mucosa and protects against breakdown and potential bacterial translocation. Glutamine levels in muscle also correlate with protein synthesis and loss of glutamine correlates with excessive protein loss. Glutamine is the substrate for production of glutathione, a major intracellular antioxidant [21]. Oxygen-induced injury due to ongoing ischemia/reperfusion and other sources of excessive oxidants in the critically ill is reduced by increased intracellular levels of antioxidants such as glutathione which may be crucial to cell survival and organ function [22]. Arginine, similar to glutamine, is an essential amino acid during stress. Arginine produces the amino group for nitric oxide production. This endogenous vasodilator is necessary for enhancing tissue perfusion during stress states. Arginine has also been shown to be a potent secretagogue causing release of growth hormone and other agents which maintain T-cell activation and other functions in the host immune response.

Finally, the use of omega-3 fatty acids (found commonly in fish oils) to modify the host response is receiving investigation in the critically ill [23, 24]. The omega-3 fatty acids replace arachidonate in the cell membrane and block production of potent arachidonic acid metabolites in response to endotoxin and other stimuli. TNF uses arachidonic acid metabolites as effector molecules for many of the pathophysiologic events occurring during stress. And as mentioned, production of PGE-2 is the major immunosuppressant following injury. All of these events are dependent on arachidonic acid levels and modulation of membrane fatty acids may well down-regulate both the excessive inflammatory and immunosuppressive events following inflammatory insults.

The ability to identify and correctly treat the specific components of immune dysfunction in the critically ill is rapidly approaching. The benefits to our ill patients will be enormous.

References

1. Maier RV (1993) The "angry" macrophage and its impact on host response mechanisms. In: Faist E, Meakins JL, Schildberg, FW (eds) Host defense dysfunction in trauma, shock and sepsis. Springer, Berlin Heidelberg New York
2. Carrico CJ, Meakins JL, Maier RV et al. (1986) Multiple-organ-failure syndrome. Arch Surg 121:196–208
3. Goris RJA, te Boekhorst TPA, Nuytinck JKS et al. (1985) Multiple organ failure: generalized autodestructive inflammation? Arch Surg 120:1109
4. Henson PM, Larsen GL, Webster RO et al. (1982) Pulmonary microvascular alterations and injury induced by complement fragments: synergistic effect of complement activation, neutrophil sequestration, and prostaglandins. Ann NY Acad Sci 384:287–300
5. Welbourn CRB, Goldman G, Paterson IS et al. (1991) Pathophysiology of ischemia reperfusion injury: central role of the neutrophil. Br J Surg 78:651–656
6. Redl H, Dinges HP, Buurman WA, van der Linden CJ et al. (1991) Expression of endothelial leukocyte adhesion molecule-1 in septic but not traumatic/hypovolemic shock in the baboon. Am J Pathol (139)2:461–466
7. Greenman RL, Schein RMH, Martin MA et al. (1991) A controlled clinical trial of E6 murine monoclonal IgM antibody to endotoxin in the treatment of gram-negative sepsis. JAMA 266:1097–1102
8. Ziegler EJ, Fisher CJ, Sprung CL et al. (1991) Treatment of gram-negative bacteremia and septic shock with HA-1A human monoclonal antibody against endotoxin. N Engl J Med 324:429–436
9. Wakabayashi G, Gelfand JA, Burke JF et al. (1991) A specific receptor antagonist for interleukin-1 prevents Escherichia coli-induced shock in rabbits. EASEBJ 5:338–343
10. Dinarello CA (1984) Interleukin-1 and pathogenesis of the acute-phase response. N Engl J Med 311:1413–1418
11. Tracey KJ, Beutler B, Lowry SF et al. (1986) Shock and tissue injury induced by recombinant human cachectin. Science 234:470–474

12. Fletcher JR, Disimone AG, Earnest MA (1990) Platelet activating factor receptor antagonist improves survival and attenuates eicosanoid release in severe endotoxemia. Ann Surg 211:312–316
13. Maier RV, Hahnel GB, Fletcher JR (1992) Platelet activating factor augments tumor necrosis factor and procoagulant activity. J Surg Res 52:258–264
14. Hershman MJ, Polk HC Jr, Pietsch JD et al. (1988) Modulation of infection by gamma interferon treatment following trauma. Infect Immun 56:2412–2416
15. Faist E, Mewes A, Strasser T et al. (1988) Aeteration of monocyte function following major injury. Arch Surg 123:287–292
16. Maier RV (1992) What's new in surgery – critical care metabolism. Bull Am Coll Surg 77:22–26
17. Wilmore DW (1991) Catabolic illness: strategies for enhancing recovery. N Engl J Med 325:695–702
18. Cerra FB (1991) Nutrient modulation of inflammatory and immune function. Am J Surg 161:230–234
19. Fisher JE, Hasselgren PO (1991) Cytokines and glucocorticoids in the regulation of the "hepato-skeletal muscle axis" in sepsis. Am J Surg 6:266–271
20. Thompson WA, Coyle SM, Lazarus D et al. (1991) The metabolic effects of a continuous infusion of insulin-like growth factor (IGF-1) in parenterally fed men. Surg Forum 42:23–25
21. Hong RW, Robinson MK, Rounds JD et al. (1991) Glutamine protects the liver following corynebacterium parvum/endotoxin-induced hepatic necrosis. Surg Forum 42:1–3
22. Robinson MK, Hong RW, Rounds JD et al. (1991) Glutathione depletion enhances bacterial translocation and alters immunologic status. Surg Forum 42:65–67
23. Sato TT, Garcia IA, Maier RV (1992) Immunomodulation of cultured human monocytes by omega-3 fatty acid. Surg Forum 43:9–10
24. Griswold JA, Grogan JB, Metcalf J et al. (1991) The impact of dietary fish oil in endotoxin-induced stress. Surg Forum 42:9–11

Effect of Clindamycin in a New Standardized Animal Model for Chronic Abscess-Forming Peritonitis

A. Woltmann, A. Lebeau, M. Schult, K. Kattenbeck, S. Gatermann, R. Broll, and H. Bruch

Introduction

To evaluate our new standardized animal model for chronic abscess-forming peritonitis we studied the effect of clindamycin. The advantages of our new model are standardization, reproducibility, and low lethality in the first 14 days [6]. As a consequence we could study the course of peritonitis with normal clinical parameters, and we did not have the disadvantage of other animal models for intraabdominal sepsis, namely uncontrollable early lethality through endotoxic shock [3–5].

Methods

We used male, 6-week-old Wistar rats with a body weight of about 270–350 g. To induce the peritonitis we inoculated 2 ml of a *Bacteroides fragilis* (American Type Culture Collection No. 25285) suspension with a concentration of 10^8 bacteria per ml. This bacterial suspension was mixed with 2 ml of a liquefied agar (Merck art. 11471). Inoculation was performed by median laparotomy under Ketanest/Rompun anesthesia and injection of the bacteria-agar mixture in all four abdominal quadrants.

In a control group we only injected 2 ml agar. In the treatment (clindamycin) group peritonitis was induced as outlined above and 15 mg clindamycin was given by intramuscular injection at 8-h intervals for a maximum of 14 days, starting 24 h after peritonitis induction.

Peritonitis was induced on day 0. The peritonitis, control, and clindamycin groups were divided into three subgroups, which were observed for 3, 7, and 14 days, respectively. After the different observation times a left-side thoracotomy was performed under the above-mentioned anesthesia. Through a sterile puncture of the heart we obtained blood samples for laboratory parameters and blood cultures. Thereafter, through relaparotomy we took one swab of every abdominal quadrant. Finally we recorded all pathological macroscopic features, took biopsies of the peritoneum, and carried out eventration of all organs for histological examination (formalin fixation, paraffin coating, 4-μm sections, staining with hematoxylin-eosin).

Results

The lethality of peritonitis was 0%. The peritonitis group comprised 19 animals, the control and clindamycin groups 15 animals each.

In the peritonitis group macroscopically we noticed adhesions as early as day 3; from day 7 on we also found intraabdominal abscesses. Peritoneal abscesses were not found in the control and clindamycin groups.

In the control group the normal bacteriological spectrum obtained by dermal swabs showed staphylococci and *Proteus*, that taken by pharyngeal swabs, *Pasteurella* and streptococci, and that obtained by anal swabs, enterococci and *Proteus*. In stool cultures we found *Bacteroides* species, *Proteus*, staphylococci, enterococci, and *Escherichia coli*.

On days 3 and 7 abdominal swabs of the peritonitis group were not only *B. fragilis* positive. Additionally we found a polyvalent, severe mixed intraabdominal infection, namely *Staph. aureus*, *E. coli*, *β*-hemolyzing streptococci, and anaerobic cocci. On day 14 we found only a few *B. fragilis*-positive swabs. In the clindamycin group only on day 3 did we obtained five *B. fragilis*-positive swabs; on days 7 and 14 all swabs were sterile (Fig. 1).

On days 3, 7, and 14 we observed *B. fragilis*-positive blood cultures in three, two, and one rats of the peritonitis group. In the clindamycin and control groups there were no *B. fragilis*-positive blood cultures.

On day 7 all groups showed a leukocytosis of about 12 000–13 000 leukocytes per ml. On day 14 leukocytosis persisted only in the peritonitis group. In contrast the number of leukocytes in the peripheral blood of the clindamycin and control groups had decreased to normal values by this time (Fig. 2).

On day 7 we saw a mild depression in the number of platelets in the peritonitis group, to below 800 000 per ml, whereas in the clindamycin and control groups platelets were in the normal range (between 900 000 and 1 200 000 per ml) during the whole observation period.

Endotoxin-positive blood levels were found only in one rat of the peritonitis group on day 3. In all other animals we did not obtain endotoxin-positive values by kinetic measurements.

In the peritonitis group the histological examination showed severe acute peritoneal inflammation on day 3. On day 7 we additionally noticed signs of chronic inflammation and multiple abscesses. On day 14 we found progressive encapsulation of the abscessing foci by connective tissue enriched with fibroblasts. There was an increase in the number of rats with histologically proven abscesses during the observation period. On day 14 the abscess rate was 100% (six/six rats). Abscesses were mainly located in the parietal peritoneum (Fig. 3). In the liver we saw an activation of the Kupffer cells. In the other organs, however, there were no metastatic septicopyemic abscesses. In the clindamycin group macroscopically and histologically there were no intraabdominal abscesses, but we found some foreign body granulomas in the abdomen due to the remaining agar.

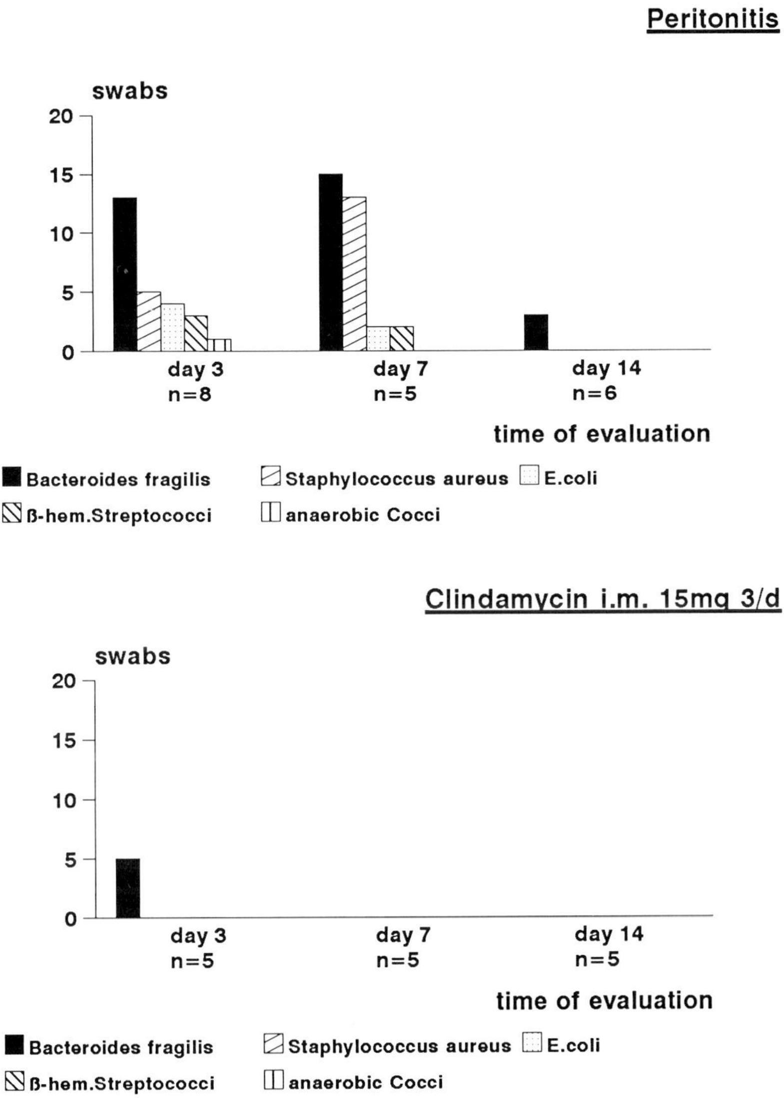

Fig. 1. Bacteriological results of abdominal swabs in the peritonitis and clindamycin groups. *n*, Number of tested animals

Discussion

Basing on the first description of Volk et al. [6] we developed a standardized animal model for chronic abscess-forming peritonitis. We obtained not only bacteriological and histological, but also reproducible laboratory blood parameter results.

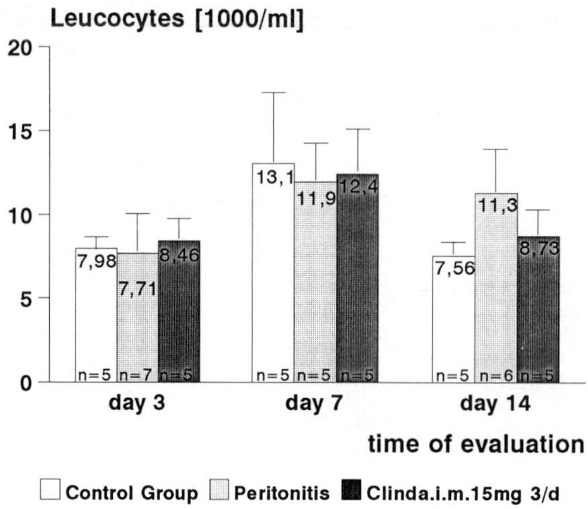

Fig. 2. Leukocytes (means + SEM) of the control, peritonitis, and clindamycin groups. *Clinda.*, Clindamycin; *n*, number of tested animals

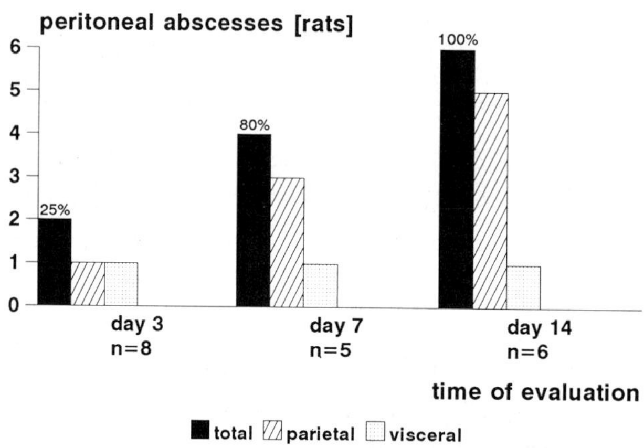

Fig. 3. Histological results in the peritonitis group: number of rats with intraabdominal abscesses at the parietal and visceral peritoneum. *n*, Number of tested animals

After intraperitoneal injection of a *B. fragilis* suspension we induced a severe intraabdominal mixed infection through translocation of gut bacteria into the peritoneal cavity in the peritonitis group. In the peritonitis group the intraabdominal abscess rate on day 14 was 100%. At this time a progressive encapsulation of the abscessing foci led to a reduction of the number of *B. fragilis*-positive abdominal swabs in the peritonitis group. However, as a sign of the abscess-forming infection, leukocytosis persisted only in this group.

In former animal model investigations, clindamycin was effective in the antibiotic treatment of peritonitis [1, 2]. In our study clindamycin reduced the number of *B. fragilis*-positive swabs on day 3. On days 7 and 14 all abdominal swabs in the clindamycin group were sterile. There was no translocation of gut bacteria into the peritoneal cavity in the clindamycin group. In blood cultures of the clindamycin group we did not find *B. fragilis*. Macroscopically and histologically we did not notice any intraabdominal abscesses in the clindamycin group. Thus antibiotic therapy with clindamycin prevented peritoneal abscesses and intraabdominal sepsis in our model.

We conclude that our results indicate the model as a qualified in vivo assay for further standardized investigations into therapy modalities in peritonitis.

References

1. Bartlett JG, Gorbach SL (1979) An animal model of intraabdominal sepsis. Scand J Infect Dis 19:26–29
2. Bartlett JG, Onderdonk AB, Louie T, Kasper DL, Gorbach SL (1978) A review. Lessons from an animal model of intra-abdominal sepsis. Arch Surg 113:853–857
3. Bohnen JMA, Matlow AG, Mustard RA, Christie NA, Kavouris B (1988) Antibiotic efficacy in intraabdominal sepsis: a clinically relevant model. Can J Microbiol 34:323–326
4. Fink MP, Heard SO (1990) Laboratory models of sepsis and septic shock. J Surg Res 49:186–196
5. Martinelli S, Falk A, Haglund U, Myrvold H (1985) Peritonitis and septic shock – an evaluation of two experimental models in the rat. Eur Surg Res 17:160–166
6. Volk HW, Schneider J, Dämmrich J, Döll W, Hörl M, Bruch H-P (1990) Animal model for chronic-abscess-forming peritonitis: Histology and microbiology. Eur Surg Res 22:347–355

GM-CSF Modulates Immune Function and Improves Survival After Thermal Injury

R.G. Molloy, R. Holzheimer, M. Nestor, K. Collins, J.R. Mannick, and M.L. Rodrick

Introduction

As a result of major advances in the care of thermally injured patients over the last two decades, mortality from hypovolemic shock, acute renal failure, and metabolic wasting has fallen dramatically. However, infection remains an important cause of morbidity and mortality in these patients [1]. The prevalence and severity of septic episodes is largely secondary to profound alterations in defence mechanisms which often characterise the host's response to major burn injury.

Defective T-cell function in particular, plays a pivotal role in mediating this increased susceptibility to infection. Thermal injury is associated with a prolonged impairment of both IL-2 production and T-cell proliferative responses in humans and animal studies [2, 3]. Although the precise mechanisms underlying impaired T-cell function have not been fully elucidated, a number of recent studies have provided direct and indirect evidence that impaired colony stimulating activity underlies many of the characteristic defects in immune function after thermal injury [4, 5]. The present study examined the potential use of GM-CSF as a immuno-restorative agent in the prevention of mortality from burn sepsis, and correlated changes in survival with alterations in T-cell proliferative responses and IL-2 production.

Materials and Methods

Seven-week-old male A/J mice (Jackson Laboratories, Bar Harbor, Maine, USA) were acclimatised for 1 week under controlled conditions with water and mouse food ad libitum. After randomisation, animals were anaesthetised and placed in a specially constructed mould which exposed 20% of their body surface area. The mould containing the animal was immersed in water at either room temp (25°C) (Sham), or 90° for 9 s (Burn) according to the treatment protocol assigned to each animal. The latter treatment resulted in a histologically proven full thickness burn to the exposed dorsum. Animals were immediately dried and resuscitated with 1 millilitre of 0.9% saline I.P. prior to re-caging.

Septic challenge was induced on day 10 post burn, as this corresponds with the point of maximum impairment in T-cell proliferative responses and maximum susceptibility to infectious challenge in this model [2]. Animals were anaesthetised and the abdomen was shaved and opened in midline. The cecum was located and ligated at its base in a non-obstructing fashion using a 4/0 silk suture. A full-thickness puncture, at two different sites in the ligated cecum, was performed using a 27-gauge needle. A small quantity of faeces was expressed from each puncture wound in order to ensure peritonitis. After ligation and puncture, the cecum was replaced in the abdomen taking care not to contaminate the wound with faeces. Wounds were closed with a continuous 5/0 nylon suture. All animals were immediately resuscitated with 1 millilitre of 0.9% saline and re-caged.

Experimental Groups

1. Sham burn groups, treated with vehicle (0.9% saline) only
2. Burn groups, treated with vehicle only
3. Burn groups, treated with GM-CSF (10, 50, 200, 500 and 1000 ng)

Both vehicle and therapy were administered on days 5–9, by subcutaneous (S.C.) injection, in a final volume of 0.5 mL for all groups. Highly purified, endotoxin-free GM-CSF was obtained as a gift (Amgen, Thousand Oaks, Calif., USA). Indomethacin (Merck Sharpe and Dohme, West Point, Pa., USA) was prepared in 0.9% saline. A fresh stock solution was prepared for each experiment.

Splenocyte Preparation

For in vitro studies of T-cell immune function, animals were sacrificed in a CO_2 chamber on day 10 after thermal injury. Splenocyte preparations were prepared and both T-cell proliferation and IL-2 production measured using standard techniques [2, 3].

Results

Low dose GM-CSF therapy (10 and 50 ng) conferred a small beneficial effect on survival, which was not significantly different to survival in burn groups treated with vehicle alone (Fig. 1). Similarly, high-dose therapy (500 and 1000 ng) did not have any beneficial effect on survival. However, burn groups treated with 200 ng GM-CSF displayed a significant improvement in survival, when compared to burn groups treated with vehicle alone (% survival, burn/vehicle – 0; burn/GM-CSF – 33; $P < 0.05$).

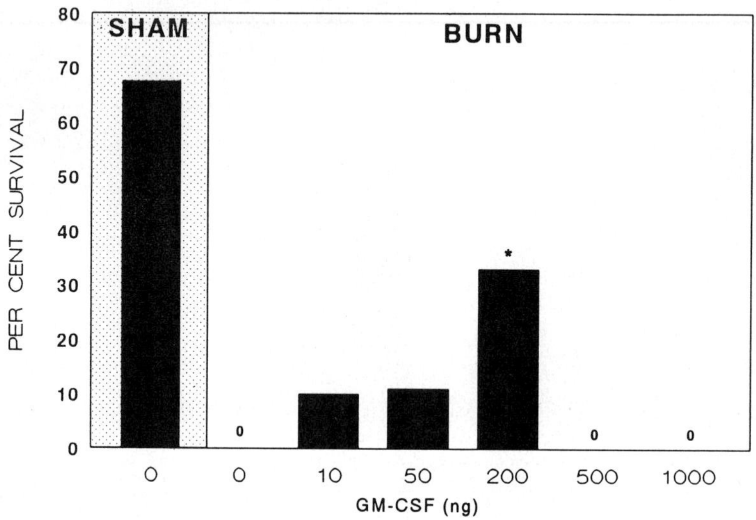

Fig. 1. Survival in sham (n = 12) and burn groups (n = 14) following cecal ligation and puncture (CLP) on day 10 post injury. Treatment groups include sham-burned animals treated with vehicle (0.9% saline), and burn groups treated with either vehicle or increasing doses of GM-CSF. ($^{*}P < 0.05$ compared to burn group treated with vehicle, Wilcoxon Gehan Survival Statistic)

Con A-stimulated T-cell proliferation was significantly lower in burn groups compared to sham-burned controls (Fig. 2). In vivo pretreatment of burn groups with GM-CSF at the dosage regimen which maximally improved survival (i.e., 200 ng from days 5–9 after injury) led to a significantly restoration in T-cell proliferative responses after thermal injury (Fig. 2).

Thermal injury was also associated with a significant reduction in the synthesis of IL-2 (Fig. 2). Splenocytes from thermally injured animals, treated in vivo with GM-CSF at the dose which maximally improved survival (200 ng/day) displayed a significant increase in synthesis of this cytokine (Fig. 2).

Discussion

The present study examined the hypothesis that deficient granulocyte macrophage-colony stimulating activity may account for aberrations in immune function which increase susceptibility to infection after thermal injury. In clinical practice, the vast majority of serious septic complications occur in the second or subsequent weeks following thermal injury. Because there is no accurate method of predicting if or when injured patients might develop a septic complication, therapy was administered right up to the point of septic challenge, which corresponded with the point of maximum immunosuppression in this model [2].

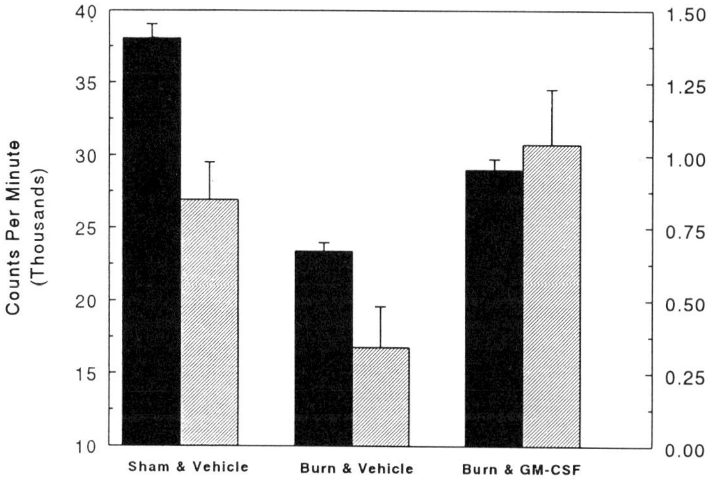

Fig. 2. Con A (■) stimulated T-cell proliferation and IL-2 (□) production in sham burn groups treated with vehicle (0.9% saline), and burn groups treated with either vehicle or GM-CSF (200 ng). Spleens were harvested on day 10 postburn. Data represent the mean (sem) proliferation within each group ($n = 12$–14/group). ($P <$ 0.05 compared to burn group treated with vehicle, Mann Whitney test)

Under these conditions, i.e., once daily S.C. injection on days 5–9 post burn, survival was significantly increased after thermal injury in groups treated with 200 ng of GM-CSF (Fig. 1). As expected from similar studies using other cytokines, GM-CSF did not display a classical dose-response curve with respect to its in vivo actions. A similar phenomenon has been reported by other investigators using both GM-CSF and IL-2 therapy [6, 7].

The present study also clearly shows that Con A-stimulated T-cell proliferation was significantly impaired in burn groups (Fig. 2). Similar findings have been reported by other investigators [2, 3]. In vivo administration of GM-CSF at the dose which maximally improved survival (i.e., 200 ng/day) was also found to significantly improve T-cell proliferation (Fig. 2).

In keeping with the findings of others [3, 7], the present study also documented a postburn reduction in synthesis of IL-2. Whereas T lymphocytes are essential for the development of an adequate response to infection, IL-2 plays a pivotal role in maintaining and amplifying this response. In vivo GM-CSF therapy was capable of restoring impaired IL-2 synthesis in burn groups (Fig. 2).

Cell-mediated immunity, a vital component of the immune response, is dependent on the T lymphocyte. T-cell dysfunction is a characteristic feature of immune response following thermal injury, and correlates with increased susceptibility to fatal infection in both clinical and experimental models [2, 3]. Although T lymphocytes are not conventionally considered to be one of the primary sites of action of GM-CSF, a number of studies have recently suggested that this cytokine may alter T-cell function via a direct action, and by modulating accessory cell function. The ability to induce growth in a T-cell line and serve as a co-factor for in vivo derived T cells suggests a possible physiological role for GM-CSF in T cell-mediated immune responses.

The present study suggests that GM-CSF therapy confers a significant survival advantage after infectious challenge in thermally injured animals. The cytokine was effective when administered right up to the point of septic challenge and appears to mediate its actions, at least in part, through a restoration in T-cell proliferation and IL-2 production. These data suggest a potential therapeutic role for the use of GM-CSF in the prevention of mortality after major thermal injury, but caution against the inappropriate use of high-dose therapy.

References

1. Pruitt BA Jr (1990) Infection and the burn patient. Br J Surg 77:1081–1082
2. Moss N, Gough DB, Jordan AL et al. (1988) Temporal correlation of impaired immune response after thermal injury with susceptibility to infection in a murine model. Surgery 104:882–887
3. Wood JJ, Rodrick ML, O'Mahony JB et al. (1984) Inadequate interleukin-2 production. A fundamental immunological deficiency in patients with major burns. Ann Surg 200:311–320
4. Peterson V, Hansbrough JF, Buerck C et al. (1983) Regulation of granulopoiesis following severe thermal injury. J Trauma 23:19–24
5. Peterson V, Robinson WA, Wallner SF, Rundus C, Hansbrough JF (1985) Granulocyte stem cells are decreased in humans with fatal burns. J Trauma 25:413–418
6. Frenck RW, Sarman G, Harper TE, Buescher ES (1990) The ability of recombinant murine granulocyte-macrophage colony-stimulating factor to protect neonatal rats from septic death due to *Staphylococcus aureus*. J Infect Dis 162:109–114
7. Gough DB, Moss NM, Jordan A et al. (1988) Recombinant interleukin-2 (rIL-2) improves immune response and host resistance to septic challenge in thermally injured mice. Surgery 104:292–300

Early-Phase Endotoxin Tolerance Enhances Survival in a Porcine Endotoxin Shock Model

K.-H. Staubach, S. Jonas, A. Kooistra, J. Eilers, U. Schade, and H.-P. Bruch

Introduction

Early-phase endotoxin (ET) tolerance is a well-known finding in mammals [1, 2], although its exact biological basis remains unclear [3]. Repeated injections of sublethal doses of any ET result in a non-specific refractoriness to ET from all other gram-negative strains [4]. The unspecific tolerant state becomes progressively greater for about 1 week before a specific immunity develops. Immunologically it seems to represent an essential protective mechanism to prevent initially unreasonable expansion of inflammatory or indiscriminate immune responses. This study was undertaken in order to investigate whether the induction of early-phase ET tolerance would enhance survival in a porcine shock model.

Material and Methods

Six pigs were immunized over a 5-day period with increasing doses of ET from *Salmonella abortus equi* (group T2). On the 5th day prior to the ET challenge they received 5 ng/kg, on the 4th day 10 ng/kg, on the 3rd day 30 ng/kg, on the 2nd day 30 ng/kg and on the day prior to the challenge, no ET. The sham-treated animals (group C2) only received saline solution at the same time intervals. All animals were mechanically ventilated under general anaesthesia with fentanyl (0.01 mg/kg h), midazolam (0.1 mg/kg h) and pancuronium (0.1 mg/kg h) medication. They received a balanced saline glucose amino acid solution at a rate of 3 ml/kg h and a continuous infusion of ET of 250 mg/kg h. A 7-French Swan-Ganz thermodilution catheter was inserted via the right jugular vein and an arterial 5-French thermodilution catheter into the left femoral artery. Mean arterial pressure (MAP), electrocardiographic tracing and body temperature were monitored continuously, and pulmonary capillary wedge pressure, cardiac output (CO) and extravascular lung water (EVLW) intermittently. Haematological studies were performed at the University laboratory using standard techniques.

In statistical analysis the Mann-Whitney U-test was used, and correlation calculations were made with linear regression: P values <0.05 were considered significant.

Results

Both groups showed signs of endotoxemia with sustained reduction in MAP and CO, while heart rate (HR) rose steadily (Fig. 1). However, in the control group C2 acute circulatory failure occurred between the 6th and 7th hour of the experiment. Survival time (Fig. 2) in the pretreated group was

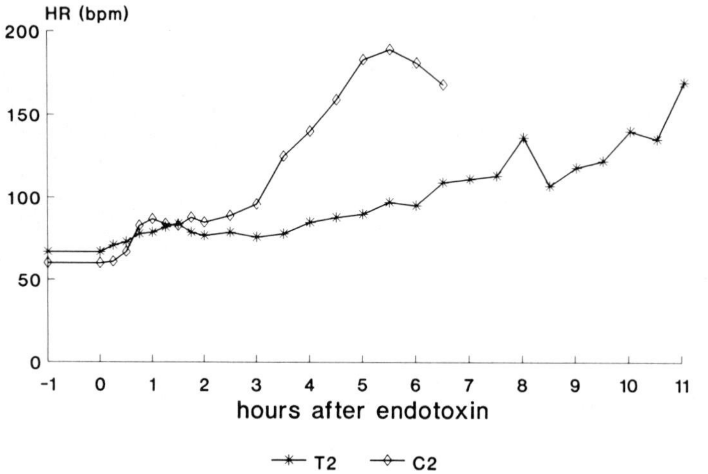

Fig. 1. Heart rate of the two groups at various times after starting the ET challenge infusion

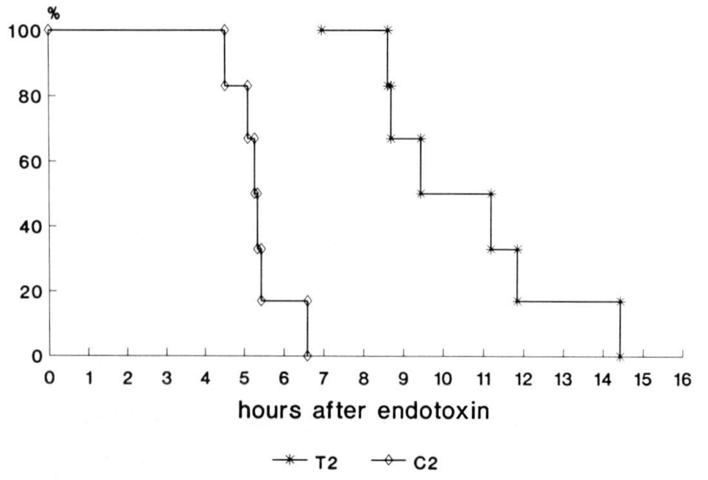

Fig. 2. Increase in survival time in the treatment group T2 during the observation period

significantly enhanced ($P = 0.0001$) by more than 100%. Haemodynamic derangements were less prominent and deterioration occurred relatively late, but then instantly. Although the HR (Fig. 1) did not show significant differences between the two groups, MAP was falling in the tolerant animals only 2 h before the animals succumbed. As a consequence urine output in the latter only decreased prior to the their death. CO also remained stable in the treatment group, as did the base excess (Fig. 3). Haematologically, the white blood count returned to normal ranges (after the initially drop)

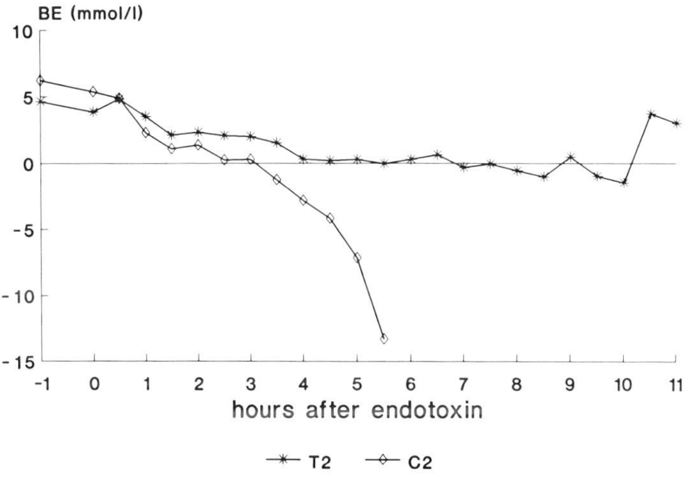

Fig. 3. Development of base excess in the two groups

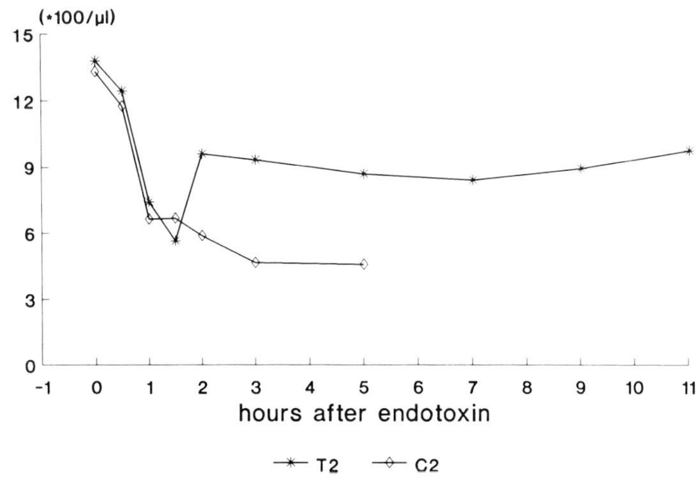

Fig. 4. Peripheral white blood count during the experiment

Table 1. Cardiorespiratory parameters at various times after ET in the two groups

Time after ET (hour)		0	1	2	3	4	5	6	7	8	9	10
CO (l/min)	C2	2.62 (0.4)	2.12 (0.4)	2.75 (0.5)	18.7 (0.3)	1.79 (0.5)	1.53 (0.8)	1.26				
	T2	2.46 (0.2)	1.91 (0.2)	2.61 (0.2)	2.45* (0.4)	2.31 (0.5)	2.10 (0.5)	1.99* (0.3)	1.97 (0.1)	2.05 (0.4)	2.36 (0.5)	1.96 (0.5)
MAP (mmHg)	C2	75 (7.2)	76 (7.4)	73 (7.7)	65 (10.9)	52 (13.1)	33 (12.4)	26				
	T2	85 (8.1)	64* (5.1)	80 (14.8)	78 (13.1)	88* (16.6)	83* (16.9)	75* (17.9)	71 (21.4)	60 (28.7)	60 (19.8)	61 (28.2)
HR (min^{-1})	C2	60 (11.2)	87 (4.9)	85 (2.4)	96 (17.0)	140 (22.8)	183 (13.2)	181				
	T2	67 (7.5)	79 (7.8)	77 (7.1)	76* (8.9)	85* (19.4)	90* (31.8)	95* (18.5)	111 (27.5)	136 (45.8)	118 (24.0)	140 (54.4)
PaO_2 (mmHg)	C2	129 (11.4)	81 (30.7)	83 (11.9)	63 (10.6)	56 (13.2)	43 (7.1)					
	T2	122 (23.2)	89 (25.8)	85 (20.6)	72 (25.8)	56 (12.6)	56 (10.7)	57 (11.7)	56 (10.1)	51 (12.1)	56 (21.6)	55 (16.5)
SVO_2 (mmHg)	C2	64 (8.5)	56 (7.2)	65 (4.2)	54 (7.3)	38 (9.2)	24 (4.4)					
	T2	54 (23.9)	51 (7.8)	63 (5.4)	50 (10.5)	44 (7.9)	44* (8.0)	42 (9.5)	42 (9.4)	41 (10.2)	40 (11.4)	44 (13.5)

within 2h, while the sham-treated animals remained leucopenic (Fig. 4). The respiratory function (Table 1) measured by the arterial PaO_2 was not significantly different but a more pronounced impairment of SVO_2 and EVLW could be observed in the control group.

Discussion

The general non-specific stimulation of host defence mechanisms by induction of ET tolerance led to a significant enhancement of survival in our porcine shock model. Impairment of all cardiorespiratory parameters was less prominent in the tolerant animals. However, the state of tolerance is relative and can be overcome by increasing the ET challenge dose [5]. Tolerance is a complex phenomenon whose induction varies with the injection schedule of ET, its antigenicity, dosage, and immunocompetence of the host. These factors and especially their interplay may explain the diverse and sometimes conflicting observations on ET tolerance. Since cytokines have been shown to induce early-phase ET tolerance as well as LPS toxicity [6, 7], we speculate that the refractoriness to ET in the tolerant state might be the result of disappearance from the plasma of the "enhancing factor". Following this hypothesis we are continuing our experiments with special emphasis on the TNF. Gifford and Lohmann-Matthes [8] also found the lowest TNF values in the primed mice after injection of non-lethal doses of ET. The highly significant enhancement of survival time in this study emphasizes the role of ET as a potent immunomodulator. Because of undesirable and even dangerous side-effects, however, it cannot be applied as a therapeutic agent: its ratio between immunostimulative and immunodepressive effects is too narrow.

Conclusion

Non-toxic synthetic lipid A analogues, because of their structural similarity, are becoming progressively more attractive. Non-specific host defence enhancement with lipid A precursors as prophylactic agents in surgical patients at risk may prove to be beneficial in the future.

References

1. Beeson PB (1947) Tolerance to bacterial pyrogens. I. Factors influencing its development. J Exp Med 86:29–38
2. Greisman SE, Young EJ, Carozza FA Jr (1969) Mechanisms of endotoxin tolerance. V. Specificity of the early and late phases of pyrogenic tolerance. J Immunol 103:1223–1236

3. Brade H, Brade L, Rietschel ET (1988) Structure-activity relationship of bacterial lipopolysaccharides (endotoxins). Zentralbl Bakteriol Hyg [A] 268:151–179
4. Flad H-D (1990) Induction of 11-1 by lipopolysaccharide (LPS) and its modulation by synthetic lipid. A precursor Ia. Lymphokine Res 9: 557–560
5. Lepe-Zungia JL, Klostergaard J (1990) Tolerance to endotoxin in vitro: independent regulation of interleukin-1, tumor necrosis factor and interferon alpha production during in vitro differentiation of human monocytes. Lymphokine Res 9:309–319
6. Dinarello CA, Morgan HR (1978) Pathogenesis of fever in man. N Engl J Med 298:607–612
7. Rietschel ET, Schade U, Jensen M, Wollenweber HW, Lüderitz O, Greisman SG (1982) Bacterial endotoxins: chemical structure, biological activity and role in septicemia. Scand J Infect Dis [Suppl 31]:8–12
8. Giffort GE, Lohmann-Matthes ML (1987) Gamma interferon priming of mouse and human macrophages for induction of tumor necrosis factor production by bacterial lipopolysaccharides. JNCI 78:121–124

Subject Index

Springer-Verlag and the Environment

We at Springer-Verlag firmly believe that an international science publisher has a special obligation to the environment, and our corporate policies consistently reflect this conviction.

We also expect our business partners – paper mills, printers, packaging manufacturers, etc. – to commit themselves to using environmentally friendly materials and production processes.

The paper in this book is made from low- or no-chlorine pulp and is acid free, in conformance with international standards for paper permanency.

Printing: Saladruck, Berlin
Binding: Buchbinderei Lüderitz & Bauer, Berlin